Mosby's
Handbook of
Anatomy &
Physiology

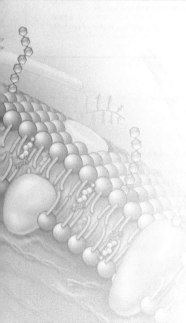

KEVIN T. PATTON, PhD

Professor Emeritus in Life Science
St. Charles Community College
Cottleville, Missouri

Professor of Human Anatomy & Physiology Instruction
New York Chiropractic College
Seneca Falls, New York

GARY A. THIBODEAU, PhD

Chancellor Emeritus and Professor Emeritus of Biology
University of Wisconsin—River Falls
River Falls, Wisconsin

ELSEVIER

3251 Riverport Lane
St. Louis, Missouri 63043

MOSBY'S HANDBOOK OF ANATOMY & PHYSIOLOGY,
SECOND EDITION   ISBN: 978-0-323-22605-9

Notices

Knowledge and best practice in this field are constantly changing. As new research and experience broaden our understanding, changes in research methods, professional practices, or medical treatment may become necessary.

Practitioners and researchers must always rely on their own experience and knowledge in evaluating and using any information, methods, compounds, or experiments described herein. In using such information or methods they should be mindful of their own safety and the safety of others, including parties for whom they have a professional responsibility.

With respect to any drug or pharmaceutical products identified, readers are advised to check the most current information provided (i) on procedures featured or (ii) by the manufacturer of each product to be administered, to verify the recommended dose or formula, the method and duration of administration, and contraindications. It is the responsibility of practitioners, relying on their own experience and knowledge of their patients, to make diagnoses, to determine dosages and the best treatment for each individual patient, and to take all appropriate safety precautions.

To the fullest extent of the law, neither the Publisher nor the authors, contributors, or editors, assume any liability for any injury and/or damage to persons or property as a matter of products liability, negligence or otherwise, or from any use or operation of any methods, products, instructions, or ideas contained in the material herein.

Library of Congress Cataloging-in-Publication Data

Patton, Kevin T., author.
   Mosby's handbook of anatomy & physiology / Kevin T. Patton, Gary A. Thibodeau. – Second edition.
      p. ; cm.
   Mosby's handbook of anatomy and physiology
   Handbook of anatomy & physiology
   Includes index.
   ISBN 978-0-323-22605-9 (pbk. : alk. paper)
   I. Thibodeau, Gary A., 1938- author.   II. Title.   III. Title: Mosby's handbook of anatomy and physiology.   IV. Title: Handbook of anatomy & physiology.
   [DNLM: 1. Anatomy–Handbooks.   2. Physiology–Handbooks.   QS 39]
   QP35
   612–dc23

                                                                                    2013033692

Vice President and Content Strategy Director: Linda Duncan
Executive Content Strategist: Kellie White
Content Development Specialist: Joe Gramlich
Content Coordinator: Nathan Wurm-Cutter
Publishing Services Manager: Catherine Jackson
Senior Project Manager: Carol O'Connell
Design Direction: Jessica Williams

Printed in the United States of America

Last digit is the print number: 9   8   7   6   5

Preface

WHO NEEDS A HANDBOOK OF THE ANATOMY AND PHYSIOLOGY OF THE HUMAN BODY?

Anatomy and physiology of the human body is a study that forms the basis of understanding the everyday workings of our own bodies. It also forms the basis of all of the clinical and applied human sciences. But because of its complexity, we don't always remember all the little details. This is true especially if we haven't reviewed them recently—or never learned them well in the first place. Well, here they are! All those little bits of handy information presented in an easy-to-interpret collection of diagrams, labeled photographs, and concise tables.

For those in direct patient care, this handbook will be a useful *mini-reference* you can carry with you as you work. It contains all of those little details that you know you know but can't seem to remember at the moment. Perhaps even more importantly, you'll have an incredibly effective tool for *patient teaching* always at your fingertips!

For those of you in related fields such as medical transcription, medical or liability insurance, health information technology, law, physical education and sports, recreation, law enforcement, teaching, human services, fiction and nonfiction writing and journalism, and so on, you will find this handbook to be an invaluable tool. It allows you to find and understand all the *basic concepts of human body structure and function* so you can do your job more easily and effectively.

Even those of you who have no professional need for such a tool as this handbook will find it to be an important part of your household or office *reference library*. We're all humans and we all have occasion to wonder about how our body is built and how it works—especially when we are sick or think we may be. Using this handbook, you will more clearly understand what your physician is saying to you. In fact, you might want to bring this handbook along next time you visit a clinic, hospital, or professional office—so that your providers can *show* you what they are trying to tell you. And what better tool is there to help you explain the structure and function of the body to an *inquisitive child*?

HOW DO I USE THIS HANDBOOK?

Because this is a handbook, you should keep it "at hand." When you have need for quickly finding information about human structure or function, simply grab it and thumb through its pages.

The first four chapters of the handbook lay out the "basic sciences" of the human body. These include the overall "Organization of the Body" (Ch. 1), "Body Chemistry" (Ch. 2), "Cells" (Ch. 3) and "Tissues" (Ch. 4). The remainder of the handbook is organized by body system: skin, skeletal, muscular, and so on. Either a quick glance at the Contents (p. vii) or simply flipping through the pages of the handbook should get you to where you want to be in a moment.

Once you've located the information you are looking for, use all the little features we have provided to make things clearer:

- **The anatomical rosette in all figures of body parts.** This rosette, like the directional compass rosette found on maps, orients you quickly to which way is "up" and which way is "down" in the body part(s) shown. We have included a handy summary of our "anatomical rosette" inside the front cover for easy reference.
- **Brief narrative explaining the content of nearly every figure, diagram, and photograph.** Thus, we "walk through" each image with you.
- **The careful use of color** to show realistic structures, to highlight different areas of important diagrams, and to contrast different concepts within tables will help you find what you are looking for quickly and easily.

This new edition features an extensively revised art program, a new and more easily usable design, content updates and clarifications in most of the tables and illustrations, and some additional illustrations and tables.

This handbook is the product of many years of teaching and writing and we can't possibly mention all of the literally hundreds who have contributed to this effort in one way or another. However, we would especially like to mention the following: Kellie White, Joe Gramlich, Nathan Wurm-Cutter, Jessica Williams, Catherine Jackson, and Carol O'Connell. Every writing team should be so fortunate as to have a support network as talented, good-humored, hard-working, professional, and fun as we have!

Kevin T. Patton
Gary A. Thibodeau

Color Key

For Select Anatomical Structures and Biochemical Compounds

BIOCHEMISTRY

Carbon

Chloride

Energy

ATP

Hydrogen

Nitrogen

Oxygen

Potassium

Sodium

Sulfur

OTHER STRUCTURES

Afferent (Sensory) Pathway

Artery

Bone

Efferent (Motor) Pathway

Hormone

Muscle

Nerve

Schwann Cell

Vein

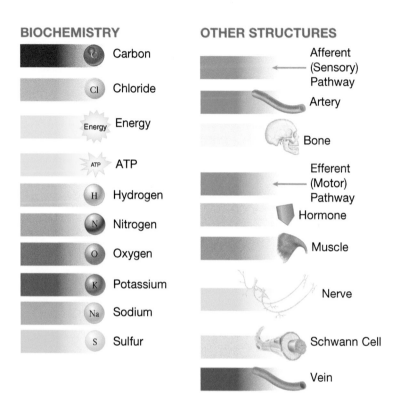

CELLULAR STRUCTURES

Cytosol

Golgi Apparatus

Mitochondrion

Na⁺ Transporter

Nucleus

Plasma Membrane

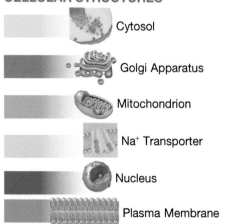

Contents

8   NERVOUS SYSTEM, 224

Organization of the Body

ANATOMY

Anatomy is often defined as the study of the structure of an organism and the relationships of its parts. The word **anatomy** is derived from two Greek words: *ana*, meaning "apart," and *temos* or *tomos*, meaning "cutting." Students of anatomy still learn about the structure of the human body by literally cutting it apart through a process called **dissection,** which remains the principal technique used to isolate and study the structural components or parts of the human body.

Biology is the study of life. Both anatomy and physiology are subdivisions of this very broad area of inquiry. Just as biology can be subdivided into specific areas of study, so can anatomy and physiology. For example, the term **gross anatomy** refers to the study of body parts that are visible to the naked eye. Before the discovery of the microscope, anatomists had to study human structure using only their eyes during dissection. These early anatomists could make only a *gross* or whole examination. With the use of modern microscopes, many anatomists now specialize in **microscopic anatomy;** this includes the study of cells, called **cytology** (sye-TOL-o-jee), and the study of *tissues*, called **histology** (his-TOL-o-jee).

Other branches of anatomy include the study of human growth and development (**developmental anatomy**) and the study of diseased body structures (**pathological anatomy**). In this handbook, the systems of the body are presented through a process called **systemic anatomy**. Systems are groups of organs that have a common function, such as the bones of the skeletal system and the muscles of the muscular system.

PHYSIOLOGY

Physiology is the science of the functions of the living organism and its parts. The term is a combination of two Greek words: *physis,* meaning "nature," and *logos,* meaning "science or study." Simply stated, it is the study of physiology that helps us to understand how the body works. Physiologists attempt to discover and understand, through active experimentation, the intricate control systems and regulatory mechanisms that permit the body to operate and survive in an often hostile environment.

As a scientific discipline, physiology can be subdivided according to the following: (1) the type of organism involved, such as **human physiology** or **plant physiology**; (2) the organizational level studied, such as **molecular physiology** or **cellular physiology**; or (3) a specific or *systemic* function being studied, such as **neurophysiology, respiratory physiology,** or **cardiovascular physiology.**

ORIENTATION TO THE BODY

This first section of the handbook provides the foundation needed to understand the rest of the handbook.

First, one must understand the basic layout of the body and become familiar with the terminology used to describe the regions of the body, the organs of the body, and directions within the body. You cannot locate something in the superior abdominal cavity if you do not know what "superior" means and do not know where the "abdominal cavity" is.

At the end of this chapter, we provide a commonly used model for understanding the "balance of functions" that keep the body alive—a concept called **homeostasis.**

ANATOMICAL POSITION AND BILATERAL SYMMETRY

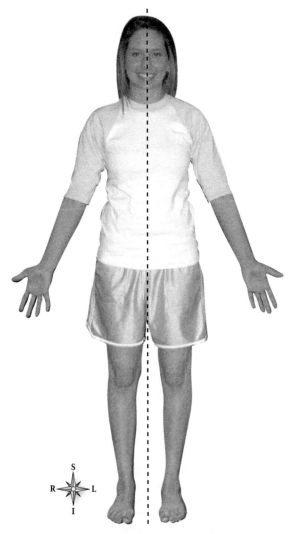

Anatomical Position and Bilateral Symmetry. In the anatomical position, the body is in an erect, or standing, posture with the arms at the sides and palms forward. The head and feet are also pointing forward. The *dotted line* shows the axis of the body's bilateral symmetry. As a result of this organizational feature, the right and left sides of the body are mirror images of each other.

BODY CAVITIES

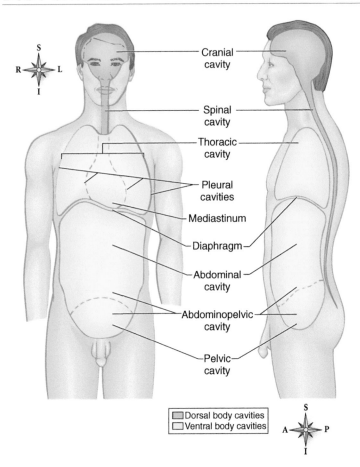

Major Body Cavities. The dorsal body cavities are in the dorsal (back) part of the body and include a cranial cavity above and a spinal cavity below. The ventral body cavities are on the ventral (front) side of the trunk and include the thoracic cavity above the diaphragm and the abdominopelvic cavity below the diaphragm. The thoracic cavity is subdivided into the mediastinum in the center and pleural cavities (surrounding the lungs) to the sides. The abdominopelvic cavity is subdivided into the abdominal cavity above the pelvis and the pelvic cavity within the pelvis.

ORGANS IN THE VENTRAL BODY CAVITIES

AREAS	ORGANS
THORACIC CAVITY	
Right pleural cavity	Right lung
Mediastinum	Heart
	Trachea
	Right and left bronchi
	Esophagus
	Thymus gland
	Aortic arch and thoracic aorta
	Venae cavae
	Various lymph nodes and nerves
	Thoracic duct
Left pleural cavity	Left lung
ABDOMINOPELVIC CAVITY	
Abdominal cavity	Liver
	Gallbladder
	Stomach
	Pancreas
	Intestines
	Spleen
	Kidneys
	Ureters
Pelvic cavity	Urinary bladder
	Female reproductive organs
	Uterus
	Uterine tubes
	Ovaries
	Male reproductive organs
	Prostate gland
	Seminal vesicles
	Part of vas deferens
	Part of large intestine (sigmoid colon and rectum)

BODY REGIONS

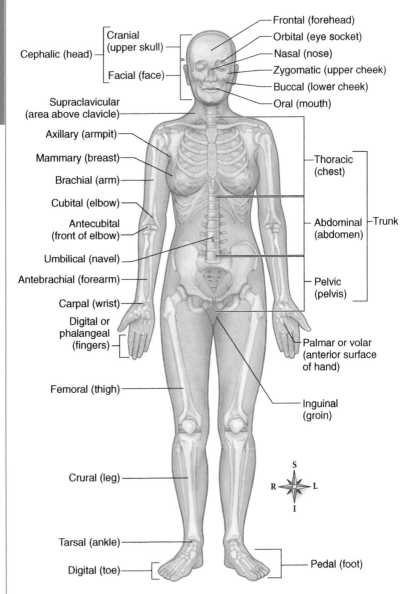

Specific Body Regions. Note that the body as a whole can be subdivided into two major portions: axial (along the middle, or *axis,* of the body) and appendicular (the arms and legs, or *appendages*). Names of specific body regions follow the Latin form, with the English equivalent in parentheses.

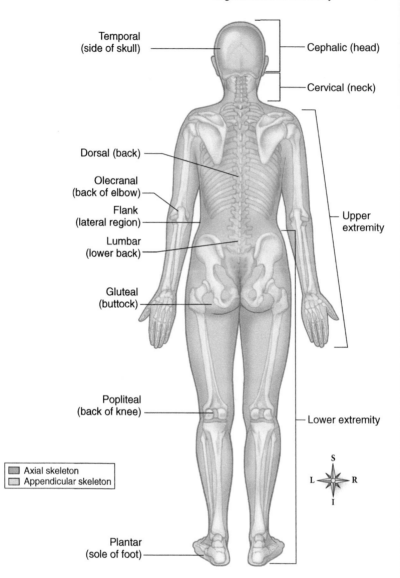

Temporal (side of skull)

Cephalic (head)

Cervical (neck)

Dorsal (back)

Olecranal (back of elbow)

Flank (lateral region)

Lumbar (lower back)

Gluteal (buttock)

Upper extremity

Popliteal (back of knee)

Lower extremity

Axial skeleton
Appendicular skeleton

Plantar (sole of foot)

S
L — R
I

LATIN-BASED DESCRIPTIVE TERMS FOR BODY REGIONS*

BODY REGION	AREA OR EXAMPLE	BODY REGION	AREA OR EXAMPLE
Abdominal (ab-DOM-in-al)	Anterior torso below diaphragm	Digital (DIJ-i-tal)	Fingers or toes
		Dorsal (DOR-sal)	Back or top
		Facial (FAY-shal)	Face
Acromial (ah-KRO-mee-al)	Shoulder	Femoral (FEM-or-al)	Thigh
Antebrachial (an-tee-BRAY-kee-al)	Forearm	Frontal (FRON-tal)	Forehead
Antecubital (an-tee-KYOO-bi-tal)	Depressed area just in front of elbow (cubital fossa)	Gluteal (GLOO-tee-al)	Buttock
		Hallux (HAL-luks)	Great toe
		Inguinal (ING-gwi-nal)	Groin
Axillary (AK-si-lair-ee)	Armpit (axilla)	Lumbar (LUM-bar)	Lower part of back between ribs and pelvis
Brachial (BRAY-kee-al)	Arm		
Buccal (BUK-al)	Cheek (inside)	Mammary (MAM-er-ee)	Breast
Calcaneal (cal-CANE-ee-al)	Heel of foot	Manual (MAN-yoo-al)	Hand
Carpal (KAR-pal)	Wrist	Mental (MEN-tal)	Chin
Cephalic (se-FAL-ik)	Head	Nasal (NAY-zal)	Nose
Cervical (SER-vi-kal)	Neck	Navel (NAY-vel)	Area around navel or umbilicus
Coxal (COX-al)	Hip		
Cranial (KRAY-nee-al)	Skull	Occipital (ok-SIP-i-tal)	Back of lower part of skull
Crural (KROOR-al)	Leg	Olecranal (o-LECK-ra-nal)	Back of elbow
Cubital (KYOO-bi-tal)	Elbow	Oral (OR-al)	Mouth
Cutaneous (kyoo-TANE-ee-us)	Skin (or body surface)	Orbital or ophthalmic (OR-bi-tal or op-THAL-mik)	Eyes

LATIN-BASED DESCRIPTIVE TERMS FOR BODY REGIONS*—cont'd

BODY REGION	AREA OR EXAMPLE	BODY REGION	AREA OR EXAMPLE
Otic (O-tick)	Ear	**Popliteal** (pop-li-TEE-al)	Area behind knee
Palmar (PAHL-mar)	Palm of hand		
Patellar (pa-TELL-er)	Front of knee	**Pubic** (PYOO-bik)	Pubis
Pedal (PED-al)	Foot	**Supraclavicular** (soo-pra-cla-VIK-yoo-lar)	Area above clavicle
Pelvic (PEL-vik)	Lower portion of torso		
Perineal (pair-i-NEE-al)	Area (perineum) between anus and genitals	**Sural** (SUR-al)	Calf
		Tarsal (TAR-sal)	Ankle
		Temporal (TEM-por-al)	Side of skull
Plantar (PLAN-tar)	Sole of foot	**Thoracic** (tho-RAS-ik)	Chest
Pollex (POL-ex)	Thumb	**Zygomatic** (zye-go-MAT-ik)	Cheek (outside)

*The left column lists English adjectives that are based on Latin terms that describe the body parts listed in English in the right column.

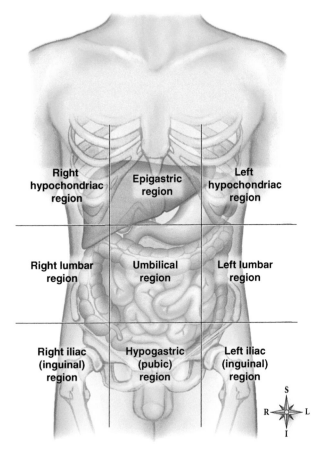

Nine Regions of the Abdominopelvic Cavity. Only the most superficial structures of the internal organs are shown here.

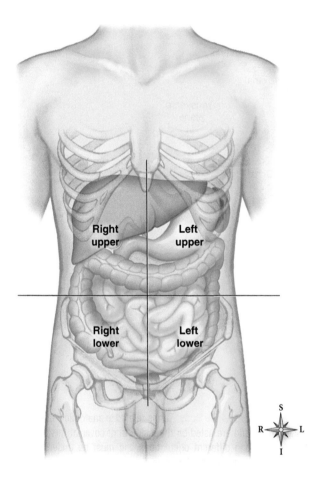

Division of the Abdomen into Four Quadrants. This diagram shows the relationship of the internal organs to the four abdominal quadrants.

DIRECTIONS AND PLANES OF THE BODY

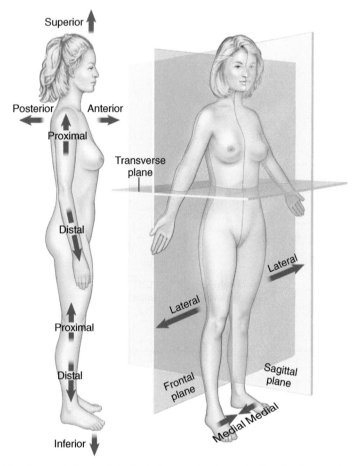

Directions and Planes of the Body. Terms related to anatomical direction are shown here using arrows and are listed on the inside front cover of this handbook. Planes divide the body along different orientations and must be understood to interpret anatomical diagrams and medical images.

Sagittal: A lengthwise plane that runs from front to back is called a *sagittal plane*. Such a plane divides the body or any of its parts into right and left sides. If a sagittal section is made in the exact midline to result in equal and symmetrical right and left halves, that plane is called a *midsagittal plane*.

Coronal: A lengthwise plane that runs from side to side and that divides the body or any of its parts into anterior and posterior portions; also called a *frontal plane*.

Transverse: A crosswise plane; divides the body or any of its parts into upper and lower parts; also called a *horizontal plane*.

Other Planes: Any individual structure within the body can be divided across the structure's long axis, producing a **cross section**. A flat division parallel to a structure's long axis is called a **longitudinal section**.

To make the reading of anatomical figures a little easier, an anatomical compass is used throughout this book. On many figures, you will notice a small compass rosette similar to those on geographical maps. Rather than being labeled N, S, E, and W, the anatomical rosette is labeled with abbreviated anatomical directions. Refer to the inside front cover of this handbook for definitions of the listed anatomical directions.

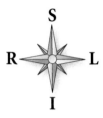

A = Anterior	**P** (opposite **A**) = Posterior
D = Distal	**P** (opposite **D**) = Proximal
I = Inferior	**S** = Superior
L (opposite **M**) = Lateral	**M** = Medial
L (opposite **R**) = Left	**R** = Right

HOMEOSTASIS

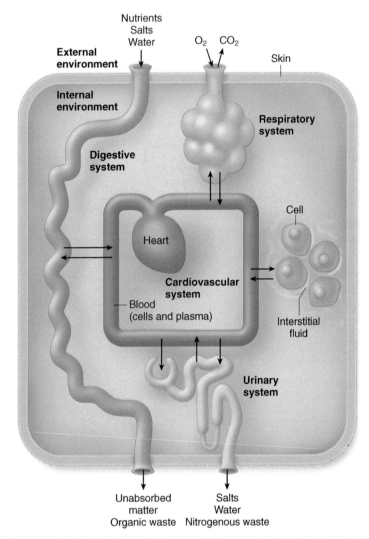

Diagram of the Body's Internal Environment. The human body is like a bag of fluid separated from the external environment. Tubes, such as the digestive tract and respiratory tract, bring the external environment to deeper parts of the bag, where substances may be absorbed into the internal fluid environment or excreted into the external environment. All of the "accessories" help to maintain a constant environment inside the bag that allows the cells that live there to survive.

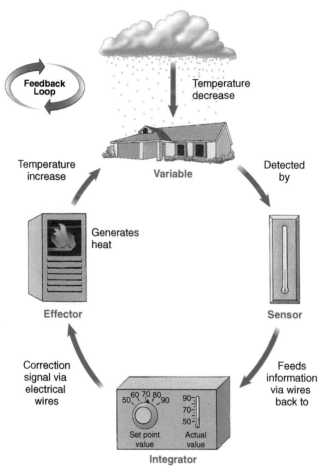

Basic Components of Homeostatic Control Mechanisms. *Heat regulation by a furnace controlled by a thermostat.* This illustration of heat from a furnace that is being controlled by a thermostat is a good analogy of the kind of feedback control mechanism that is also found in the human body.

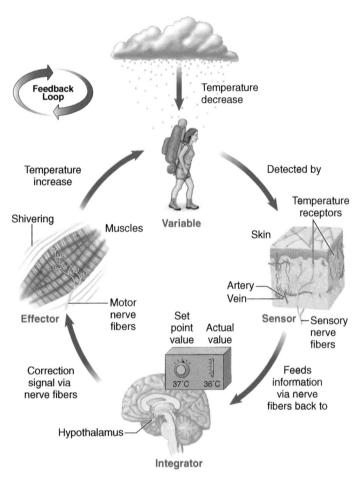

Basic Components of Homeostatic Control Mechanisms. *Homeostasis of body temperature.* This illustrates the body's mechanism for maintaining homeostasis of body temperature. Note that in both this illustration and the one before it, a stimulus (drop in temperature) activates a sensor mechanism (thermostat or body temperature receptor) that sends input to an integrating, or control, center (on/off switch or hypothalamus), which then sends input to an effector mechanism (furnace or contracting muscle). The resulting heat that is produced maintains the temperature in a "normal range." Feedback of effector activity to the sensor mechanism completes the control loop.

METRIC MEASUREMENTS AND THEIR EQUIVALENTS

Units of Measurement

BASIC UNIT	METRIC	ENGLISH	ENGLISH/ METRIC
Time	second (sec)	second (sec)	Same
Length	meter (m)	yard (yd)	1.09 yards/1 meter
Volume	liter (l or L)	quart (qt)	1.06 quarts/1 liter
Mass	gram (g)	ounce (oz)	0.035 ounce/ 1 gram
Temperature	degree Celsius (°C)	degree Fahrenheit (°F)	1.8°F/1°C

PREFIXES

LESS THAN ONE BASIC UNIT		
nano-	one billionth	0.000000001
micro-	one millionth	0.000001
milli-	one thousandth	0.001
centi-	one hundredth	0.01
deci-	one tenth	0.1
MORE THAN ONE BASIC UNIT		
deka-	ten	10
hecto-	one hundred	100
kilo-	one thousand	1000
mega-	one million	1,000,000

COMMON CONVERSIONS

MULTIPLY	BY	TO GET
TIME		
Seconds	1000	Milliseconds
Seconds	0.00167	Minutes
Minutes	60	Seconds
Milliseconds	0.001	Seconds
LENGTH		
Meters	1.09	Yards
Meters	3.28	Feet
Meters	100	Centimeters
Meters	1000	Millimeters
Centimeters	0.01	Meters
Centimeters	10	Millimeters
Centimeters	100000	Micrometers
Millimeters	0.001	Meters
Millimeters	0.1	Centimeters
VOLUME		
Liters	1.06	Quarts
Liters	0.26	Gallons
Liters	1000	Milliliters
Liters	100	Centiliters
Liters	10	Deciliters
Centiliters	0.01	Liters
Centiliters	10	Milliliters
Centiliters	0.1	Deciliters
Deciliters	0.1	Liters
Deciliters	10	Centiliters
MASS		
Grams	0.35	Ounces
Grams	0.001	Kilograms
Grams	1000	Milligrams
Milligrams	0.001	Grams
Kilograms	1000	Grams
Kilograms	2.21	Pounds

As you can see from the Units of Measurement table, one "degree" in Celsius is a larger unit than one degree in Fahrenheit. In fact, a Celsius degree is ⅝ (1.8) times the size of a Fahrenheit degree. When you convert temperature readings from one form to another, this discrepancy in size must be taken into account. The 32° is added during the conversion to Fahrenheit to account for the fact that, in the Fahrenheit scale, the freezing point of water is 32°, not 0°, as it is in Celsius.

TEMPERATURE CONVERSIONS

To Convert °C to °F
Multiply °C by $\frac{9}{5}$ and add 32:
_____°C × $\frac{9}{5}$ + 32 = _____°F
For example, to convert 35°C to °F:
35°C × $\frac{9}{5}$ + 32 = 95°F

To Convert °F to °C
Subtract 32 from °F and multiply by $\frac{5}{9}$:
(_____°F − 32) × $\frac{5}{9}$ = °C
For example, to convert 101°F to °C:
(101°F − 32) × $\frac{5}{9}$ = 38.3°C

BODY TEMPERATURES IN DEGREES CELSIUS AND DEGREES FAHRENHEIT

°C	°F	°C	°F
35.0	95.0	37.8	100.0
35.1	95.2	37.9	100.2
35.2	95.4	38.0	100.4
35.3	95.6	38.1	100.6
35.4	95.8	38.2	100.8
35.5	96.0	38.3	101.0
35.7	96.2	38.4	101.2
35.8	96.4	38.6	101.4
35.9	96.6	38.7	101.6
36.0	96.8	38.8	101.8
36.1	97.0	38.9	102.0
36.2	97.2	39.0	102.2
36.3	97.4	39.1	102.4
36.4	97.6	39.2	102.6
36.6	97.8	39.3	102.8
36.7	98.0	39.4	103.0
36.8	98.2	39.6	103.2
36.9	98.4	39.7	103.4
37.0	98.6	39.8	103.6
37.1	98.8	39.9	103.8
37.2	99.0	40.0	104.0
37.3	99.2	40.1	104.2
37.4	99.4	40.2	104.4
37.6	99.6	40.3	104.6
37.7	99.8	40.4	104.8

2

Body Chemistry

Anatomy and physiology are subdivisions of biology—the study of life. To best understand the characteristics of life, what living matter is, how it is organized, and what it can do, we must appreciate and understand certain basic principles of **chemistry** that apply to the life process.

Life itself depends on proper levels and proportions of chemical substances in the cytoplasm of cells. The various structural levels of organization described in Chapter 1 are ultimately based on the existence and interrelationships of atoms and molecules. Chemistry, like biology, is a very broad scientific discipline. It deals with the structure, arrangement, and composition of substances and the reactions they undergo. Just as biology may be subdivided into many sub-disciplines or branches, like anatomy and physiology, chemistry may also be divided into focused areas.

Biochemistry is the field of chemistry that deals with living organisms and the life processes we collectively called **metabolism**. It deals directly with the chemical composition of living matter and the metabolic processes that underlie life activities such as growth, muscle contraction, and transmission of nervous impulses.

ELEMENTS AND COMPOUNDS

Periodic Table of Elements

Legend:
- 6 — Atomic number (number of protons)
- C — Chemical symbol
- 12.011 — Atomic mass (number of protons plus average number of neutrons)
- ☐ Major elements
- ☐ Trace elements

1	2	3	4	5	6	7	8	9	10	11	12	13	14	15	16	17	18
1 H [1.007; 1.009]																	2 He 4.002
3 Li [6.938; 6.997]	4 Be 9.012											5 B [10.80; 10.83]	6 C [12.00; 12.02]	7 N [14.00; 14.01]	8 O [15.99; 16.00]	9 F 18.998	10 Ne 20.180
11 Na 22.990	12 Mg 24.305											13 Al 26.982	14 Si [28.08; 28.09]	15 P 30.974	16 S [32.05; 32.08]	17 Cl [35.44; 35.46]	18 Ar 39.948
19 K 39.098	20 Ca 40.078	21 Sc 44.956	22 Ti 47.867	23 V 50.942	24 Cr 51.996	25 Mn 54.931	26 Fe 55.845	27 Co 58.933	28 Ni 58.963	29 Cu 63.546	30 Zn 65.39	31 Ga 69.723	32 Ge 72.61	33 As 74.922	34 Se 78.96(3)	35 Br 79.904	36 Kr 83.80
37 Rb 85.468	38 Sr 87.62	39 Y 88.906	40 Zr 91.224	41 Nb 92.906	42 Mo 95.94	43 Tc (98)	44 Ru 101.07	45 Rh 102.906	46 Pd 106.42	47 Ag 107.868	48 Cd 112.411	49 In 114.818	50 Sn 118.710	51 Sb 121.760	52 Te 127.60	53 I 126.904	54 Xe 131.29
55 Cs 132.905	56 Ba 137.327	57 La 138.905	72 Hf 178.49	73 Ta 180.948	74 W 183.84	75 Re 186.207	76 Os 190.23	77 Ir 192.217	78 Pt 195.08	79 Au 196.967	80 Hg 200.59	81 Tl [204.3; 204.4]	82 Pb 207.2	83 Bi 208.980	84 Po (209)	85 At (210)	86 Rn (222)
87 Fr (223)	88 Ra 226.025	89 Ac 227.028	104 Rf (263.113)	105 Db (262.114)	106 Sg (266.122)	107 Bh (264.125)	108 Hs (269.134)	109 Mt (268.139)	110 Ds (272.146)	111 Rg (272.154)	112 Cn (285)	113 Uut (284)	114 Fl (289)	115 Uup (288)	116 Lv (293)	117 Uus (292)	118 Uuo (294)

58 Ce 140.115	59 Pr 140.907	60 Nd 144.24	61 Pm (145)	62 Sm 150.36	63 Eu 151.965	64 Gd 157.25	65 Tb 158.925	66 Dy 162.50	67 Ho 164.930	68 Er 167.26	69 Tm 168.939	70 Yb 173.04	71 Lu 174.967
90 Th 232.038	91 Pa 231.036	92 U 238.029	93 Np 237.048	94 Pu (244)	95 Am (243)	96 Cm (247)	97 Bk (247)	98 Cf (251)	99 Es (252)	100 Fm (257)	101 Md (258)	102 No (259)	103 Lr (260)

Periodic Table of Elements. The major elements found in the body are highlighted in pink. The trace elements, found in very tiny quantities in the body, are highlighted in orange. (Atomic mass numbers in brackets show the natural range of isotopes; those in parentheses are uncertain or theoretical.)

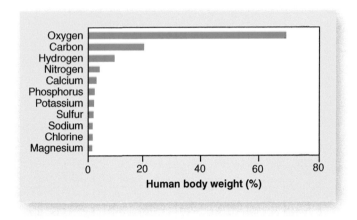

Major Elements of the Body. These elements are found in great quantity in the body. The graph shows the relative abundance of each in the body. Notice that oxygen (O), carbon (C), hydrogen (H), and nitrogen (N) predominate.

ELEMENTS IN THE HUMAN BODY

ELEMENT	SYMBOL	HUMAN BODY WEIGHT (%)	IMPORTANCE OR FUNCTION
MAJOR ELEMENTS			
Oxygen	O	65.0	Necessary for cellular respiration; component of water
Carbon	C	18.5	Backbone of organic molecules
Hydrogen	H	9.5	Component of water and most organic molecules; necessary for energy transfer and respiration
Nitrogen	N	3.3	Component of all proteins and nucleic acids
Calcium	Ca	1.5	Component of bones and teeth; triggers muscle contraction
Phosphorus	P	1.0	Principal component in the backbone of nucleic acids; important in energy transfer
Potassium	K	0.4	Principal positive ion within cells; important in nerve function
Sulfur	S	0.3	Component of many energy-transferring enzymes
Sodium	Na	0.2	Important positive ion surrounding cells

ELEMENT	SYMBOL	HUMAN BODY WEIGHT (%)	IMPORTANCE OR FUNCTION
Chlorine	Cl	0.2	Important negative ion surrounding cells
Magnesium	Mg	0.1	Component of many energy-transferring enzymes
TRACE ELEMENTS			
Silicone	Si	<0.1	Uncertain
Aluminum	Al	<0.1	Uncertain
Iron	Fe	<0.1	Critical component of hemoglobin in the blood
Manganese	Mn	<0.1	Component of many energy-transferring enzymes
Fluorine	F	<0.1	Hardens crystals that form teeth and bones
Vanadium	V	<0.1	Uncertain
Chromium	Cr	<0.1	Alters insulin (hormone) effects, which regulate carbohydrate, lipid, and protein metabolism
Copper	Cu	<0.1	Key component of many enzymes
Boron	B	<0.1	May strengthen cell membranes; plays a role in brain and bone development
Cobalt	Co	<0.1	Component of vitamin B_{12}
Zinc	Zn	<0.1	Key component of some enzymes
Selenium	Se	<0.1	Component of an antioxidant enzyme
Molybdenum	Mo	<0.1	Key component of some enzymes
Tin	Sn	<0.1	Uncertain
Iodine	I	<0.1	Component of thyroid hormone

INORGANIC SALTS IMPORTANT FOR BODY FUNCTIONS

INORGANIC SALT	CHEMICAL FORMULA	ELECTROLYTES
Sodium chloride	$NaCl$	$Na^+ + Cl^-$
Calcium chloride	$CaCl_2$	$Ca^{++} + 2Cl^-$
Magnesium chloride	$MgCl_2$	$Mg^{++} + 2Cl^-$
Sodium bicarbonate	$NaHCO_3$	$Na^+ + HCO^- + Cl^-$
Potassium chloride	KCl	$K^+ + Cl^-$
Sodium sulfate	Na_2SO_4	$2Na^+ + SO_4^=$
Calcium carbonate	$CaCO_3$	$Ca^{++} + CO_3^=$
Calcium phosphate	$Ca_3(PO_4)_2$	$3Ca^{++} + 2PO_4^{\equiv}$

ORGANIC MOLECULES

EXAMPLES OF IMPORTANT BIOMOLECULES

MACROMOLECULE	SUBUNIT	FUNCTION	EXAMPLE
CARBOHYDRATES			
Glucose	Simple sugar (hexose: $C_6H_{12}O_6$)	Stores energy	Blood glucose
Ribose	Simple sugar (pentose: $C_5H_{10}O_5$)	Plays role in expression of hereditary information	Component of RNA
Deoxyribose	Simple sugar (pentose: $C_5H_{10}O_4$)	Plays role in storage and transmission of hereditary information	Component of DNA
Glycogen	Glucose	Stores energy	Liver glycogen
LIPIDS			
Triglycerides	Glycerol + 3 fatty acids	Store energy	Body fat
Phospholipids	Glycerol + phosphate + 2 fatty acids	Make up cell membranes	Plasma membrane of cell
Steroids	Steroid nucleus (4-carbon ring)	Make up cell membranes Hormone synthesis	Cholesterol, various steroid hormones, estrogens
Prostaglandins	20-carbon unsaturated fatty acid containing 5-carbon ring	Regulate hormone action; enhance immune system; affect inflammatory response	Prostaglandin E, prostaglandin A

PROTEINS

Functional proteins	Amino acids	Regulate chemical reactions	Hemoglobin, antibodies, enzymes
Structural proteins	Amino acids	Component of body support tissues	Muscle filaments, tendons, ligaments

NUCLEIC ACIDS

DNA	Nucleotides (sugar, phosphate, base)	Encodes hereditary information	Chromatin, chromosomes
RNA	Nucleotides (sugar, phosphate, base)	Helps decode hereditary information; acts as "RNA enzyme"; silencing of gene expression	Transfer RNA (tRNA), messenger RNA (mRNA), double-stranded RNA (dsRNA)

NUCLEOTIDES AND RELATED MOLECULES

Adenosine triphosphate (ATP)	Phosphorylated nucleotide (adenine + ribose + 3 phosphates)	Transfers energy from fuel molecules to working molecules	ATP present in every cell of the body
Creatine phosphate (CP)	Amino acid derivative + phosphate	Transfers energy from fuel to ATP	CP present in muscle fiber as "backup" to ATP
Nicotinic adenine dinucleotide (NAD)	Combination of two ribonucleotides	Acts as coenzyme to transfer high-energy particles from one chemical process to another	NAD present in every cell of the body

Continued

EXAMPLES OF IMPORTANT BIOMOLECULES—cont'd

MACROMOLECULE	SUBUNIT	FUNCTION	EXAMPLE
COMBINED OR ALTERED FORMS			
Glycoproteins	Large proteins with small carbohydrate groups attached	Similar to functional proteins	Some hormones, antibodies, enzymes, cell membrane components
Proteoglycans	Large polysaccharides with small polypeptide chains attached	Lubrication; increases thickness of fluid	Component of mucous fluid and many tissue fluids in the body
Lipoproteins	Protein complex containing lipid groups	Transport lipids in the blood	Low-density lipoproteins (LDLs) and high-density lipoproteins (HDLs)
Glycolipids	Lipid molecule with carbohydrate group attached	Component of cell membranes	Component of membranes of nerve cells
Ribonucleoprotein	Combination of RNA nucleotide and protein	Enzyme-like actions, such as splicing mRNA	Small nuclear ribonucleoproteins (snRNPs or "snurps") that make up the spliceosome structure in a cell

MAJOR FUNCTIONS OF HUMAN PROTEIN COMPOUNDS

FUNCTION	EXAMPLE
Provide structure	Structural proteins include keratin of skin, hair, and nails; parts of cell membranes; tendons
Catalyze chemical reactions	Lactase (enzyme in intestinal digestive juice) catalyzes chemical reaction that changes lactose to glucose and galactose
Transport substances in blood	Proteins classified as albumins combine with fatty acids to transport them in form of lipoproteins
Communicate information to cells	Insulin, a protein hormone, serves as chemical message from islet cells of the pancreas to cells all over the body
Act as receptors	Binding sites of certain proteins on surfaces of cell membranes serve as receptors for insulin and various other hormones
Defend body against many harmful agents	Proteins called *antibodies* or *immunoglobulins* combine with various harmful agents to render those agents harmless
Provide energy	Proteins can be metabolized for energy

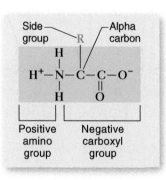

Basic Structural Formula for an Amino Acid. Note the relationship of the side group (R), amino group, and carboxyl group to the alpha carbon. The amino group (NH_2) is depicted in the figure as H_2N to show that the nitrogen atom of the group bonds to the alpha carbon.

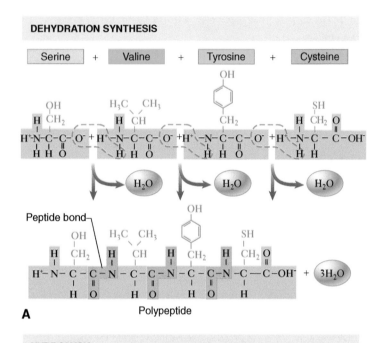

Formation (Dehydration Synthesis) and Decomposition (Hydrolysis) of a Polypeptide. A, Linkage of four amino acids by three peptide bonds resulting in the dehydration synthesis of a polypeptide chain and three molecules of water. **B,** Decomposition (hydrolysis) reaction resulting from the addition of three molecules of water. Peptide bonds are broken and individual amino acids are released.

Primary (first level)
Protein structure is a sequence of amino acids in a chain.

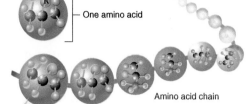

One amino acid

Amino acid chain

Secondary (second level)
Protein structure is formed by folding and twisting of amino acid chain.

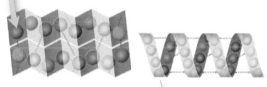

Folded sheet

Twisted helix

Tertiary (third level)
Protein structure is formed when the twists and folds of the secondary structure fold again to form a larger 3-dimensional structure.

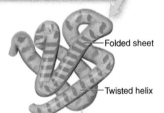

Folded sheet

Twisted helix

Quaternary (fourth level)
Protein structure is a protein consisting of more than one folded amino acid chain.

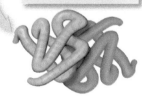

Protein. Protein molecules are large, complex molecules formed by one or more strands of amino acids. Each amino acid is connected to the next by a type of covalent bond called a **peptide bond**. Additional weak forces between atoms of the larger molecule then cause the strand to twist or fold into a **secondary** (second-level) protein structure. New relationships among the atoms then cause the molecule to fold again on itself to form a three-dimensional **tertiary** (third-level) protein structure. Several tertiary proteins may join to form a **quaternary** (fourth-level) protein structure.

MAJOR FUNCTIONS OF HUMAN LIPID COMPOUNDS

FUNCTION	EXAMPLE
Energy	Lipids can be stored and broken down later for energy; they yield more energy per unit of weight than carbohydrates or proteins do
Structure	Phospholipids and cholesterol are required components of cell membranes
Vitamins	Fat-soluble vitamins: vitamin A forms retinal (necessary for night vision); vitamin D increases calcium uptake; vitamin E promotes wound healing; and vitamin K is required for the synthesis of blood-clotting proteins
Protection	Fat surrounds and protects organs
Insulation	Fat under the skin minimizes heat loss; fatty tissue (myelin) covers nerve cells and electrically insulates them
Regulation	Steroid hormones regulate many physiological processes; for example, estrogen and testosterone are responsible for many of the differences between females and males; prostaglandins help regulate inflammation and tissue repair

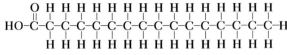

Palmitic acid (saturated)

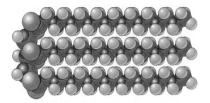

A

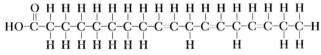

α-Linolenic acid (unsaturated)

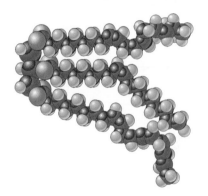

B

Types of Fatty Acids. A, Palmitic acid, a **saturated** fatty acid. Note that it contains no double bonds; its hydrocarbon chain is filled with hydrogen atoms. The lower three-dimensional model shows three molecules of palmitic acid joined to a molecule of glycerol to form a triglyceride. **B,** The upper structural formula shows the **unsaturated** fatty acid α-linolenic acid (double bonds shown in *red*). The lower three-dimensional model shows triglycerides that are exhibiting "kinks" caused by the presence of double bonds in the component fatty acids.

BLOOD LIPOPROTEINS

A lipid such as cholesterol can travel in the blood only after it has attached to a protein molecule—forming a **lipoprotein.** Some of these molecules are called **high-density lipoproteins (HDLs)** because they have a high density due to having more protein than cholesterol. Another type of molecule contains less protein than cholesterol, so it is called **low-density lipoprotein (LDL).** The composite nature of a lipoprotein molecule is shown in the figure.

The cholesterol in LDLs is often called "bad" cholesterol because high blood levels of LDL are associated with **atherosclerosis,** a life-threatening blockage of arteries. LDLs carry cholesterol to cells, including the cells that line blood vessels. HDLs, on the other hand, carry so-called "good" cholesterol *away from cells* and toward the liver for elimination from the body. A high proportion of HDL in the blood is associated with a low risk for atherosclerosis.

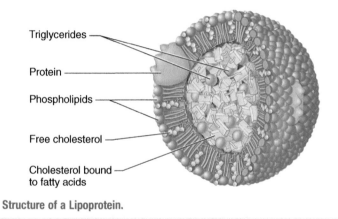

Triglycerides

Protein

Phospholipids

Free cholesterol

Cholesterol bound to fatty acids

Structure of a Lipoprotein.

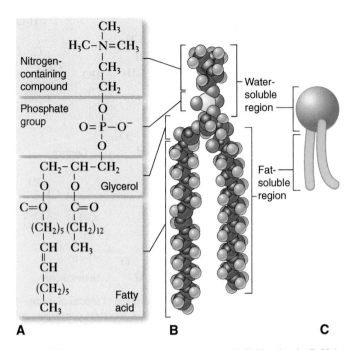

Phospholipid Molecule. A, Chemical formula of a phospholipid molecule. **B,** Molecular model showing water- and fat-soluble regions. **C,** Cartoon often used to represent the double-tailed phospholipid molecule.

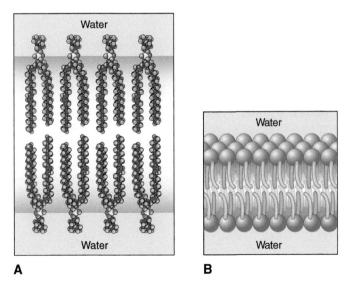

Phospholipid Bilayer. A, Orientation of phospholipid molecules when surrounded by water and forming a bilayer. **B,** Cartoon commonly used to depict a phospholipid bilayer.

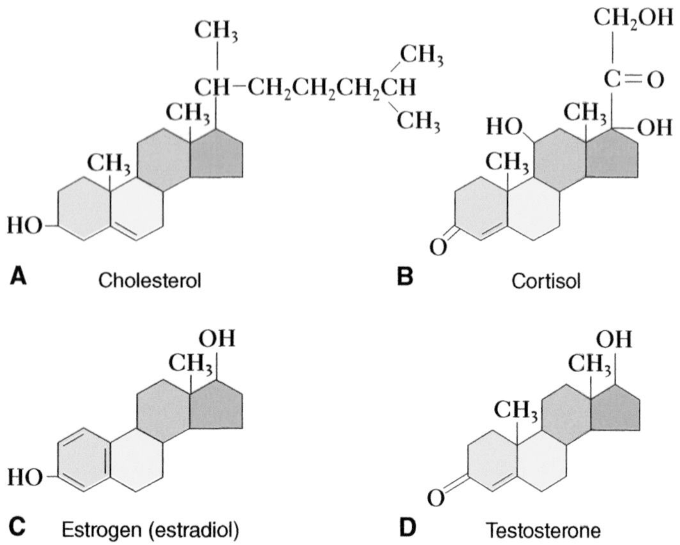

A Cholesterol

B Cortisol

C Estrogen (estradiol)

D Testosterone

Steroid Compounds. The steroid nucleus—*highlighted in shades of yellow*—found in cholesterol **(A)** forms the basis for many other important compounds such as cortisol **(B),** estradiol (an estrogen) **(C)**, and testosterone **(D)**.

COMPARISON OF DNA AND RNA STRUCTURE

	DNA	RNA
Polynucleotide strands	Double; very long	Single or double; short
Sugar	Deoxyribose	Ribose
Base pairing	Adenine–thymine (A–T)	Adenine–uracil (A–U)
	Guanine–cytosine (G–C)	Guanine–cytosine (G–C)

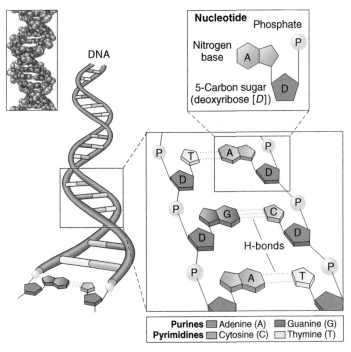

The DNA Molecule. Representation of the **DNA double helix** showing the general structure of a nucleotide and the two kinds of *base pairs:* adenine (A) *(blue)* with thymine (T) *(yellow)* and guanine (G) *(purple)* with cytosine (C) *(red).* Note that the G–C base pair has three hydrogen bonds and the A–T base pair has two. Hydrogen bonds are extremely important in maintaining the structure of this molecule.

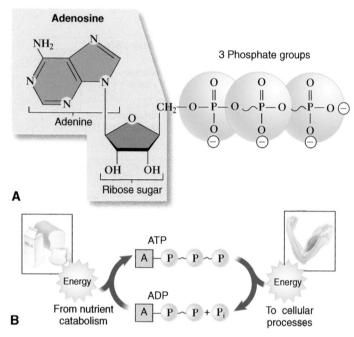

Adenosine Triphosphate (ATP). A, Structure of ATP. A single adenosine group (A) has three attached **phosphate groups (P).** High-energy bonds between the phosphate groups can release chemical energy to do cellular work. **B,** General scheme of the ATP energy cycle. ATP stores energy in its last high-energy phosphate bond. When that bond is later broken, energy is transferred as important intermediate compounds are formed. **The adenosine diphosphate (ADP)** and phosphate groups that result can be resynthesized into ATP, thereby capturing additional energy from nutrient catabolism. Note that energy is transferred from nutrient catabolism to ADP, thus converting it to ATP, and energy is transferred *from* ATP to provide the energy required for anabolic reactions or cellular processes as it reverts back to ADP.

Cells

The **cell theory** states simply that the cell is the fundamental organizational unit of life; all living things are composed of cells.

Almost all human cells are microscopic in size. Their diameters range from 7.5 micrometers (μm) (example, red blood cells) to about 150 μm (example, female sex cell or ovum). The period at the end of this sentence measures about 100 μm—roughly 13 times as large as our smallest cells and two thirds the size of the human ovum.

Like other anatomical structures, cells exhibit a particular size or form because they perform a certain activity. A nerve cell, for example, may have threadlike extensions over a meter in length to transmit nervous impulses from one area of the body to another. Muscle cells are adapted to contract, that is, to shorten or lengthen with pulling strength. Other types of cells may serve protective or secretory function.

Despite their distinctive anatomical characteristics and specialized functions, the cells of your body have many similarities. The so-called *typical* or **composite cell**—one that exhibits the most important characteristics of many different human cell types—is shown on the next page. Keep in mind that no such "typical" cell actually exists in the body; it is a composite structure created for reference purposes.

ANATOMY OF CELLS

Typical, or Composite, Cell. Artist's interpretation of cell structure. Note the mitochondria, known as the "power plants of the cell." Also note the innumerable dots bordering the endoplasmic reticulum. These are ribosomes, the cell's "protein factories." The magnified view in the inset better shows the microfilaments and microtubules of the cell's cytoskeleton.

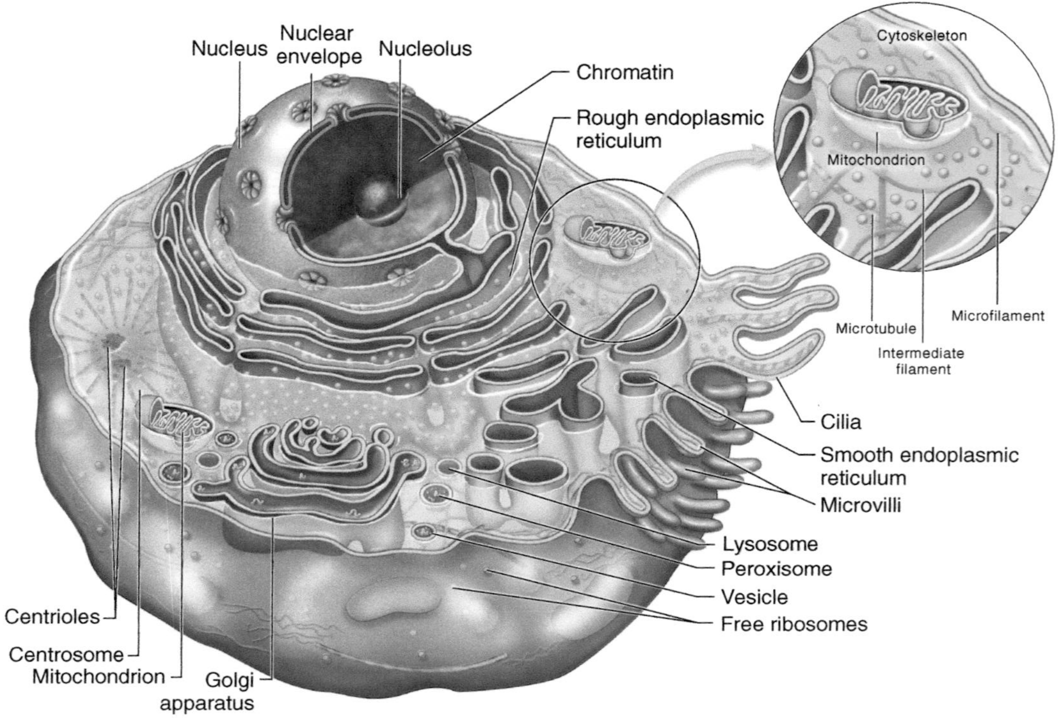
Nucleus
Nuclear envelope
Nucleolus
Chromatin
Rough endoplasmic reticulum
Cytoskeleton
Mitochondrion
Microtubule
Intermediate filament
Microfilament
Cilia
Smooth endoplasmic reticulum
Microvilli
Lysosome
Peroxisome
Vesicle
Free ribosomes
Centrioles
Centrosome
Mitochondrion
Golgi apparatus

SOME MAJOR CELL STRUCTURES AND THEIR FUNCTIONS

CELL STRUCTURE	DESCRIPTION	FUNCTIONS
MEMBRANOUS		
Plasma membrane	Phospholipid bilayer reinforced with cholesterol and embedded with proteins and other organic molecules	Serves as the boundary of the cell, maintains its integrity; protein molecules embedded in plasma membrane perform various functions; for example, they serve as markers that identify cells of each individual, as receptor molecules for certain hormones and other molecules, and as transport mechanisms
Endoplasmic reticulum (ER)	Network of canals and sacs extending from the nuclear envelope; may have ribosomes attached	Ribosomes attached to rough ER synthesize proteins that leave cells via the Golgi apparatus; smooth ER synthesizes lipids incorporated in cell membranes, steroid hormones, and certain carbohydrates used to form glycoproteins—also removes and stores Ca^{++} from the cell's interior
Golgi apparatus	Stack of flattened sacs (cisternae) surrounded by vesicles	Synthesizes carbohydrate, combines it with protein, and packages the product as globules of glycoprotein
Vesicles	Tiny membranous bags	Temporarily contain molecules for transport or later use
Lysosomes	Tiny membranous bags containing enzymes	Digestive enzymes break down defective cell parts and ingested particles; a cell's "digestive system"
Peroxisomes	Tiny membranous bags containing enzymes	Enzymes detoxify harmful substances in the cell

Continued

SOME MAJOR CELL STRUCTURES AND THEIR FUNCTIONS—cont'd

CELL STRUCTURE	DESCRIPTION	FUNCTIONS
Mitochondria	Tiny membranous capsule surrounding an inner, highly folded membrane embedded with enzymes; has small, ringlike chromosome (DNA)	Catabolism; adenosine triphosphate (ATP) synthesis; a cell's "power plants"
Nucleus	A usually central, spherical double-membrane container of chromatin (DNA); has large pores	Houses the genetic code, which in turn dictates protein synthesis, thereby playing an essential role in other cell activities, namely, cell transport, metabolism, and growth
NONMEMBRANOUS		
Ribosomes	Small particles assembled from two tiny subunits of rRNA and protein	Site of protein synthesis; a cell's "protein factories"
Proteasomes	Hollow protein cylinders with embedded enzymes	Destroys misfolded or otherwise abnormal proteins manufactured by the cell; a "quality control" mechanism for protein synthesis
Cytoskeleton	Network of interconnecting flexible filaments, stiff tubules, and molecular motors within the cell	Supporting framework of the cell and its organelles; functions in cell movement (using molecular motors); forms cell extensions (microvilli, cilia, flagella)

SOME MAJOR CELL STRUCTURES AND THEIR FUNCTIONS—cont'd

CELL STRUCTURE	DESCRIPTION	FUNCTIONS
Centrosome	Region of cytoskeleton that includes two cylindrical groupings of microtubules called *centrioles*	Acts as the microtubule-organizing center (MTOC) of the cell; centrioles assist in forming and organizing microtubules
Microvilli	Short, fingerlike extensions of plasma membrane; supported internally by microfilaments	Tiny, fingerlike extensions that increase a cell's absorptive surface area
Cilia and flagella	Moderate (cilia) to long (flagella) hairlike extensions of plasma membrane; supported internally by cylindrical formation of microtubules, sometimes with attached molecular motors	Cilia move substances over the cell surface or detect changes outside the cell; flagella propel sperm cells
Nucleolus	Dense area of chromatin and related molecules within nucleus	Site of formation of ribosome subunits

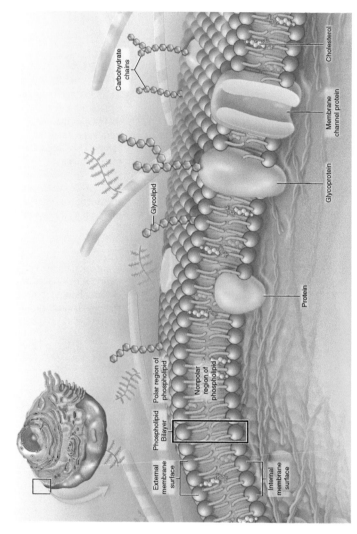

Plasma Membrane. The plasma membrane is made of a bilayer of phospholipid molecules arranged with their nonpolar "tails" pointing toward each other. Cholesterol molecules help stabilize the flexible bilayer structure to prevent breakage. Protein molecules (integral membrane proteins or IMPs) and protein—hybrid molecules may be found on the outer or inner surface of the bilayer or extending all the way through the membrane.

FUNCTIONAL ANATOMY OF CELL MEMBRANES

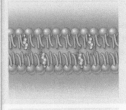

Structure: Sheet (bilayer) of phospholipids stabilized by cholesterol
Function: Maintains boundary (integrity) of a cell or membranous organelle

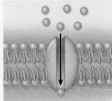

Structure: Integral membrane proteins that act as channels or carriers of molecules
Function: Controlled transport of water-soluble molecules from one compartment to another

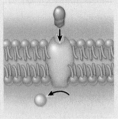

Structure: Receptor molecules that trigger metabolic changes in membrane (or on other side of membrane)
Function: Sensitivity to hormones and other regulatory chemicals; involved in signal transduction

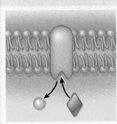

Structure: Enzyme molecules that catalyze specific chemical reactions
Function: Regulation of metabolic reactions

Continued

FUNCTIONAL ANATOMY OF CELL MEMBRANES—cont'd

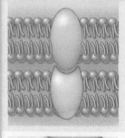

Structure: Integral membrane proteins that bind to molecules outside the cell
Function: Form connections between one cell and another

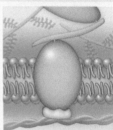

Structure: Integral membrane proteins that bind to support structures
Function: Support and maintain the shape of a cell or membranous organelle; participate in cell movement; bind to fibers of the extracellular matrix (ECM)

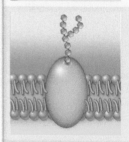

Structure: Glycoproteins or proteins in the membrane that act as markers
Function: Recognition of cells or organelles

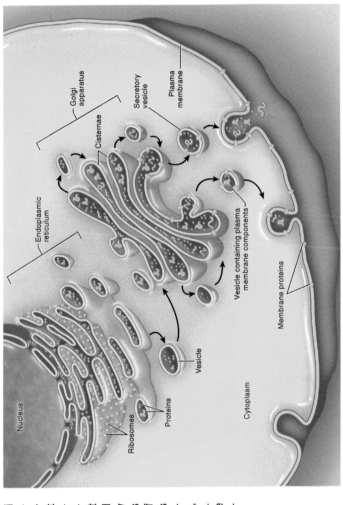

The Cell's Protein Export System. The **Golgi apparatus** processes and packages protein molecules delivered from the **endoplasmic reticulum** by small **vesicles**. After entering the first *cisterna* of the Golgi apparatus, a protein molecule undergoes a series of chemical modifications, is sent (by means of a vesicle) to the next cisterna for further modification, and so on, until it is ready to exit the last cisterna. When it is ready to exit, a molecule is packaged in a membranous secretory vesicle that migrates to the surface of the cell and "pops open" to release its contents into the space outside the cell. The vesicle membrane, including any integral membrane proteins, then becomes part of the plasma membrane. Some vesicles remain inside the cell for some time and serve as storage vessels for the substance to be secreted.

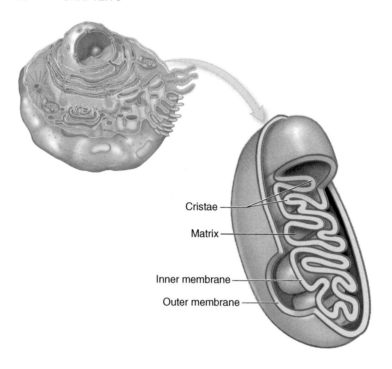

Mitochondrion. Cutaway sketch showing outer and inner membranes. Note the many folds (cristae) of the inner membrane.

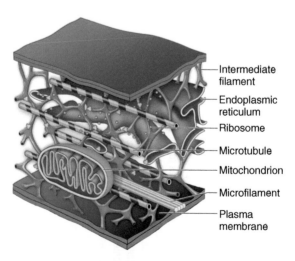

The Cytoskeleton. Artist's interpretation of the cell's internal framework. Notice that the "free" ribosomes and other organelles are not really freely floating in the cell.

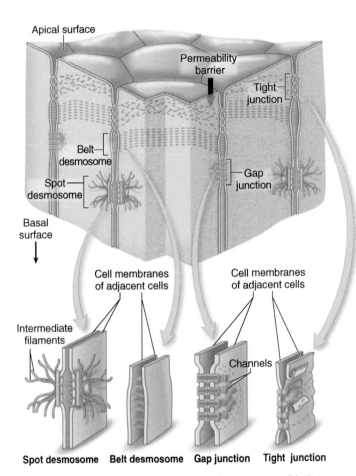

Apical surface

Permeability
barrier

Tight
junction

Belt
desmosome

Spot
desmosome

Gap
junction

Basal
surface

Cell membranes
of adjacent cells

Cell membranes
of adjacent cells

Intermediate
filaments

Channels

Spot desmosome | **Belt desmosome** | **Gap junction** | **Tight junction**

Cell Connections. A few of the major types of junctions possible between cells. Many cells are linked by more than one type of junction.

PHYSIOLOGY OF CELLS

PASSIVE TRANSPORT PROCESSES

PROCESS	DESCRIPTION	EXAMPLES
Simple diffusion	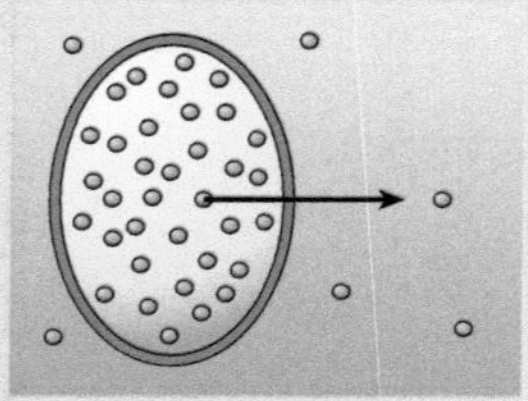	Movement of particles through the phospholipid bilayer or through channels from an area of high concentration to an area of low concentration—that is, down the concentration gradient	Movement of carbon dioxide out of all cells
Osmosis	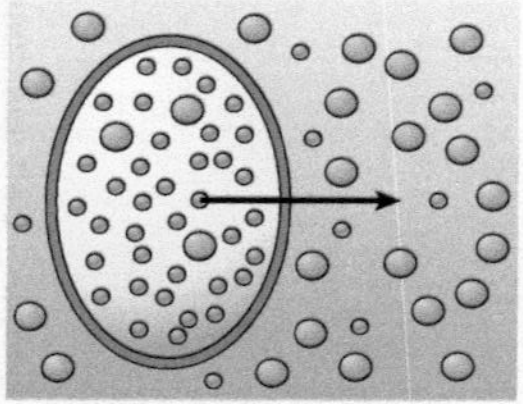	Diffusion of water through a selectively permeable membrane in the presence of at least one impermeant solute (often involves both simple and channel-mediated diffusion)	Diffusion of water molecules into and out of cells to correct imbalances in water concentration

		Description	Example
Channel-mediated passive transport (facilitated diffusion)	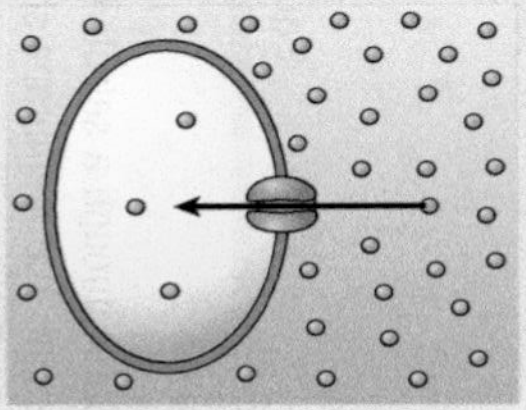	Diffusion of particles through a membrane by means of channel structures in the membrane (particles move down their concentration gradient)	Diffusion of sodium ions into nerve cells during a nerve impulse
Carrier-mediated passive transport (facilitated diffusion)	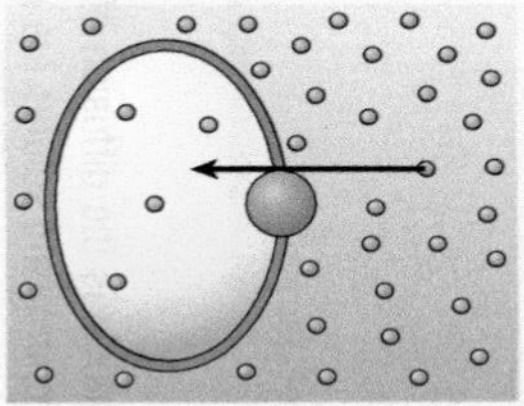	Diffusion of particles through a membrane by means of carrier structures in the membrane (particles move down their concentration gradient)	Diffusion of glucose molecules into most cells

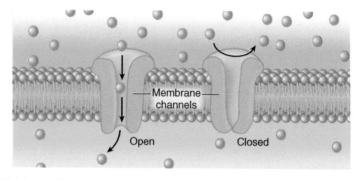

Membrane Channels. Gated channel proteins form tunnels through which only specific molecules may pass—as long as the "gates" are open. Molecules that do not have a specific shape and charge are never permitted to pass through the channel. Notice that the transported molecules move from an area of high concentration to an area of low concentration. The cell membrane is said to be **permeable** to the type of molecule in question.

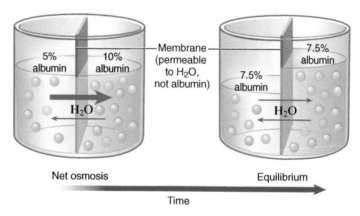

Osmosis. Osmosis is the diffusion of water through a selectively permeable membrane when impermeant solutes are present. The membrane shown in this diagram is permeable to water but not to albumin. Because there are relatively more water molecules in 5% albumin than 10% albumin, more water molecules osmose from the more dilute into the more concentrated solution (as indicated by the *larger arrow* in the left diagram) than osmose in the opposite direction. The overall direction of osmosis, in other words, is toward the more concentrated solution. Net osmosis produces the following changes in these solutions: (1) their concentrations equilibrate, (2) the volume and pressure of the originally more concentrated solution increase, and (3) the volume and pressure of the other solution decrease proportionately.

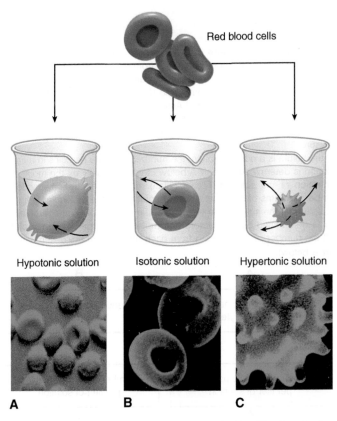

Red blood cells

Hypotonic solution   Isotonic solution   Hypertonic solution

A   **B**   **C**

Effects of Osmosis on Cells. **A,** Normal red blood cells placed in a **hypotonic** solution may swell (as the scanning electron micrograph shows) or even burst (as the drawing shows). This change results from the inward diffusion of water (osmosis). **B,** Cells placed in an **isotonic** solution maintain constant volume and pressure because the potential osmotic pressure of the intracellular fluid matches that of the extracellular fluid. **C,** Cells placed in a solution that is **hypertonic** lose volume and pressure as water osmoses out of the cell into the hypertonic solution. The "spikes" seen in the scanning electron micrograph are rigid microtubules of the cytoskeleton. These supports become visible as the cell "deflates," giving each cell a bumpy or *crenated* appearance.

DETERMINING THE POTENTIAL OSMOTIC PRESSURE OF A SOLUTION

Potential osmotic pressure is the maximum osmotic pressure that could develop in a solution if it were separated from distilled water by a selectively permeable membrane. (**Actual osmotic pressure** is a pressure that already has developed, not just one that could develop.) What determines a solution's potential osmotic pressure? Answer: the number of solute particles in a unit volume of solution directly determines its potential osmotic pressure– the more solute particles per unit volume, the greater the potential osmotic pressure.

If the solute is a nonelectrolyte, the number of solute particles in a liter of solution is determined, as part A below indicates, solely by the molar concentration of the solution. (To calculate molar concentration, divide the number of grams of solute in a liter of solution by the molecular weight of the solute.) If the solute is an electrolyte, the number of solute particles per liter is determined by two factors: the molar concentration of the solution and the number of ions formed from each molecule of the electrolyte (see part B below).

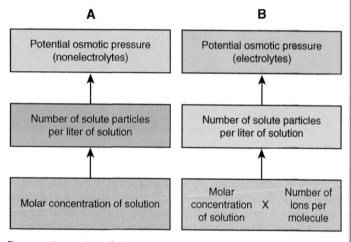

Because the number of solute particles per unit volume directly determines a solution's potential osmotic pressure, one might jump to the conclusion that all solutions having the same percent concentration also have the same potential osmotic pressure. Obviously it is true that all solutions containing the same percent concentration of the same solute do also have the same potential osmotic pressures. All 5% glucose solutions, for example, have a potential osmotic pressure at body temperature of somewhat more than 5300 mm Hg pressure. But all solutions with the same percent concentrations of different solutes do not have the same molar concentrations. And since it is molar concentration, not percent concentration, that determines potential osmotic pressure, solutions with the same percent concentration of different solutes have different potential osmotic pressures. For example, 5% NaCl at body temperature has a potential osmotic pressure of approximately 33,000 mm Hg–quite different from 5% glucose's potential osmotic pressure of about 5300 mm Hg. You can calculate these potential osmotic pressures using the formulas given in the following box.

FORMULAS FOR DETERMINING OSMOTIC PRESSURE

Potential osmotic pressure of nonelectrolyte (in mm Hg)	=	Molar concentration of solution	X	19,300*		

Potential osmotic pressure of electrolyte (in mm Hg)	=	Molar concentration of solution	X	Number of ions per molecule	X	19,300

*Experimentation has shown that a solution with a 1.0 molar concentration of any nonelectrolyte has a potential osmotic pressure of 19,300 mm Hg pressure (at body temperature, 37° C).

Molar concentration	=	Grams solute in 1 liter solution divided by molecular weight of solute

Example: Two solutions commonly used in hospitals are 0.85% NaCl and 5% glucose. What is the potential osmotic pressure of 0.85% NaCl at body temperature? (0.85 NaCl = 8.5 g NaCl in 1 liter solution)

(Molecular weight of NaCl = 58 [NaCl yields two ions per molecule in solution].)

Using the formula given for computing potential osmotic pressure of an electrolyte:

Potential osmotic pressure of 0.85% NaCl	=	8.5/58 × 2 × 19,300 = 5656.8 mm Hg pressure

Using the formula given for computing potential osmotic pressure of an electrolyte:

Problem: What is potential osmotic pressure of 5% glucose solution at body temperature? Molecular weight glucose = 180. Glucose does not ionize. It is a nonelectrolyte.**

**5% glucose solution has potential osmotic pressure of 5359.6 mg Hg pressure.

ACTIVE TRANSPORT PROCESSES

PROCESS	DESCRIPTION		EXAMPLES
Pumping		Movement of solute particles from an area of low concentration to an area of high concentration (up the concentration gradient) by means of an energy-consuming pump structure in the membrane	In muscle cells, pumping of nearly all calcium ions to special compartments—or out of the cell
Phagocytosis (endocytosis)		Movement of cells or other large particles into cell by trapping it in a section of plasma membrane that pinches off to form an intracellular vesicle; a type of *vesicle-mediated transport*	Trapping of bacterial cells by phagocytic white blood cells

Pinocytosis (endocytosis)	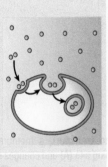	Movement of fluid and dissolved molecules into a cell by trapping them in a section of plasma membrane that pinches off to form an intracellular vesicle; a type of *vesicle-mediated transport*	Trapping of large protein molecules by some body cells
Exocytosis	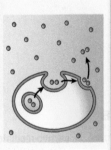	Movement of proteins or other cell products out of the cell by fusing a secretory vesicle with the plasma membrane; a type of *vesicle-mediated transport*	Secretion of the hormone prolactin by pituitary cells

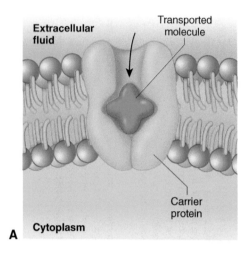

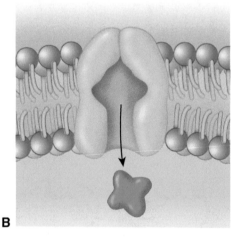

Membrane Carrier. In **carrier-mediated transport,** a membrane-bound carrier protein attracts a solute molecule to a binding site **(A)** and changes shape in a manner that allows the solute to move to the other side of the membrane **(B)**. Passive carriers may transport molecules in either direction, depending on the concentration gradient.

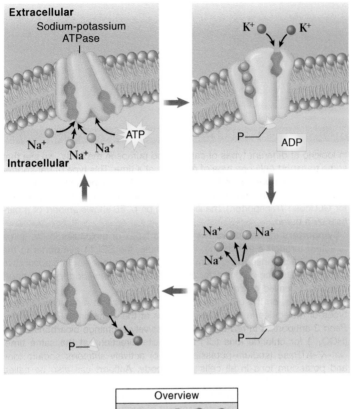

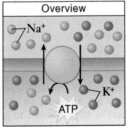

Sodium–Potassium Pump. Three sodium ions (Na^+) bind to sodium-binding sites on the pump's inner face. At the same time, an energy-containing adenosine triphosphate (ATP) molecule produced by the cell's mitochondria binds to the pump. The ATP breaks apart, and its stored energy is transferred to the pump. The pump then changes shape, releases the three Na^+ ions to the outside of the cell, and attracts two potassium ions (K^+) to its potassium-binding sites. The pump then returns to its original shape, and the two K^+ ions and the remnant of the ATP molecule are released to the inside of the cell. The pump is now ready for another pumping cycle. *ATPase,* Adenosine triphosphatase. The *inset* is a simplified overview of Na^+–K^+ pump activity.

TRANSPORT OF DIFFERENT SOLUTES

In looking at different types of carriers and pumps in the body, we see that some transport only one type of molecule at a time. This type of transporter is often called a **uniporter.** For example, the GLUT uniporters in many cells passively move glucose from blood plasma into cells. (*GLUT* is an acronym for *GLU*cose *T*ransporter.) The illustration on p. 56 shows *uniport* of a particle by a pump.

Symporters instead move two or more types of molecules in the same direction through a membrane. For example, the SGLT1 symporter in the digestive tract transports sodium ions and glucose together into absorptive cells. (*SGLT1* is an acronym for *S*odium-*GL*ucose *T*ransporter *1*.) *Symport* can also be called **cotransport.**

Antiporters, on the other hand, are transporters that move two different types of molecules in opposite directions at the same time. For example, *Band 3* antiporters in red blood cells passively exchange bicarbonate ions (HCO_3^-) for chloride ions (Cl^-) in opposite directions at the same time. Na^+-K^+-ATPase (sodium-potassium pump) actively *antiports* sodium ions and potassium ions in all cells of the body. Antiport can also be called **countertransport.**

Sometimes, active transport of one type of solute creates a concentration gradient that drives the passive transport of another solute. For example, in part B of the figure the active transport of sodium ions creates a concentration gradient that drives the cotransport of glucose along with sodium by a symport mechanism. In this case, the movement of sodium is an example of **primary active transport.** The movement of glucose, which depends on the sodium concentration gradient created by primary active transport, is an example of **secondary active transport.** This particular example of secondary active transport is often referred to as *sodium cotransport of glucose.*

TRANSPORT OF DIFFERENT SOLUTES—cont'd

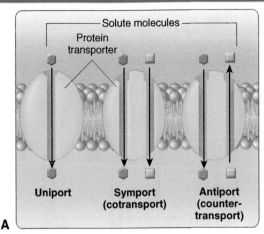

A

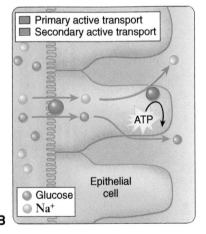

B

A, Direction of transport. Movement of one solute (uniport), movement of two or more solute types in the same direction (symport or cotransport), and movement of two or more solute types in opposite directions (antiport or countertransport). **B, Primary and secondary active transport.** In this example, primary active transport of sodium by a sodium pump creates a concentration gradient that drives the passive cotransport of glucose along with sodium. Because it depends on the sodium gradient, sodium cotransport of glucose is an example of secondary active transport. *ATP,* Adenosine triphosphate.

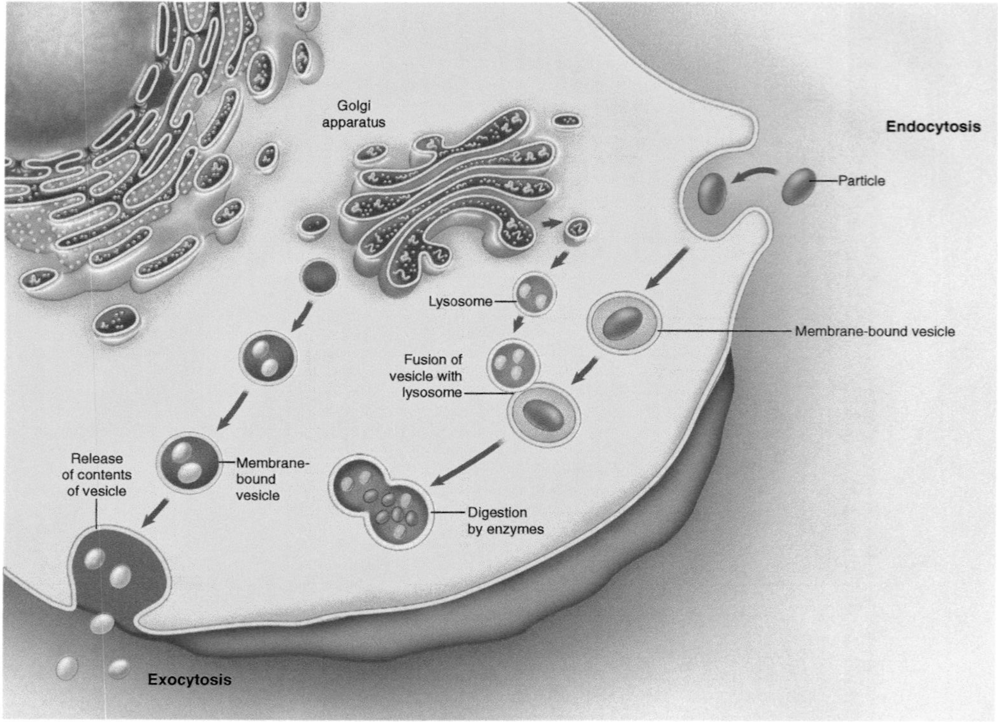

Bulk Transport by Vesicles. This sketch summarizes the essential difference between **endocytosis,** which moves substances into the cell by means of a vesicle, and **exocytosis,** which moves substances out of the cell by means of a vesicle. The type of endocytosis shown here is **phagocytosis,** in which the endocytic vesicle fuses with a lysosome to allow digestive enzymes to break down the ingested material.

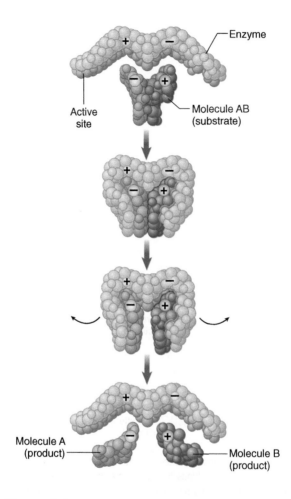

Model of Enzyme Action. Enzymes are functional proteins whose molecular shape allows them to catalyze chemical reactions. Substrate molecule AB is acted on by a digestive enzyme to yield simpler molecules A and B as products of the reaction. Notice how the active site of the enzyme chemically fits the substrate—the lock-and-key model of biochemical interaction. Notice also how the enzyme molecule bends its shape in performing its function.

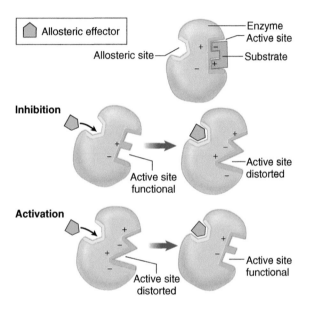

Allosteric Effect. The allosteric effect occurs when some agent, in this case an allosteric effector molecule, binds to the enzyme at an allosteric site and thereby changes the shape of the enzyme's active site. Such an allosteric effect may inhibit enzyme action (by distorting the active site) or activate the enzyme (by giving the active site its functional shape).

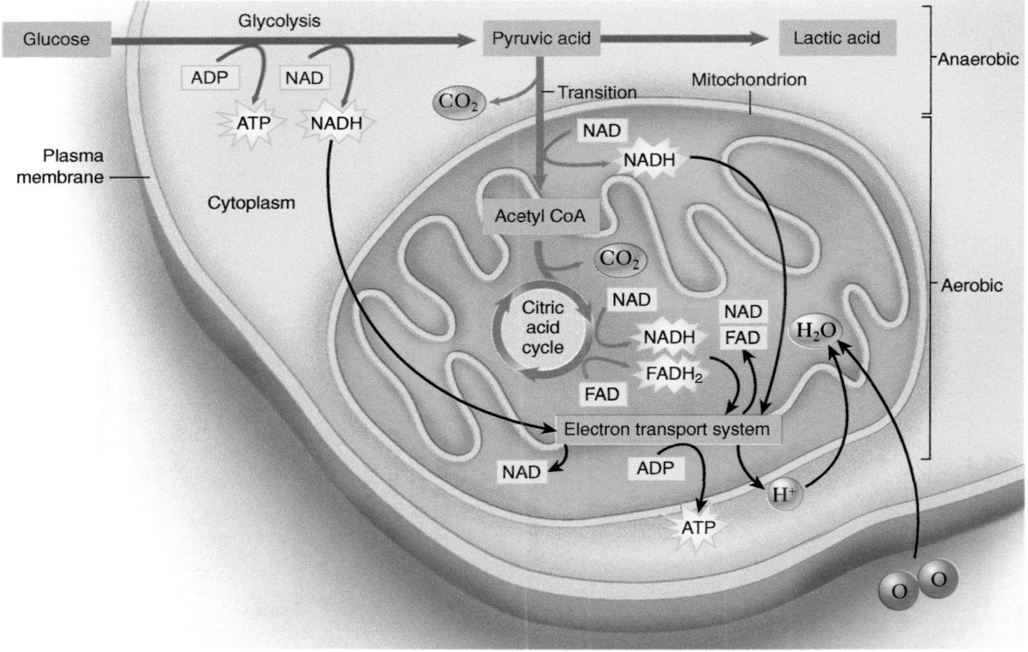

Summary of Cellular Respiration. This simplified outline of cellular respiration represents one of the most important catabolic pathways in the cell. Note that one phase **(glycolysis)** occurs in the cytosol, but that the two remaining phases **(citric acid cycle** and **electron transport system)** occur within a mitochondrion. Note also the divergence of the **anaerobic** and **aerobic** pathways of cellular respiration. *ADP,* Adenosine diphosphate; *ATP,* adenosine triphosphate; *CoA,* coenzyme A; *CO₂,* carbon dioxide; *FAD,* flavin adenine dinucleotide; *FADH₂,* form of flavin adenine dinucleotide; *H,* hydrogen; *H₂O,* water; *NAD,* nicotinamide adenine dinucleotide; *NADH,* form of nicotinamide adenine dinucleotide; *O,* oxygen.

CELL GROWTH AND REPRODUCTION

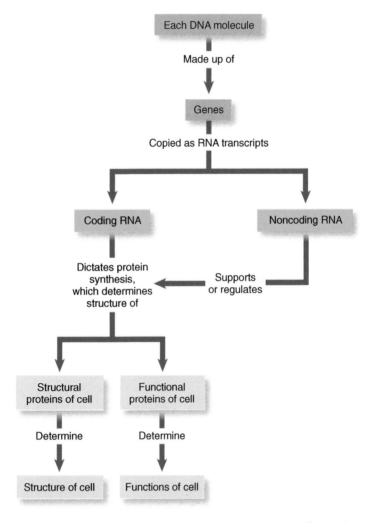

Function of Genes. Genes copied from DNA are copied to RNA molecules, which use the code to determine a cell's structural and functional characteristics. There are approximately 24,000 genes in the human genome (all the DNA molecules together).

MAJOR TYPES OF RNA

ACRONYM	NAME	DESCRIPTION	ROLE IN CELL FUNCTION
RNA INVOLVED IN PROTEIN SYNTHESIS			
mRNA	Messenger RNA	Single, unfolded strand of nucleotides	Serves as working copy of one protein-coding gene
rRNA	Ribosomal RNA	Single, folded strand of nucleotides	Component of the ribosome (along with proteins); attaches to mRNA and participates in translation
tRNA	Transfer RNA	Single, folded strand of nucleotides; has an anticodon at one end and an amino acid–binding site at the other end	Carries a specific amino acid to a specific codon of mRNA at the ribosome during translation
snRNP	Small nuclear ribonucleo-protein	Single, folded strand of RNA (combined with polypeptide chains)	Component of the spliceosome (see box on p. 59); attaches to an mRNA transcript to facilitate editing (removal of introns; splicing of exons) into the final version of mRNA
RNA INVOLVED IN GENE SILENCING			
dsRNA	Double-stranded RNA	Double strand of nucleotides (may be up to several hundred nucleotides long)	Involved in RNA interference; see siRNA, which is a type of dsRNA
siRNA	Short interfering RNA	Short segment of double-stranded RNA (only 20-25 nucleotides long)	Forms part of the RNA-induced silencing complex (RISC) during RNA interference

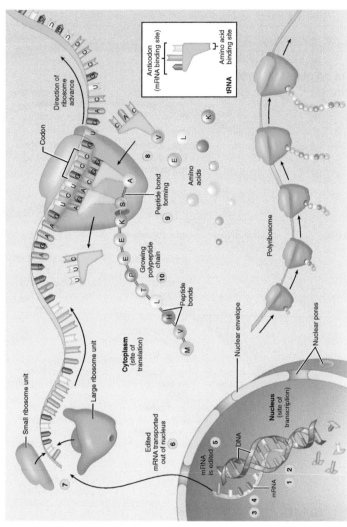

Protein Synthesis. Each of the numbered steps in the figure is further summarized in the following table. Protein synthesis begins with transcription, a process in which an mRNA molecule forms along one gene sequence of a DNA molecule within the cell's nucleus (1-3). As it is formed, the mRNA molecule separates from the DNA molecule (4), is edited (5), and leaves the nucleus through the large nuclear pores (6). Outside the nucleus, ribosome subunits attach to the beginning of the mRNA molecule and begin the process of translation (7). In translation, transfer RNA (tRNA) molecules bring specific amino acids—encoded by each mRNA codon—into place at the ribosome site (8). As the amino acids are brought into the proper sequence, they are joined together by peptide bonds (9) to form long strands called polypeptides (10). Several polypeptide chains may be needed to make a complete protein molecule. Amino acids are identified by color codes and abbreviations.

SUMMARY OF PROTEIN SYNTHESIS

STEP	LOCATION IN THE CELL	DESCRIPTION
TRANSCRIPTION		
1	Nucleus	One region, or gene, of a DNA molecule "unzips" to expose its bases
2	Nucleus	According to the principles of complementary base pairing, RNA nucleotides already present in the nucleoplasm temporarily attach themselves to the exposed bases along one side of the DNA molecule
3	Nucleus	As RNA nucleotides align themselves along the DNA strand, they bind to each other and thus form a chainlike strand called *messenger RNA* (mRNA); this binding of RNA nucleotides is controlled by the enzyme RNA polymerase
PREPARATION OF mRNA		
4	Nucleus	As the preliminary mRNA strand is formed, it peels away from the DNA strand; this mRNA strand is a copy or *transcript* of a gene
5	Nucleus	The spliceosome edits the mRNA molecule by removing noncoding portions of the strand (introns) and splicing the remaining pieces (exons)
6	Nuclear pores	The edited mRNA strand is transported out of the nucleus through pores in the nuclear envelope
TRANSLATION		
7	Cytoplasm	Two subunits sandwich the end of the mRNA molecule to form a ribosome
8	Cytoplasm	Specific transfer RNA (tRNA) molecules bring specific amino acids into place at the ribosome, which acts as a sort of "holder" for the mRNA strand and tRNA molecules; the kind of tRNA (and thus the kind of amino acid) that moves into position is determined by complementary base pairing: each mRNA codon exposed at the ribosome site will permit only a tRNA with a complementary *anticodon* to attach

Continued

SUMMARY OF PROTEIN SYNTHESIS—cont'd

STEP	LOCATION IN THE CELL	DESCRIPTION
9	Cytoplasm	As each amino acid is brought into place at the ribosome, an enzyme in the ribosome binds it to the amino acid that arrived just before it; the chemical bonds formed, called *peptide bonds,* link the amino acids together to form a long chain called a *polypeptide*
10	Cytoplasm	As the ribosome moves along the mRNA strand, more and more amino acids are added to the growing polypeptide chain in the sequence dictated by the mRNA codons (each codon represents a specific amino acid to be placed in the polypeptide chain); when the ribosome reaches the end of the mRNA molecule, it drops off the end and separates into large and small subunits again; often, enzymes later link two or more polypeptides together to form a whole protein molecule

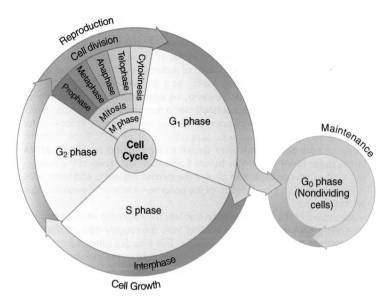

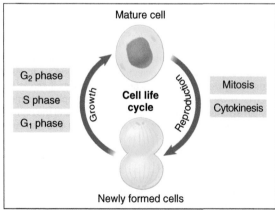

Life Cycle of the Cell. The processes of growth and reproduction of successive generations of cells exhibit a cyclic pattern. Newly formed cells grow to maturity by synthesizing new molecules and organelles (*G₁* and *G₂ phases*), including the replication of an extra set of DNA molecules (*S phase*) in anticipation of reproduction. Mature cells reproduce (*M phase*) by first distributing the two identical sets of DNA (produced during the S phase) in the orderly process of mitosis, then by splitting the plasma membrane, cytoplasm, and organelles of the parent cell into two distinct daughter cells (cytokinesis). Daughter cells that do not go on to reproduce are in a maintenance phase (*G₀*).

THE RNA REVOLUTION

For nearly a half century after the discovery of DNA and its central role in heredity in 1953, scientific understanding of cellular physiology focused primarily on DNA—that "most golden of molecules." RNA was seen as the "go between" molecule, acting mainly as a temporary working copy of a segment of DNA code (gene). However, we soon learned that **tRNA (transfer RNA)** and **rRNA (ribosomal RNA)** play a functional role other than direct coding for proteins. This discovery sparked some interest in looking for possible additional regulatory or supportive roles of RNA. Soon, catalytic forms of **noncoding RNA** were shown to be involved in editing **mRNA (messenger RNA)** transcripts before translation. The dawn of the twenty-first century saw an explosion of new discoveries regarding additional roles of RNA in regulating the function of the genome—a scientific revolution that still continues.

One aspect of the RNA revolution involves the surprising treasure trove of noncoding RNA molecules transcribed from the roughly 98% of the DNA genome that does not code for proteins. This includes **introns** (noncoding segments) that are removed from transcribed (mRNA) protein-coding genes during the editing process before translation. Current scientific databases are chock full of thousands of such regulatory RNA sequences. To cell scientists, it is becoming clear that an extensive RNA regulatory system manages the human genome.

One of the more interesting and useful recent discoveries of the current RNA revolution involves a cellular process of "gene silencing" called **RNA interference (RNAi).** Stated simply, RNAi is a process in which certain genes are silenced and thus synthesis of a particular protein is halted. RNAi occurs naturally in every cell, and scientists are still working to discover the mechanisms that govern the process and the purposes it serves in the cell. In human cells, RNAi is thought to be part of a complex scheme of "fine-tuning" protein synthesis. RNAi plays a variety of roles in the normal regulation of gene expression—what proteins we make and when we make them. For example, the cell could use RNAi to inhibit replication of virus components within the cell during a viral infection—thus protecting the cell. When the RNAi system fails, it may lead to disease.

How does RNAi work? A special form of RNA with two strands—**double-stranded RNA (dsRNA)**—seems to be the key, as the figure shows. A small segment of dsRNA, only about 20 or so nucleotides long, called **short interfering RNA (siRNA),** begins the process by combining with protein subunits to form an **RNA-induced silencing complex (RISC).** The siRNA within the RISC unwinds and exposes anticodons that allow the RISC to attach to a particular mRNA transcript. After the RISC attaches to its target mRNA, the mRNA breaks apart and therefore fails to translate its encoded protein. Of course, this effectively silences the gene encoded in the target mRNA. RNAi has also been shown to remodel chromatin, thus changing the "master code" in the DNA molecule!

Scientists are especially excited about using RNAi as a research tool. Researchers can synthesize a particular siRNA double strand and insert it into a cell that they want to study. The siRNA will induce the silencing of a particular gene so that researchers can see what happens to the cell. Knocking out the activity of just one gene at a time allows scientists to test hypotheses regarding how particular genes or particular proteins function in the cell.

The therapeutic possibilities of RNAi are also very exciting. Work is already underway to find an effective means of using RNAi for creating antiviral creams containing siRNA to protect against the human immunodeficiency virus (HIV) and other viruses. Some researchers are using RNAi to knock out genes that permit permanent tissue damage during heart attacks, kidney failure, and stroke. Researchers are also attempting to harness the power of RNAi to treat cancer and many types of infections.

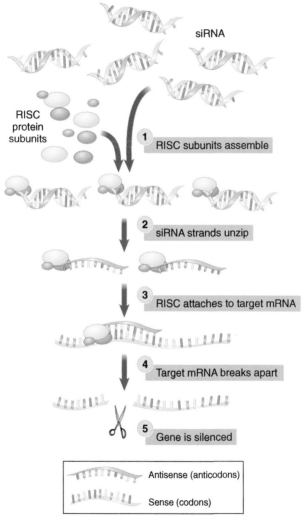

RNA Interference. *1,* Short, double-stranded siRNA (short interfering RNA) segments combine with protein subunits to form an RNA-induced silencing complex (RISC). *2,* The siRNA within the RISC unwinds to expose anticodons. *3,* The activated RISC attaches to target mRNA possessing complementary codons. *4,* The RISC causes the mRNA molecule to break apart. *5,* The mRNA can no longer code for a polypeptide, and thus the gene is effectively silenced. Eventually, the mRNA is broken down into its component nucleotides, which can be reused by the cell to build other RNA molecules.

SUMMARY OF DNA REPLICATION

STEP	DESCRIPTION
1	DNA molecules uncoil and "unzip" to expose their bases
2	Nucleotides already present in the intracellular fluid of the nucleus attach to the exposed bases according to the principle of obligatory base pairing
3	As nucleotides attach to complementary bases along each DNA strand, the enzyme *DNA polymerase* causes them to bind to each other
4	As new nucleotides fill in the spaces left open on each DNA strand, two identical *daughter molecules* are formed; as the parent DNA molecule completely unzips, the two daughter molecules coil to become distinct, but genetically identical, DNA double helices called *chromatids*

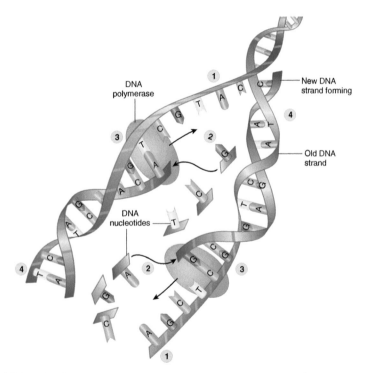

DNA Replication. When a DNA molecule makes a copy of itself, it "unzips" to expose its nucleotide bases. Through the mechanism of **obligatory base pairing,** coordinated by the enzyme *DNA polymerase,* new DNA nucleotides bind to the exposed bases (in an opposite direction on each strand). This forms a new "other half" to each half of the original molecule. After all the bases have new nucleotides bound to them, two identical DNA molecules will be ready for distribution to the two daughter cells. Numbers refer to steps described in the table above.

THE MAJOR EVENTS OF MITOSIS

PROPHASE

1. Chromosomes shorten and thicken (from coiling of the DNA molecules that compose them); each chromosome consists of two chromatids attached at the centromere

2. Centrosomes move to opposite poles of the cell; spindle fibers appear and begin to orient between opposing poles

3. Nucleoli and the nuclear membrane disappear

METAPHASE

1. Chromosomes align across the equator of the spindle fiber at its centromere

ANAPHASE

1. Each centromere splits, thereby detaching two chromatids that compose each chromosome from each other, elongating in the process (DNA molecules start uncoiling)

2. Sister chromatids (now called *chromosomes*) move to opposite poles; there are now twice as many chromosomes as there were before mitosis started

TELOPHASE

1. Changes occurring during telophase essentially reverse those taking place during prophase; new chromosomes start elongating (DNA molecules start uncoiling)

2. A nuclear envelope forms again to enclose each new set of chromosomes

3. Spindle fibers disappear

Interphase — Nucleus; Centrioles, Aster — Centrosome; Centromere

Prophase — Centrosome; Spindle fibers; Chromatids

Metaphase

Anaphase — Sister chromatids

Telophase — Nuclear envelope

SUMMARY OF THE CELL LIFE CYCLE

PHASE OF CELL LIFE CYCLE	DESCRIPTION
CELL GROWTH	**INTERPHASE**
Protein synthesis	Proteins are manufactured according to the cell's genetic code; functional proteins, the enzymes, direct the synthesis of other molecules in the cells and thus the production of more and larger organelles and plasma membrane; sometimes called the *first growth phase* or G_1 *phase* of interphase
DNA replication	Nucleotides, influenced by newly synthesized enzymes, arrange themselves along the open sides of an "unzipped" DNA molecule, thereby creating two identical daughter DNA molecules; produces two identical sets of the cell's genetic code, which enables the cell to later split into two different cells, each with its own complete set of DNA; sometimes called the *(DNA) synthesis* stage or *S phase* of interphase
Protein synthesis	After DNA is replicated, the cell continues to grow by means of protein synthesis and the resulting synthesis of other molecules and various organelles; this *second growth phase* is also called the G_2 *phase*
CELL REPRODUCTION	**M PHASE**
Mitosis or meiosis	The parent cell's replicated set of DNA is divided into two sets and separated by an orderly process into distinct cell nuclei; mitosis is subdivided into at least four phases: *prophase, metaphase, anaphase,* and *telophase*
Cytokinesis	The plasma membrane of the parent cell "pinches in" and eventually separates the cytoplasm and two daughter nuclei into two genetically identical daughter cells

CHANGES IN CELL GROWTH, REPRODUCTION, AND SURVIVAL

Cells have the ability to adapt to changing conditions. Cells may alter their size, reproductive rate, or other characteristics to adapt to changes in the internal environment. Such adaptations usually allow cells to work more efficiently. However, sometimes cells alter their characteristics abnormally—thereby decreasing their efficiency and threatening the health of the body. Common types of changes in cell growth and reproduction are summarized on the next couple of pages.

Cells may respond to changes in function, hormone signals, or the availability of nutrients by increasing or decreasing in size. The term **hypertrophy** (hye-PER-tro-fee) refers to an increase in cell size, and the term **atrophy** (AT-ro-fee) refers to a decrease in cell size. Either type of adaptive change can occur easily in muscle tissue. When a person continually uses muscle cells to pull against heavy resistance, as in weight training, for example, the cells respond by increasing in size. Body builders thus increase the size of their muscles by hyper-trophy—increasing the size of muscle cells. Atrophy often occurs in underused muscle cells. For example, when a broken arm is immobilized in a cast for a long period, muscles that move the arm often atrophy. Because the muscles are temporarily out of use, muscle cells decrease in size. Atrophy may also occur in tissues whose nutrient or oxygen supply is diminished. Sometimes cells respond to changes in the internal environment by increasing their rate of reproduction—a process called **hyperplasia** (hye-per-PLAY-zha). The ending –*plasia* comes from a Greek word that means "shape" or "formation"—referring to the formation of new cells. Because *hyper-* means "excessive," *hyperplasia* means "excessive cell reproduction." Like hypertrophy, hyperplasia causes an increase in the size of a tissue or organ. However, hyperplasia is an increase in the *number of cells* rather than an increase in the size of each cell. A common example of hyperplasia occurs in the milk-producing glands of the female breast during pregnancy. In response to hormone signals, the glandular cells reproduce rapidly to prepare the breast for milk production and nursing.

If the body loses its ability to control mitosis normally, abnormal hyperplasia may occur. The new mass of cells thus formed is a tumor or **neoplasm** (NEE-o-plazm). Neoplasms may be relatively harmless growths called **benign** (be-NYNE) tumors. If tumor cells can break away and travel through the blood or lymphatic vessels to other parts of the body, the neoplasm is a **malignant tumor,** or cancer. Cells in malignant neoplasms often exhibit a characteristic called **anaplasia** (an-ah-PLAY-zha). Anaplasia is a condition in which cells fail to differentiate into a specialized cell type. **Dysplasia** (diss-PLAY-zha) is an abnormal change in shape, size, or organization of cells in a tissue and is often associated with neoplasms.

Part A of the figure summarizes a few of the changes that can occur in cell growth and reproduction.

Cells also die sometimes. In **necrosis** (ne-KROH-sis), cells die because of an injury or pathological condition, often causing nearby cells to die and triggering an immune response called *inflammation,* which removes the debris if possible. Nonpathological cell death, often called **apoptosis** (ap-po-TOH-sis *or* ap-op-TOH-sis), occurs frequently in the cells of your body. Apoptosis is a type of programmed cell death in which organized biochemical steps within the cell lead to fragmentation of the cell and removal of the pieces by phagocytic cells. Apoptosis occurs when cells are no longer needed or when they have certain malfunctions that could lead to cancer or some other potential problem. Apoptosis is the normal process by which our tissues and other groups of cells remodel themselves throughout the life span. Although apoptosis is a normal cell function, it can be abnormally triggered in some conditions.

Continued

CHANGES IN CELL GROWTH, REPRODUCTION, AND SURVIVAL—cont'd

A, Alterations in cell growth and reproduction. **B,** Apoptosis. *1,* Early in apoptosis, the cell begins making the enzymes needed to break down the cell, but no structural changes yet occur. *2,* As apoptosis proceeds, surface features such as microvilli and cell junctions are lost, and nuclear DNA condenses and is broken into fragments. *3,* The cell then rapidly splits into apoptotic bodies. Notice that the nucleus has also fragmented. *4,* Apoptotic bodies may then be digested by adjacent cells, by extracellular enzymes, or (not shown) by nearby phagocytic cells.

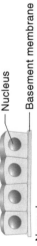

Normal

Atrophy

Hypertrophy

A

Hyperplasia

Dysplasia

Nucleus

Basement membrane

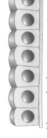

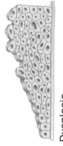

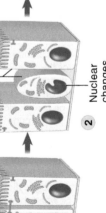

1

2 Nuclear changes

Loss of microvilli and junctions

3 Fragmentation

Apoptotic body

4 Phagocytosis

Apoptotic body

B

Changes in Cell Growth, Reproduction, and Survival—cont'd

Tissues

A *tissue* is a group of similar cells that perform a common function. Tissues can be thought of as the fabric of the body, which is "sewn together" to form the organs of the body and to hold all the organs together as a whole.

Each tissue specialized in performing at least one unique function that helps maintain homeostasis, assuring the survival of the whole body. The branch of anatomy that studies tissues is called **histology.**

Regardless of the size, shape, or arrangement of cells in a tissue, they are all surrounded by or embedded in a nonliving intercellular material that is often simply called **matrix.** The matrix, illustrated on p. 79, is not simply supportive packing material—it is a dynamic system of molecules and fibers that carry out some of the body's most important homeostatic functions.

All tissues in the human body can be classified by their structure and function into four principal types:

(1) **epithelial tissue,**
(2) **connective tissue,**
(3) **muscle tissue,** and
(4) **nervous tissue.**

These tissue types originate from the three primary **germ layers.** These primary germ layers appear on p. 78.

TYPES OF TISSUE

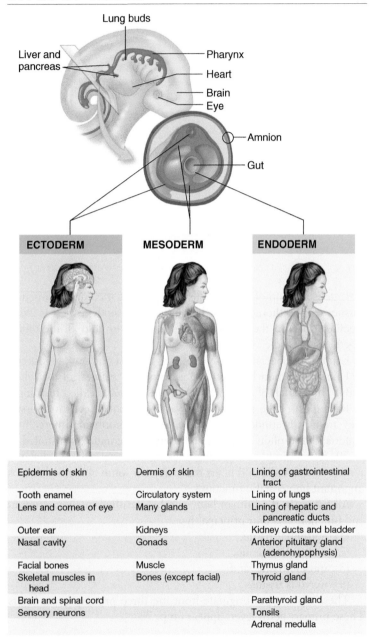

The Primary Germ Layers. Illustration shows the primary germ layers and the body systems into which they develop.

Extracellular Matrix (ECM).
A, The extracellular matrix is made up of water, proteins/glycoproteins, and proteoglycans that often form large bundles or complexes that bind together and to the cells of the tissue. Although the makeup of ECM varies from tissue to tissue, it usually includes some connections to integrins in the plasma membranes, thereby allowing for structural integrity, as well as communication and coordination within the tissue. B, A detailed view of a proteoglycan complex shows many proteoglycans, each with a protein backbone and attached carbohydrate subunits—all held together by a polysaccharide chain. C, Detailed view of a collagen bundle showing the individual collagen fibers within it.

COMPONENTS OF THE EXTRACELLULAR MATRIX*

COMPONENT	EXAMPLE	DESCRIPTION	FUNCTION	EXAMPLE OF LOCATION
Water		Water molecules along with a small number of ions (mostly Na+ and Cl-)	Solvent for dissolved ECM components; provides fluidity of ECM	All tissues of the body
Proteins and glycoproteins	Collagen	Strong, flexible structural protein fiber	Provides flexible strength to tissues	Tendons, ligaments, bones, cartilage, many tissues
	Elastin	Flexible, elastic structural protein fiber	Allows flexibility and elastic recoil of tissues	Skin, cartilage of ear, walls of arteries
	Fibronectin	Rodlike glycoprotein	Binds ECM to cells; communicates with cells through integrins	Many tissues of the body, for example, connective tissues
	Laminin	Glycoproteins arranged as a three-pronged fork	Binds ECM components together and to cells; communicates with cells through integrins	In basal lamina (basement membrane) of epithelial tissues
Proteoglycans	Various types	Protein backbone with attached chains of various polysaccharides:		
		Chondroitin sulfate	Shock absorber	Cartilage, bone, heart valves
		Heparin	Reduces blood clotting	Lining of some arteries
		Hyaluronate	Thickens fluid; lubricates	Loose fibrous connective tissue, joint fluids

ECM, Extracellular matrix.

*Not all components are present in all ECM; examples of only some of the many major ECM components are provided.

MAJOR TISSUES OF THE BODY

TISSUE TYPE	STRUCTURE	FUNCTION	EXAMPLES IN THE BODY
Epithelial tissue	One or more layers of densely arranged cells with very little extracellular matrix May form either sheets or glands	Covers and protects the body surface Lines body cavities Transport of substances (absorption, secretion, excretion) Glandular activity	Outer layer of skin Lining of the respiratory, digestive, urinary, reproductive tracts Glands of the body
Connective tissue	Sparsely arranged cells surrounded by a large proportion of extracellular matrix Often containing structural fibers (and sometimes mineral crystals)	Supports body structures Transports substances throughout the body	Bones Joint cartilage Tendons and ligaments Blood Fat

Continued

MAJOR TISSUES OF THE BODY—cont'd

TISSUE TYPE	STRUCTURE	FUNCTION	EXAMPLES IN THE BODY
Muscle tissue 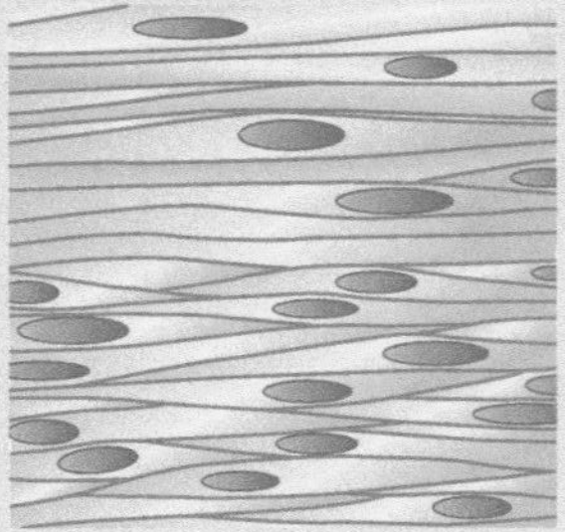	Long fiberlike cells, sometimes branched, capable of pulling loads; extracellular fibers sometimes hold muscle fiber together	Produces body movements Produces movements of organs such as the stomach, heart Produces heat	Heart muscle Muscles of the head/neck, arms, legs, trunk Muscles in the walls of hollow organs such as the stomach, intestines
Nervous tissue 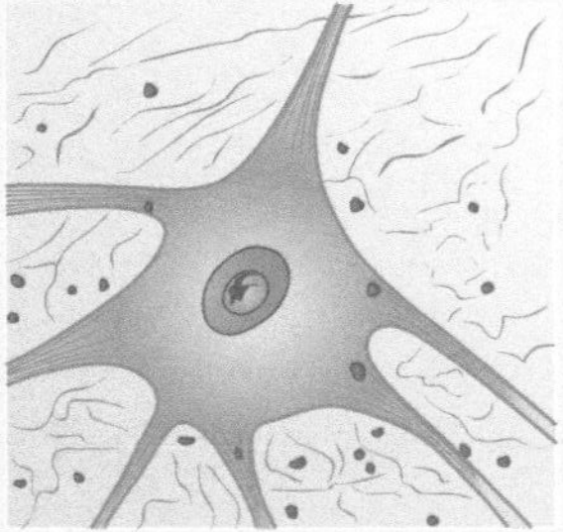	Mixture of many cell types, including several types of neurons (conducting cells) and neuroglia (support cells)	Communication between body parts Integration/regulation of body functions	Tissue of brain and spinal cord Nerves of the body Sensory organs of the body

EPITHELIAL TISSUE

CLASSIFICATION SCHEME FOR MEMBRANOUS EPITHELIAL TISSUES

	SHAPE OF CELLS*	TISSUE TYPE
One layer	Squamous	Simple squamous
	Cuboidal	Simple cuboidal
	Columnar	Simple columnar
	Pseudostratified columnar	Pseudostratified columnar
Several layers	Squamous	Stratified squamous
	Cuboidal	Stratified cuboidal
	Columnar	Stratified columnar
	Various shapes	Transitional

*In the top layer (if more than one layer in the tissue).

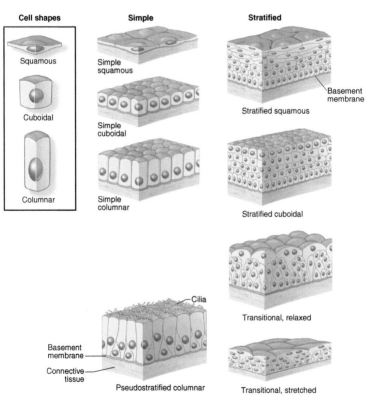

Classification of Epithelial Tissues. The tissues are classified according to the shape and arrangement of cells. The color scheme of these drawings is based on a common staining technique used by histologists called *hematoxylin and eosin (H&E)* staining. H&E staining usually renders the cytoplasm pink and the chromatin inside the nucleus a purplish color. The cellular membranes, including the plasma membrane and nuclear envelope, do not usually pick up any stain and thus may be transparent.

EPITHELIAL TISSUES

TISSUE	LOCATION	FUNCTION
MEMBRANOUS		
Simple squamous	Alveoli of lungs	Absorption by diffusion of respiratory gases between alveolar air and blood
	Lining of blood and lymphatic vessels (called *endothelium*; classified as connective tissue by some histologists)	Absorption by diffusion, filtration, and osmosis
	Surface layer of the pleura, pericardium, and peritoneum (called *mesothelium*; classified as connective tissue by some histologists)	Absorption by diffusion and osmosis; also, secretion
Stratified squamous Keratinized Nonkeratinized	Surface of the mucous membrane lining the mouth, esophagus, and vagina	Protection
	Surface of the skin (epidermis)	

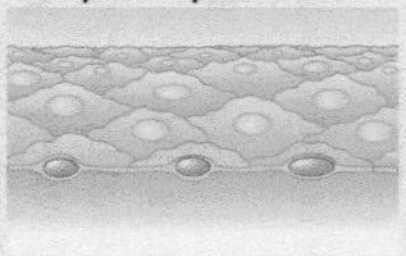

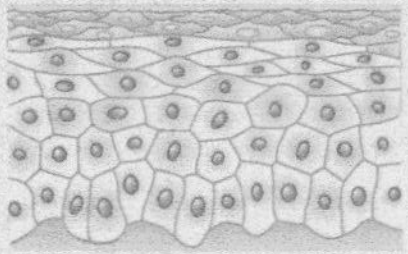

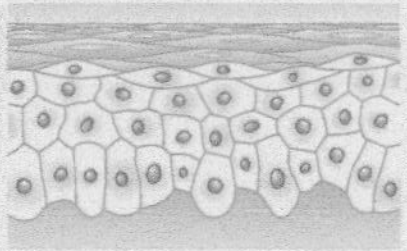

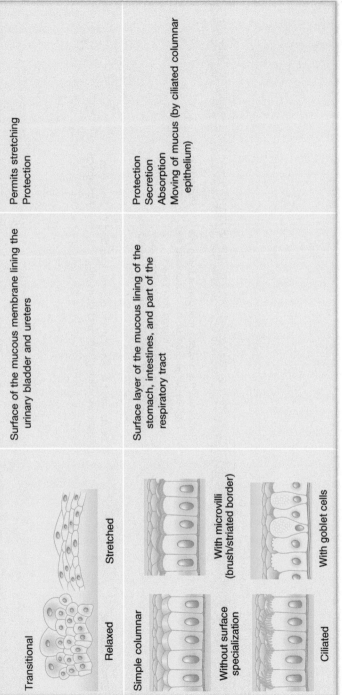Transitional Relaxed Stretched	Surface of the mucous membrane lining the urinary bladder and ureters	Permits stretching Protection
Simple columnar Without surface specialization With microvilli (brush/striated border) Ciliated With goblet cells	Surface layer of the mucous lining of the stomach, intestines, and part of the respiratory tract	Protection Secretion Absorption Moving of mucus (by ciliated columnar epithelium)

Continued

EPITHELIAL TISSUES—cont'd

TISSUE	LOCATION	FUNCTION
Pseudostratified columnar 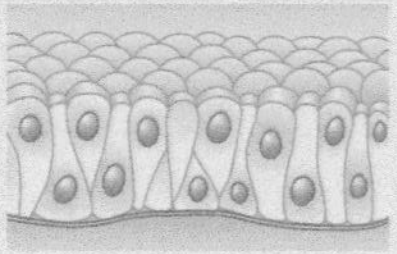	Surface of the mucous membrane lining the trachea, large bronchi, nasal mucosa, and parts of the male reproductive tract (epididymis and vas deferens); lines the large ducts of some glands (e.g., parotid)	Protection
Simple cuboidal 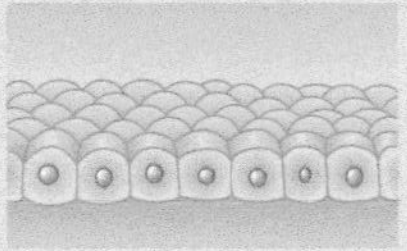	Ducts and tubules of many organs, including the exocrine glands and kidneys	Secretion Absorption

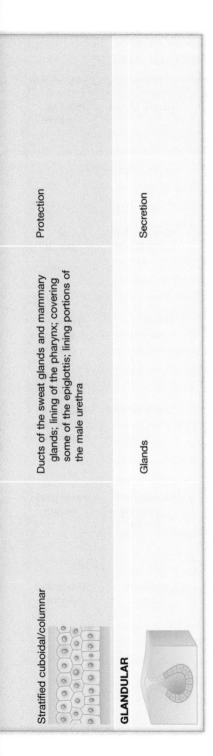

| Stratified cuboidal/columnar | Ducts of the sweat glands and mammary glands; lining of the pharynx; covering some of the epiglottis; lining portions of the male urethra | Protection |

GLANDULAR

| Glands | Secretion |

STRUCTURAL CLASSIFICATION OF MULTICELLULAR EXOCRINE GLANDS

SHAPE*	COMPLEXITY†	TYPE	EXAMPLE
Tubular (single, straight) 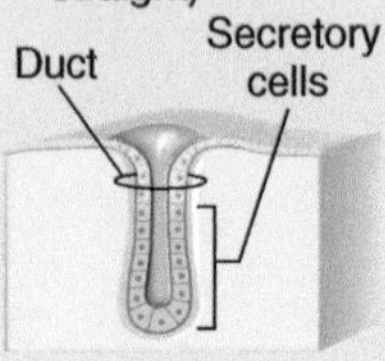 Duct / Secretory cells	Simple	Simple tubular	Intestinal glands
Tubular (coiled) 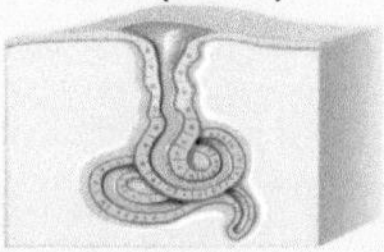	Simple	Simple coiled tubular	Sweat glands
Tubular (multiple) 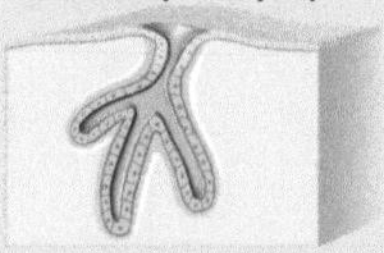	Simple	Simple branched tubular	Gastric (stomach) glands
Alveolar (single) 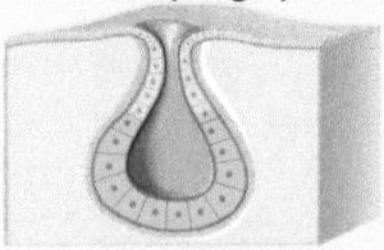	Simple	Simple alveolar	Sebaceous (skin oil) glands
Alveolar (multiple) 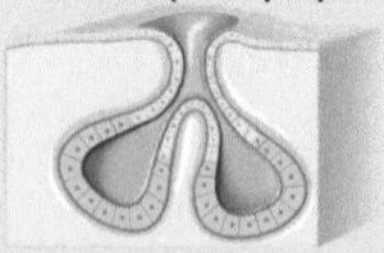	Simple	Simple branched alveolar	Sebaceous glands
Tubular (multiple) 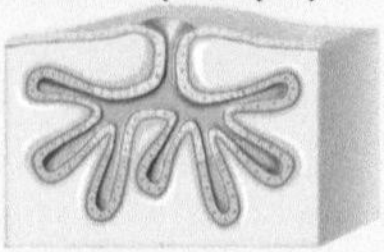	Compound	Compound tubular	Mammary glands

SHAPE*	COMPLEXITY†	TYPE	EXAMPLE
Alveolar (multiple) 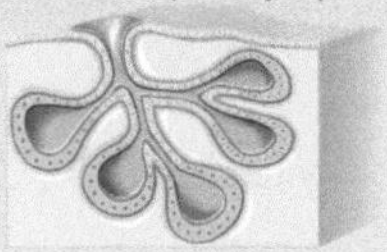	Compound	Compound alveolar	Mammary glands
Some tubular; some alveolar 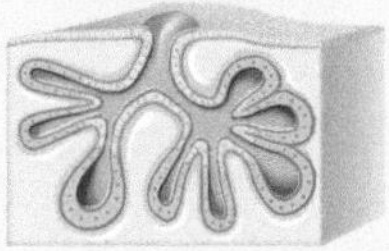	Compound	Compound tubuloalveolar	Salivary glands

*Shape of the distal secreting units of the gland.
†Number of ducts reaching the surface.

CONNECTIVE TISSUES

CLASSIFICATION OF CONNECTIVE TISSUE

1. Fibrous (connective tissue proper)
   a. Loose fibrous (areolar)
   b. Adipose
   c. Reticular
   d. Dense
      (1) Irregular
      (2) Regular
         (a) Collagenous
         (b) Elastic
2. Bone
   a. Compact
   b. Cancellous (spongy)
3. Cartilage
   a. Hyaline
   b. Fibrocartilage
   c. Elastic
4. Blood

CONNECTIVE TISSUES

TISSUE	LOCATION	FUNCTION
FIBROUS		
Loose fibrous (areolar) 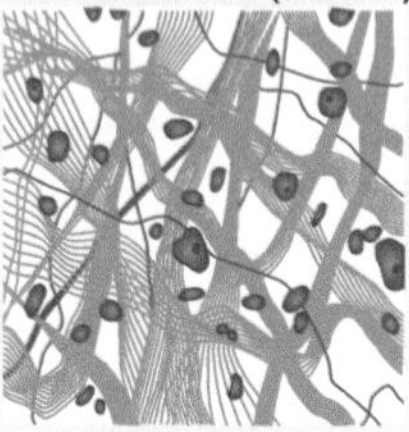	Between other tissues and organs Superficial fascia	Connection
Adipose (fat) 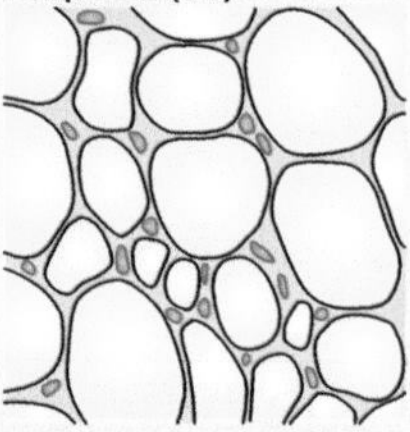	Under skin Padding at various points	Protection Insulation Support Energy reserves Regulation of other tissues
Reticular 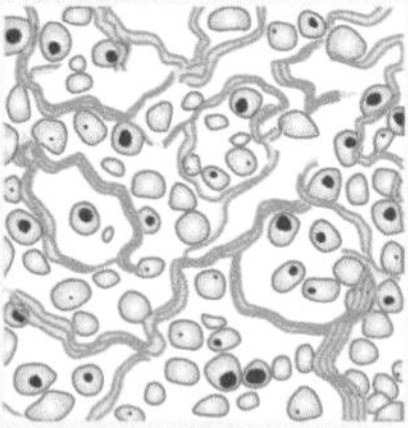	Inner framework of spleen, lymph nodes, bone marrow	Support Filtration Blood production Immunity
DENSE FIBROUS		
Irregular 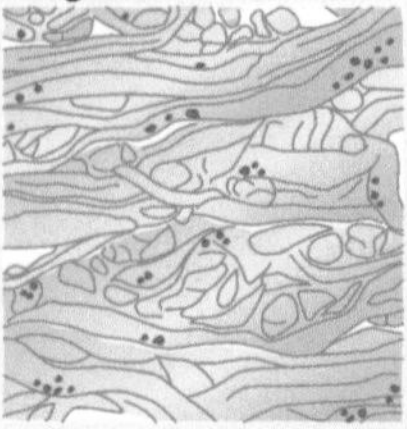	Deep fascia Dermis Scars Capsule of kidney, spleen, lymph nodes, etc.	Connection Support

CONNECTIVE TISSUES—cont'd

TISSUE	LOCATION	FUNCTION
Regular collagenous 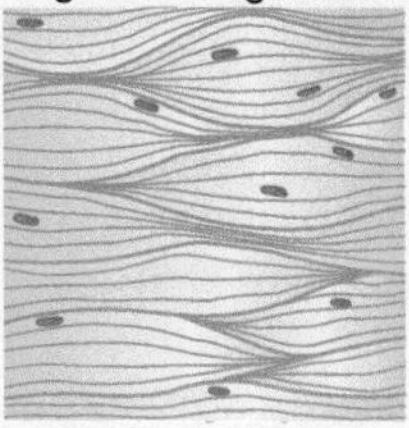	Tendons Ligaments Aponeuroses	Flexible but strong connection
Elastic 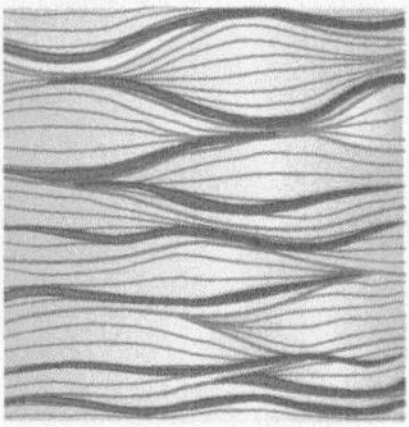	Walls of some arteries	Flexible, elastic support
BONE		
Compact bone 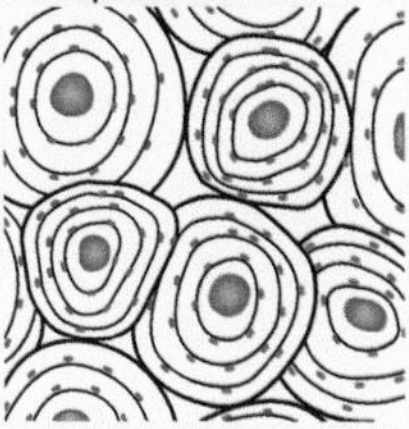	Skeleton (outer shell of bones)	Support Protection Calcium reservoir
Cancellous (spongy) bone 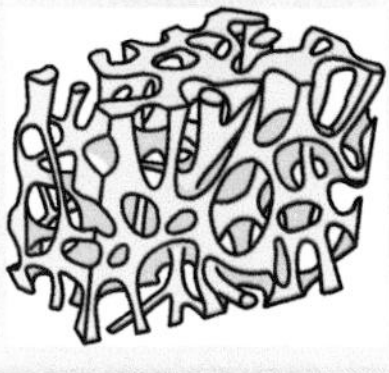	Skeleton (inside bones)	Support Provides framework for blood production

Continued

CONNECTIVE TISSUES—cont'd

TISSUE	LOCATION	FUNCTION
CARTILAGE		

Hyaline 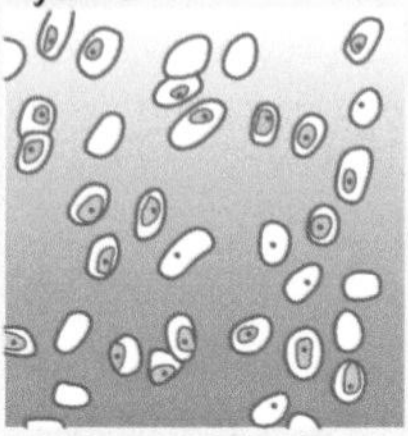	Part of nasal septum
	Covering articular
	  surfaces of bones
	Larynx
	Rings in trachea and
	  bronchi
		Firm but flexible
		  support;
		  connection
		  between
		  structures

Fibrocartilage 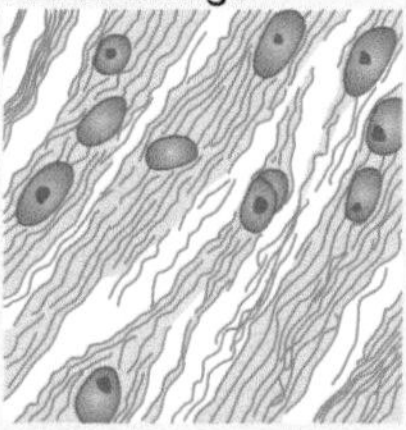	Disks between vertebrae Pubic symphysis	
Elastic 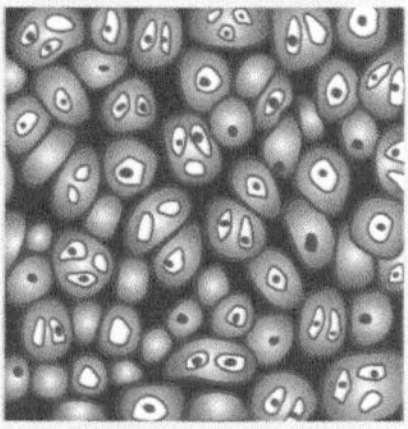	External ear Eustachian or auditory tube	
BLOOD		
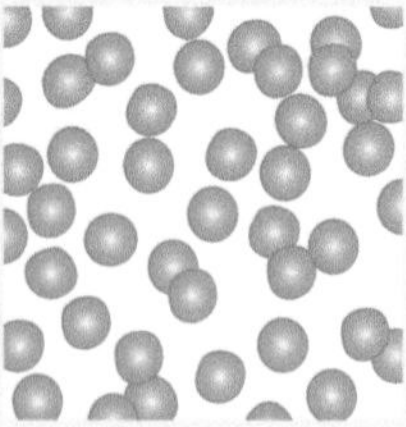	In the blood vessels	Transportation Protection

MUSCLE AND NERVOUS TISSUES

TISSUE	LOCATION	FUNCTION
MUSCLE		
Skeletal (striated voluntary)	Muscles that attach to bones Extrinsic eyeball muscles Upper third of the esophagus	Movement of bones Heat production Eye movements First part of swallowing
Smooth (nonstriated, involuntary, or visceral)	In the walls of tubular viscera of the digestive, respiratory, and genitourinary tracts In the walls of blood vessels and large lymphatic vessels In the ducts of glands Intrinsic eye muscles (iris and ciliary body) Arrector muscles of hairs	Movement of substances along the respective tracts Change diameter of blood vessels, thereby aiding in regulation of blood pressure Movement of substances along ducts Change diameter of pupils and shape of the lens Erection of hairs (gooseflesh)
Cardiac (striated involuntary)	Wall of the heart	Contraction of the heart
NERVOUS		
	Brain Spinal cord Nerves	Excitability Conduction

BODY MEMBRANES

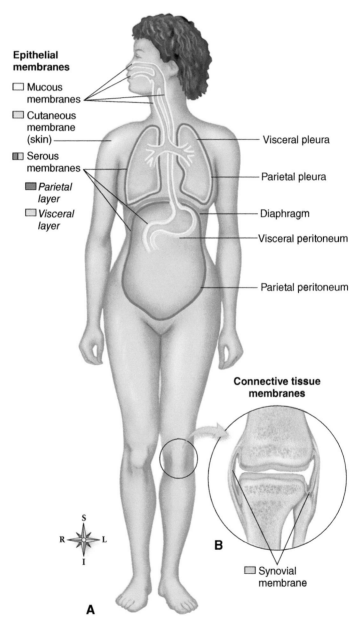

Epithelial membranes

☐ Mucous membranes

☐ Cutaneous membrane (skin)

☐☐ Serous membranes

  ☐ *Parietal layer*

  ☐ *Visceral layer*

Visceral pleura

Parietal pleura

Diaphragm

Visceral peritoneum

Parietal peritoneum

Connective tissue membranes

☐ Synovial membrane

A

B

Types of Body Membranes. A, Epithelial membranes, including cutaneous membrane (skin), serous membranes (parietal and visceral pleura and peritoneum), and mucous membranes. **B,** Connective tissue membranes, including synovial membranes.

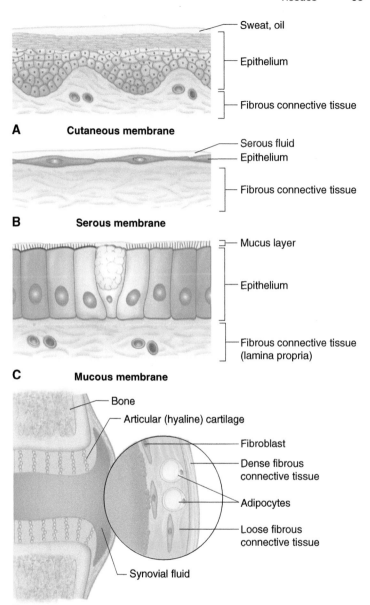

A   **Cutaneous membrane**

- Sweat, oil
- Epithelium
- Fibrous connective tissue

B   **Serous membrane**

- Serous fluid
- Epithelium
- Fibrous connective tissue

C   **Mucous membrane**

- Mucus layer
- Epithelium
- Fibrous connective tissue (lamina propria)

D   **Synovial membrane**

- Bone
- Articular (hyaline) cartilage
- Fibroblast
- Dense fibrous connective tissue
- Adipocytes
- Loose fibrous connective tissue
- Synovial fluid

Structure of Body Membranes.

MEMBRANES OF THE BODY

TYPE	SUPERFICIAL LAYER	DEEP LAYER	LOCATION	FLUID SECRETION	FUNCTION
EPITHELIAL					
Cutaneous (skin)	Keratinized stratified squamous epithelium (epidermis)	Dense irregular fibrous connective tissue (dermis)	Directly exposed to external environment	Sweat; sebum (skin oil)	Protection, sensation, thermoregulation
Serous	Simple squamous epithelium	Fibrous connective tissue	Lines body cavities that are not open to the external environment	Serous fluid	Lubrication
Mucous	Various types of epithelium	Fibrous connective tissue (lamina propria)	Lines tracts that open to the external environment	Mucus	Protection, lubrication
CONNECTIVE					
Synovial	Dense fibrous connective tissue	Loose fibrous connective tissue	Lines joint cavities (in movable joints)	Synovial fluid	Helps hold joints together, lubricates, cushions

Skin

The skin forms a self-repairing and protective boundary between the internal environment of the body and an often hostile external world. **Integument** is another name for the skin; **integumentary system** is a term used to denote the skin and its appendages—hair, nails, and skin glands.

The skin is a thin, relatively flat organ classified as a membrane— the **cutaneous membrane.** The skin surface is as large as the body, an area in average-sized adults of roughly 1.6 to 1.9 m^2 (17 to 20 square feet). Its thickness varies from slightly less than 0.05 cm (1/50 inch) to slightly more than 0.3 cm (1/8 inch).

Two main layers compose the skin: an outer, thinner layer called the **epidermis** and an inner, thicker layer named the **dermis.**

The skin surface is as large as the body, an area in average-sized adults of roughly 1.6 to 1.9 m^2 (17 to 20 square feet). Its thickness varies from slightly less than 0.05 cm (1/50 inch) to slightly more than 0.3 cm (1/8 inch).

The epidermis is an epithelial layer made up of *keratinized stratified epithelium* and derived from the *ectodermal germ layer* of the embryo (see p. 78). By the seventeenth week of gestation, the epidermis of the developing baby has all the essential characteristics of the adult.

The deeper dermis is derived from the *mesoderm.* The dermis is mostly *irregular dense fibrous connective tissue* with an extensive network of blood vessels and nerves. It may average more than 4 mm in thickness in some body areas.

The gluelike *basement membrane* located where the cells of the epidermis meet the connective tissue cells of the dermis is called the **dermoepidermal junction (DEJ).** Beneath the dermis lies a loose **hypodermis** rich in *adipose* and *loose fibrous connective tissue.*

STRUCTURE AND FUNCTION OF THE SKIN

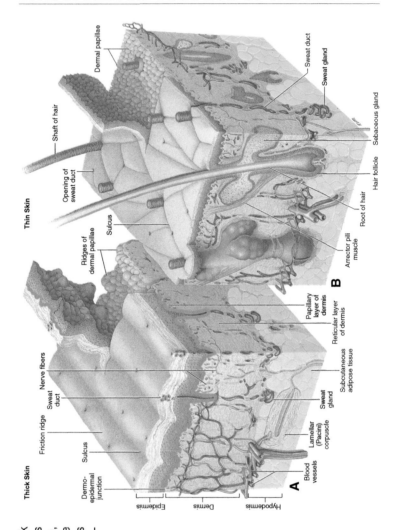

Diagram of Skin Structure. A, Thick skin, found on surfaces of the palms and soles of the feet. **B,** Thin skin, found on most surface areas of the body. In each diagram, the epidermis is raised at one corner to reveal the papillae of the dermis.

FUNCTIONS OF THE SKIN

FUNCTION	EXAMPLE	MECHANISM
Protection	Against microorganisms	Surface film/ mechanical barrier
	Against dehydration	Keratin
	Against ultraviolet radiation	Melanin
	Against mechanical trauma	Tissue strength
Sensation	Pain	Somatic sensory receptors
	Heat and cold	
	Pressure	
	Touch	
Permits movement and growth without injury	Body growth and change in body contours during movement	Elastic and recoil properties of skin and subcutaneous tissue
Endocrine	Vitamin D production	Activation of precursor compound in skin cells by ultraviolet light
Excretion	Water	Regulation of sweat volume and content
	Urea	
	Ammonia	
	Uric acid	
Immunity	Destruction of microorganisms and interaction with immune system cells (helper T cells)	Phagocytic cells and epidermal dendritic cells
Temperature regulation	Heat loss or retention	Regulation of blood flow to the skin and evaporation of sweat

STRUCTURE OF THE SKIN

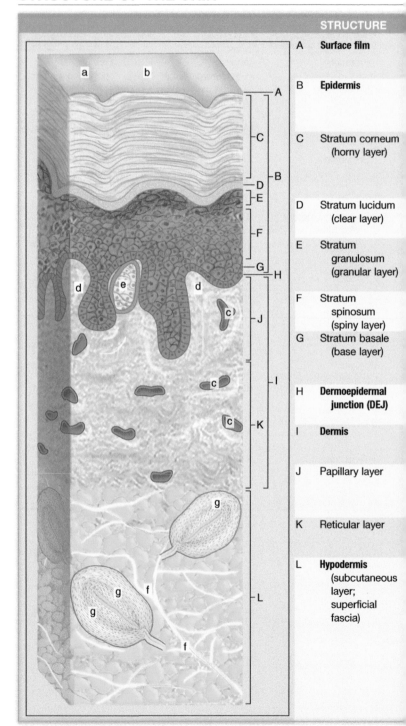

	STRUCTURE
A	**Surface film**
B	**Epidermis**
C	Stratum corneum (horny layer)
D	Stratum lucidum (clear layer)
E	Stratum granulosum (granular layer)
F	Stratum spinosum (spiny layer)
G	Stratum basale (base layer)
H	**Dermoepidermal junction (DEJ)**
I	**Dermis**
J	Papillary layer
K	Reticular layer
L	**Hypodermis** (subcutaneous layer; superficial fascia)

Thin film coating the skin; made up of a mixture of sweat, sebum, desquamated cells/fragments, various chemicals; protects the skin

Superficial primary layer of the skin; made up entirely of keratinized stratified squamous epithelium; derived from the ectoderm; also includes hairs, sweat glands, sebaceous glands

Several layers of flakelike dead cells (or *corneocytes*) mostly made up of dense networks of *keratin* fibers cemented by *glycophospholipids* and forming a tough, waterproof barrier; the keratinized layer *a,* sulcus (groove*)* b, friction ridge

A few layers of squamous cells filled with *eleidin*—a keratin precursor that gives this layer a translucent quality (not visible in thin skin)

2-5 layers of dying, somewhat flattened cells filled with darkly staining keratohyalin granules and multilayered bodies of glycophospholipids; nuclei disappear in this layer

8-10 layers of cells pulled by desmosomes into a spiny appearance

Single layer of mostly columnar cells capable of mitotic cell division; it is from this layer that all cells of superficial layers are derived; includes keratinocytes and some melanocytes

The basement membrane, a unique and complex arrangement of adhesive components that glue the epidermis and dermis together

Deep primary layer of the skin; made up of fibrous tissue; also includes some blood vessels *(c),* muscles, and nerves; derived from mesoderm

Loose fibrous tissue with collagenous and elastic fibers; forms nipplelike bumps *(papillae, d)*; includes tactile corpuscles (touch receptors, *e)* and other sensory receptors

Tough network (reticulum) of collagenous dense irregular fibrous tissue (with some elastic fibers); forms most of the dermis

Loose fibrous (areolar) connective tissue and adipose tissue; under the skin (not part of the skin); includes fibrous bands or *skin ligaments (f)* that connect the skin strongly to underlying structures; includes lamellar corpuscles (pressure receptors, *g)* and other sensory receptors

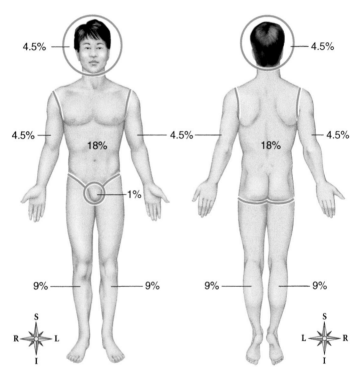

"Rule of Nines." The "rule of nines" is one method used to estimate amount of skin surface burned in an adult.

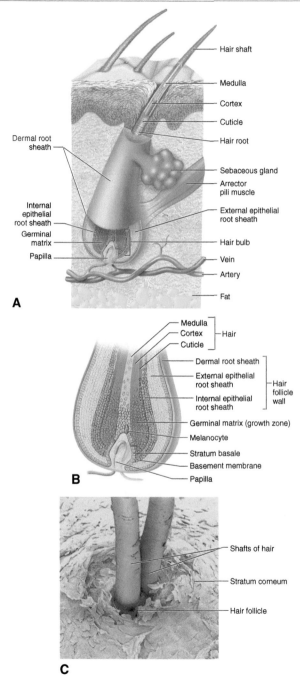

Hair Follicle. A, Relationship of a hair follicle and related structures to the epidermal and dermal layers of the skin. **B,** Enlargement of a hair follicle wall and hair bulb. **C,** Scanning electron micrograph showing shafts of hair extending from their follicles.

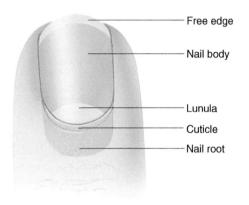

Free edge

Nail body

Lunula

Cuticle

Nail root

A

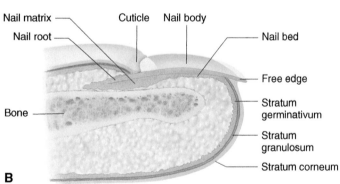

Nail matrix

Nail root

Cuticle

Nail body

Bone

Nail bed

Free edge

Stratum germinativum

Stratum granulosum

Stratum corneum

B

Structure of Nails. A, Fingernail viewed from above. **B,** Sagittal section of a fingernail and associated structures.

Skeletal System

Structurally, there are four types of bones in the human skeleton: long bones, short bones, flat bones, and irregular bones. Bones differ in size and shape and also in the amount and proportion of two different types of bone tissue that comprise them: **compact bone,** solid in appearance, and **trabecular** (also *cancellous* or *spongy*) **bone. Ligaments** are fibrous bands that help hold the various bones together into an organized skeleton.

The main functions of the bones and ligaments of the skeletal system include:

1. **Support.** Bones serve as the supporting framework of the body, much as steel girders are the supporting framework of our modern buildings.

2. **Protection.** Hard, bony "boxes" serve to protect the delicate structures they enclose. One can also use the arm or leg bones to help defend against injuries.

3. **Movement.** Bones and their joints form lever systems operated by skeletal muscles.

4. **Mineral storage.** Bone tissue is a reservoir for calcium, phosphorus, and certain other minerals.

5. **Hematopoiesis.** *Hematopoiesis*, or blood cell formation, is a vital process carried on by red bone marrow, or *myeloid tissue*.

SKELETAL TISSUE

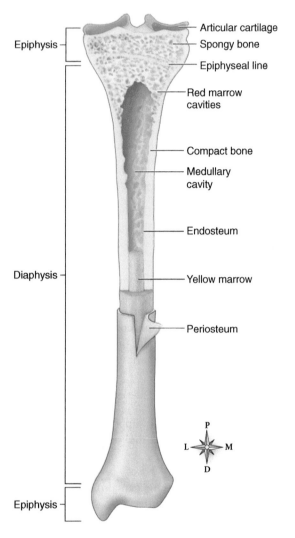

Long Bone. Partial frontal section of a long bone (tibia) showing cancellous and compact bone.

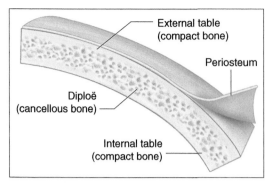

Flat Bone. Horizontal section of a flat bone of the skull (frontal bone) showing cancellous and compact bone.

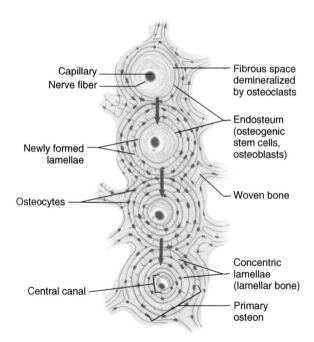

Primary Osteon Formation. First, a tubelike passage in the woven bone surrounding a blood vessel is demineralized by osteoblasts. Osteoblasts then begin laying down one layer (lamella) after another along the endosteal lining of the tube. As layers build up, they eventually fill most of the demineralized tube—thus forming the concentric lamellae around a central canal that characterize an osteon.

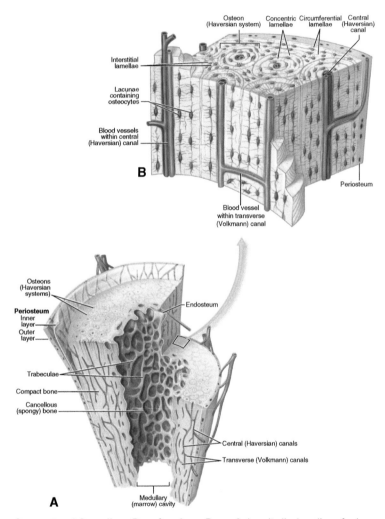

Compact and Cancellous Bone in a Long Bone. A, Longitudinal section of a long bone showing both cancellous and compact bone. **B,** Magnified view of compact bone.

SKELETAL SYSTEM

Divisions of the Skeleton

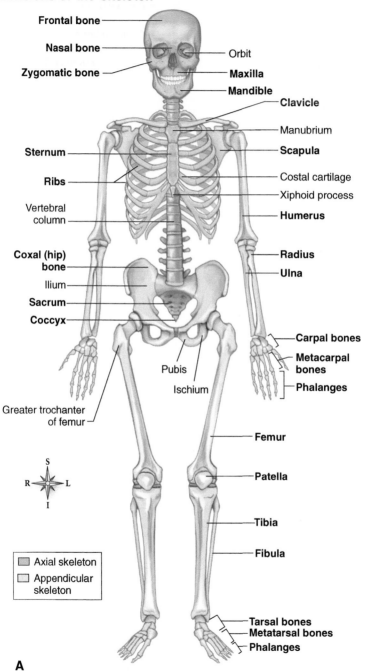

Frontal bone

Nasal bone

Zygomatic bone

Orbit

Maxilla

Mandible

Clavicle

Manubrium

Sternum

Scapula

Ribs

Costal cartilage

Xiphoid process

Vertebral column

Humerus

Coxal (hip) bone

Radius

Ilium

Ulna

Sacrum

Coccyx

Carpal bones

Metacarpal bones

Pubis

Phalanges

Ischium

Greater trochanter of femur

Femur

Patella

S

R —★— L

I

Tibia

Fibula

☐ Axial skeleton

☐ Appendicular skeleton

Tarsal bones

Metatarsal bones

Phalanges

A

Skeleton. A, Anterior view.

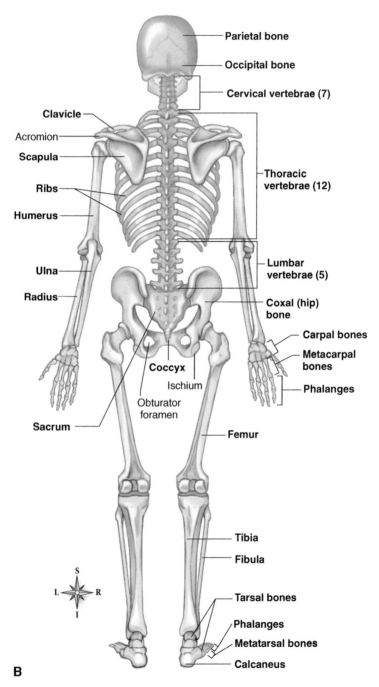

Parietal bone

Occipital bone

Cervical vertebrae (7)

Clavicle

Acromion

Scapula

Ribs

Humerus

Ulna

Radius

Thoracic vertebrae (12)

Lumbar vertebrae (5)

Coxal (hip) bone

Carpal bones

Metacarpal bones

Phalanges

Coccyx

Ischium

Obturator foramen

Sacrum

Femur

Tibia

Fibula

Tarsal bones

Phalanges

Metatarsal bones

Calcaneus

S

L R

I

B

Skeleton—cont'd. B, Posterior view.

BONES OF THE SKELETON (206 TOTAL)*

PART OF BODY	NAME OF BONE
AXIAL SKELETON (80 BONES TOTAL)	
Skull (28 bones total)	
Cranium (8 bones)	Frontal (1) Parietal (2) Temporal (2) Occipital (1) Sphenoid (1) Ethmoid (1)
Face (14 bones)	Nasal (2) Maxillary (2) Zygomatic (malar) (2) Mandible (1) Lacrimal (2) Palatine (2) Inferior nasal conchae (turbinates) (2) Vomer (1)
Ear bones (6 bones)	Malleus (hammer) (2) Incus (anvil) (2) Stapes (stirrup) (2)
Hyoid bone (1)	
Spinal column (26 bones)	Cervical vertebrae (7) Thoracic vertebrae (12) Lumbar vertebrae (5) Sacrum (1) Coccyx (1)
Sternum and ribs (25 bones)	Sternum (1) True ribs (14) False ribs (10)

Continued

BONES OF THE SKELETON
(206 TOTAL)*—cont'd

PART OF BODY	NAME OF BONE
APPENDICULAR SKELETON (126 BONES TOTAL)	
Upper extremities (including shoulder girdle) (64 bones)	Clavicle (2) Scapula (2) Humerus (2) Radius (2) Ulna (2) Carpal bones (16) Metacarpal bones (10) Phalanges (28)
Lower extremities (including hip girdle) (62 bones)	Innominate (2) Fibula (2) Femur (2) Patella (2) Tibia (2) Tarsal bones (14) Metatarsal bones (10) Phalanges (28)

*An inconstant number of small, flat, round bones known as *sesamoid bones* (because of their resemblance to sesame seeds) are found in various tendons in which considerable pressure develops. Because the number of these bones varies greatly between individuals, only two of them, the patellae, have been counted among the 206 bones of the body. Generally, two of them can be found in each thumb (in the flexor tendon near the metacarpophalangeal and interphalangeal joints) and great toe, plus several others in the upper and lower extremities. *Sutural bones (wormian bones),* the small islets of bone frequently found in some of the cranial sutures, have not been counted in this list of 206 bones because of their variable occurrence. The numeral following each bone name is the typical number of bones found in the adult skeleton.

TERMS USED TO DESCRIBE BONE MARKINGS

TERM	MEANING
Angle	A corner
Body	The main portion of a bone
Border	Edge of a bone
Condyle	Rounded bump; usually fits into a fossa on another bone to form a joint
Crest	Moderately raised ridge; generally a site for muscle attachment
Epicondyle	Bump near a condyle; often gives the appearance of a "bump on a bump"; for muscle attachment
Facet	Flat surface that forms a joint with another facet or flat bone
Fissure	Long, cracklike hole for blood vessels and nerves
Foramen	Round hole for vessels and nerves (*pl.,* foramina)
Fossa	Depression; often receives an articulating bone (*pl.,* fossae)
Head	Distinct epiphysis on a long bone, separated from the shaft by a narrowed portion (or neck)
Line	Similar to a crest but not raised as much (is often rather faint)
Margin	Edge of a flat bone or flat portion of the edge of a flat area
Meatus	Tubelike opening or channel (*pl.,* meatus or meatuses)
Neck	A narrowed portion, usually at the base of a head
Notch	A V-like depression in the margin or edge of a flat area
Process	A raised area or projection
Ramus	Curved portion of a bone, like a ram's horn (*pl.,* rami)
Sinus	Cavity within a bone
Spine	Similar to a crest but raised more; a sharp, pointed process; for muscle attachment
Sulcus	Groove or elongated depression (*pl.,* sulci)
Trochanter	Large bump for muscle attachment (larger than a tubercle or tuberosity)
Tuberosity	Oblong, raised bump, usually for muscle attachment; also called a *tuber*; a small tuberosity is called a *tubercle*

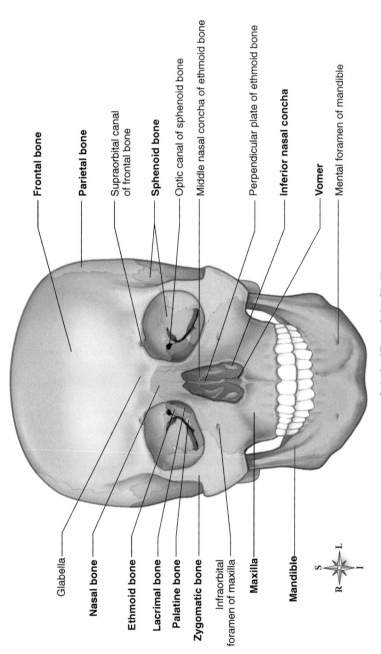

Frontal bone

Parietal bone

Supraorbital canal of frontal bone

Sphenoid bone

Optic canal of sphenoid bone

Middle nasal concha of ethmoid bone

Perpendicular plate of ethmoid bone

Inferior nasal concha

Vomer

Mental foramen of mandible

Glabella

Nasal bone

Ethmoid bone

Lacrimal bone

Palatine bone

Zygomatic bone

Infraorbital foramen of maxilla

Maxilla

Mandible

Anterior View of the Skull.

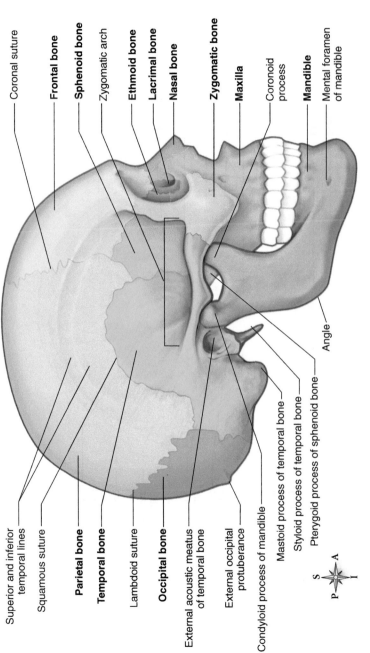

Coronal suture

Frontal bone

Sphenoid bone

Zygomatic arch

Ethmoid bone

Lacrimal bone

Nasal bone

Zygomatic bone

Maxilla

Coronoid process

Mandible

Mental foramen of mandible

Superior and inferior temporal lines

Squamous suture

Parietal bone

Temporal bone

Lambdoid suture

Occipital bone

External acoustic meatus of temporal bone

External occipital protuberance

Condyloid process of mandible

Mastoid process of temporal bone

Styloid process of temporal bone

Pterygoid process of sphenoid bone

Angle

Skull Viewed from the Right Side.

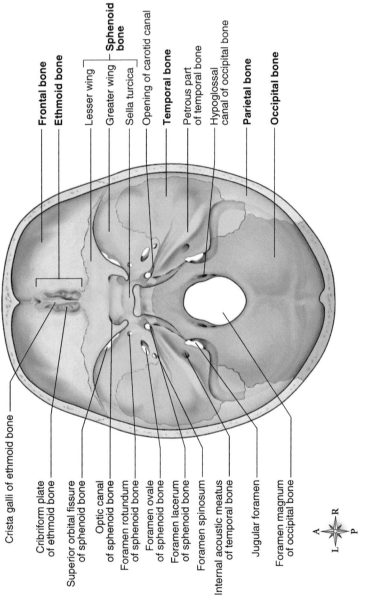

Frontal bone

Ethmoid bone

Lesser wing ⎤
Greater wing ⎦ **Sphenoid bone**

Sella turcica

Opening of carotid canal

Temporal bone

Petrous part of temporal bone

Hypoglossal canal of occipital bone

Parietal bone

Occipital bone

Crista galli of ethmoid bone

Cribriform plate of ethmoid bone

Superior orbital fissure of sphenoid bone

Optic canal of sphenoid bone

Foramen rotundum of sphenoid bone

Foramen ovale of sphenoid bone

Foramen lacerum of sphenoid bone

Foramen spinosum

Internal acoustic meatus of temporal bone

Jugular foramen

Foramen magnum of occipital bone

Floor of the Cranial Cavity viewed from Above.

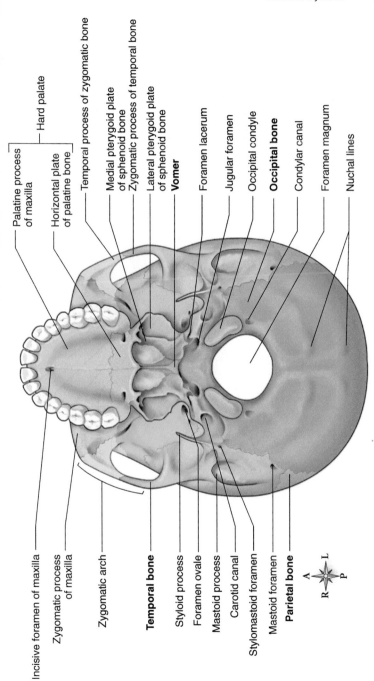

Palatine process of maxilla
Hard palate
Horizontal plate of palatine bone
Temporal process of zygomatic bone
Medial pterygoid plate of sphenoid bone
Zygomatic process of temporal bone
Lateral pterygoid plate of sphenoid bone
Vomer
Foramen lacerum
Jugular foramen
Occipital condyle
Occipital bone
Condylar canal
Foramen magnum
Nuchal lines

Incisive foramen of maxilla
Zygomatic process of maxilla
Zygomatic arch
Temporal bone
Styloid process
Foramen ovale
Mastoid process
Carotid canal
Stylomastoid foramen
Mastoid foramen
Parietal bone

Skull Viewed from Below.

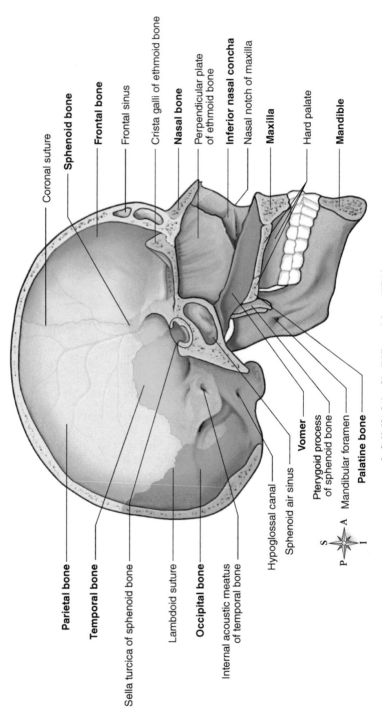

Coronal suture

Sphenoid bone

Frontal bone

Frontal sinus

Crista galli of ethmoid bone

Nasal bone

Perpendicular plate of ethmoid bone

Inferior nasal concha

Nasal notch of maxilla

Maxilla

Hard palate

Mandible

Parietal bone

Temporal bone

Sella turcica of sphenoid bone

Lambdoid suture

Occipital bone

Internal acoustic meatus of temporal bone

Hypoglossal canal

Sphenoid air sinus

Vomer

Pterygoid process of sphenoid bone

Mandibular foramen

Palatine bone

Left Half of the Skull Viewed from Within.

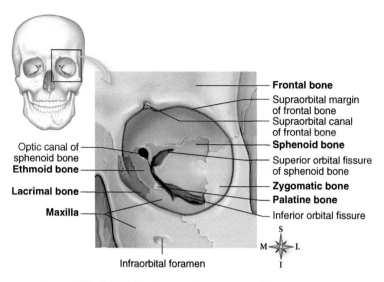

Bones of the Left Orbit. Diagram showing detail of the orbital bones.

CRANIAL BONES AND THEIR MARKINGS

BONES AND MARKINGS	DESCRIPTION
PARIETAL	Prominent, bulging bones behind the frontal bone; form the top sides of the cranial cavity
TEMPORAL	Form the lower sides of the cranium and part of the cranial floor; contain the middle and inner ear structures
Squamous portion	Thin, flaring upper part of the bone
Mastoid portion	Rough-surfaced lower part of the bone posterior to the external acoustic meatus
Petrous portion	Wedge-shaped process that forms part of the center section of the cranial floor between the sphenoid and occipital bones; name derived from the Greek word meaning "stone" because of the extreme hardness of this process; houses the middle and inner ear structures
Mastoid process	Protuberance just behind the ear
Mastoid air cells	Mucosa-lined, air-filled spaces within the mastoid process
External acoustic meatus (or canal)	Tube extending into the temporal bone from the external ear opening to the tympanic membrane

Continued

CRANIAL BONES AND THEIR MARKINGS—cont'd

BONES AND MARKINGS	DESCRIPTION
Zygomatic process	Projection that articulates with the zygomatic (or malar) bone
Internal acoustic meatus	Fairly large opening on the posterior surface of the petrous part of the bone; transmits the eighth cranial nerve to the inner ear and the seventh cranial nerve on its way to the facial structures
Mandibular fossa	Oval-shaped depression anterior to the external acoustic meatus; forms the socket for the condyle of the mandible
Styloid process	Slender spike of bone extending downward and forward from the undersurface of the bone anterior to the mastoid process; often broken off in a dry skull; several neck muscles and ligaments attach to the styloid process
Stylomastoid foramen	Opening between the styloid and mastoid processes where the facial nerve emerges from the cranial cavity
Jugular fossa	Depression on the undersurface of the petrous part; dilated beginning of the internal jugular vein lodged here
Jugular foramen	Opening in the suture between the petrous part and occipital bone; transmits the lateral sinus and ninth, tenth, and eleventh cranial nerves
Carotid canal (or foramen)	Channel in the petrous part; best seen from the undersurface of the skull; transmits the internal carotid artery
FRONTAL	Forehead bone; also forms most of the roof of the orbits (eye sockets) and the anterior part of the cranial floor
Supraorbital margin	Arched ridge just below eyebrow; forms the upper edge of the orbit
Frontal sinuses	Cavities inside the bone just above supraorbital margin; lined with mucosa; contain air
Frontal tuberosities (tubers or eminences)	Bulge above each orbit; most prominent part of forehead
Superciliary arches (ridges)	Curved ridges caused by projection of the frontal sinuses; eyebrows lie superficial to these ridges
Supraorbital foramen (sometimes notch)	Foramen or notch in the supraorbital margin slightly medial to its midpoint; transmits supraorbital nerve and blood vessels
Glabella	Smooth area between the superciliary ridges and above the nose

BONES AND MARKINGS	DESCRIPTION
OCCIPITAL	Forms the posterior part of the cranial floor and walls
Foramen magnum	Hole through which the spinal cord enters the cranial cavity
Occipital condyles	Convex, oval processes on either side of the foramen magnum; articulate with depressions on the first cervical vertebra
External occipital protuberance	Prominent projection on the posterior surface in the midline a short distance above the foramen magnum; can be felt as a definite bump
Superior nuchal line	Curved ridge extending laterally from the external occipital protuberance
Inferior nuchal line	Less well defined ridge paralleling the superior nuchal line a short distance below it
Internal occipital protuberance	Projection in the midline on the inner surface of the bone; grooves for the lateral sinuses extend laterally from this process, and one for sagittal sinus extends upward from it
SPHENOID	Keystone of the cranial floor; forms its midportion; resembles a bat with wings outstretched and legs extended downward posteriorly; lies behind and slightly above the nose and throat; forms part of the floor and sidewalls of the orbit
Body	Hollow, cubelike central portion
Greater wings	Lateral projections from the body; form part of the outer wall of the orbit
Lesser wings	Thin, triangular projections from the upper part of the sphenoid body; form the posterior part of the roof of the orbit
Sella turcica	Saddle-shaped depression on the upper surface of the sphenoid body; contains the pituitary gland; literally means "Turkish saddle"
Sphenoid sinuses	Irregular mucosa-lined, air-filled spaces within the central part of the sphenoid
Pterygoid processes	Downward projections on either side, where the body and greater wing unite; comparable to the extended legs of a bat if the entire bone is likened to this animal; form part of the lateral nasal wall
Optic canal	Passage that transmits the optic nerve into the orbit (at the base of the lesser wing)
Superior orbital fissure	Slitlike opening into the orbit; lateral to the optic foramen; transmits the third, fourth, and part of the fifth cranial nerves

Continued

CRANIAL BONES AND THEIR MARKINGS—cont'd

BONES AND MARKINGS	DESCRIPTION
Foramen rotundum	Opening in the greater wing that transmits the maxillary division of the fifth cranial nerve
Foramen ovale	Opening in the greater wing that transmits the mandibular division of the fifth cranial nerve
Foramen lacerum	Opening at the junction of the sphenoid, temporal, and occipital bones; transmits a branch of the ascending pharyngeal artery
Foramen spinosum	Opening in the greater wing that transmits the middle meningeal artery to supply the meninges
ETHMOID	Complex irregular bone that helps make up the anterior portion of the cranial floor, medial wall of the orbits, upper parts of the nasal septum, and sidewalls and part of the nasal roof; lies anterior to the sphenoid and posterior to the nasal bones
Cribriform plate	Olfactory nerves pass through numerous holes in this horizontal plate
Crista galli	Meninges (membranes around the brain) attach to this process
Perpendicular plate	Forms the upper part of the nasal septum
Ethmoid sinuses	Honeycombed, mucosa-lined air spaces within the lateral masses of the bone
Superior and middle nasal conchae (turbinates)	Help form the lateral walls of the nose
Ethmoidal labyrinth	Hollow lateral masses of the ethmoid; contain many air spaces (ethmoid cells or sinuses); the inner surface forms the superior and middle conchae

FACIAL BONES AND THEIR MARKINGS

BONES AND MARKINGS	DESCRIPTION
VOMER	Forms lower and posterior part of nasal septum; shaped like the blade of a plow
MAXILLA	Upper jawbones; form part of the floor of the orbit, anterior part of the roof of the mouth, and floor of the nose and part of the sidewalls of the nose
Alveolar process	Archlike process that holds the tooth sockets
Maxillary sinus	Large, air-filled cavity within body of maxilla; lined with mucous membranes; largest of paranasal sinuses

FACIAL BONES AND THEIR MARKINGS—cont'd

BONES AND MARKINGS	DESCRIPTION
Palatine process	Horizontal plate that projects inward from the alveolar process; forms anterior and larger part of hard palate
Infraorbital foramen	Hole on external surface of orbit; transmits vessels and nerves
Lacrimal groove	Groove on inner surface; joined by similar groove on lacrimal bone to form bony space for the nasolacrimal duct
ZYGOMATIC	Cheekbones; form part of floor and sidewall of eye orbit
PALATINE	Form the posterior part of the hard palate, floor, and part of the sidewalls of the nasal cavity and floor of orbit
Horizontal plate	Joined to the palatine processes of the maxillae to complete part of the hard palate
LACRIMAL	Thin platelike bones; posterior and lateral to nasal bones in medial wall of eye orbit; help form sidewall of nasal cavity (often missing in dry skull specimen)
NASAL	Pair of small bones that form the upper part of bridge of nose
INFERIOR NASAL CONCHAE (TURBINATES)	Thin scroll of bone forming shelf along inner surface of sidewall of nasal cavity; lies above roof of mouth
MANDIBLE	Lower jawbone; largest, strongest bone of the face
Body	Main part of the bone; forms the chin
Ramus	Process, one on either side, that projects upward from the posterior part of the body
Condylar process	Part of each ramus that articulates with the mandibular fossa of the temporal bone
Neck	Constricted part just below the condyles
Alveolar process	Teeth set into this arch
Mandibular foramen	Opening on the inner surface of the ramus; transmits nerves and vessels to the lower teeth
Mental foramen	Opening on the outer surface below the space between the two bicuspids; transmits the terminal branches of the nerves and vessels that enter the bone through the mandibular foramen; dentists inject anesthetics through these foramina
Coronoid process	Projection upward from the anterior part of each ramus; the temporal muscle inserts here
Angle	Juncture of posterior and inferior margins of ramus

SPECIAL FEATURES OF THE SKULL

FEATURE	DESCRIPTION
SUTURES	Immovable joints between skull bones
Squamous	Line of articulation along the top curved edge of the temporal bone
Coronal	Joint between the parietal bones and frontal bone
Lambdoid	Joint between the parietal bones and occipital bone
Sagittal	Joint between the right and left parietal bones
FONTANELS	"Soft spots" where ossification is incomplete at birth; allow some compression of the skull during birth; also important in determining the position of the head before delivery; six such areas located at angles of the parietal bones
Anterior (or frontal)	At the intersection of the sagittal and coronal sutures (juncture of the parietal bones and frontal bone); diamond shaped; largest of the fontanels; usually closed by 11.2 years of age
Posterior (or occipital)	At the intersection of the sagittal and lambdoid sutures (juncture of the parietal bones and occipital bone); triangular; usually closed by the second month
Sphenoid (or anterolateral)	At the juncture of the frontal, parietal, temporal, and sphenoid bones
Mastoid (or posterolateral)	At the juncture of the parietal, occipital, and temporal bones; usually closed by the second year
AIR SINUSES	Spaces, or cavities, within bones; those that communicate with the nose are called *paranasal sinuses* (frontal, sphenoidal, ethmoidal, and maxillary); mastoid cells communicate with the middle ear rather than the nose, so not included among the paranasal sinuses
ORBITS FORMED BY	
Frontal bone	Roof of the orbit
Ethmoid bone	Medial wall
Lacrimal bone	Medial wall
Sphenoid bone	Lateral wall
Zygomatic bone	Lateral wall
Maxilla	Floor
Palatine bone	Floor

SPECIAL FEATURES OF THE SKULL—cont'd

FEATURE	DESCRIPTION
NASAL SEPTUM FORMED BY	Partition in the midline of the nasal cavity; separates the cavity into right and left halves
Perpendicular plate of the ethmoid bone	Forms the upper part of the septum
Vomer	Forms the lower, posterior part of the septum
Cartilage	Forms the anterior part of the septum
SUTURAL (WORMIAN) BONES	Small islets of bone in sutures; vary greatly from person to person
MALLEUS, INCUS, STAPES	Tiny bones, referred to as *auditory ossicles,* in the middle ear cavity in the temporal bones; resemble, respectively, a miniature hammer, anvil, and stirrup

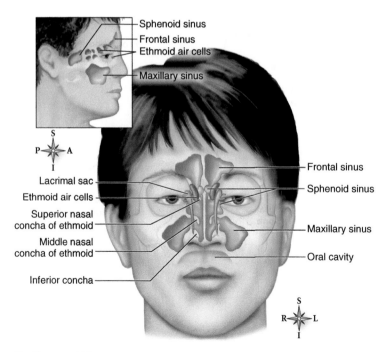

The Paranasal Sinuses. The anterior view shows the anatomical relationship of the paranasal sinuses to each other and to the nasal cavity. The *inset* is a lateral view of the position of the sinuses.

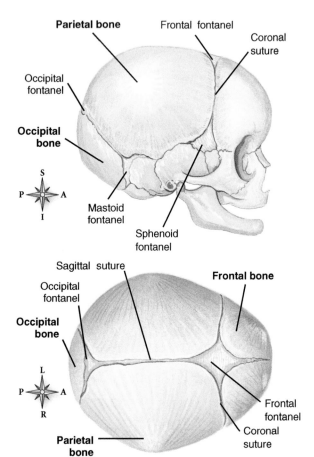

The Skull at Birth.

Hyoid Bone

HYOID, VERTEBRAE, AND THORACIC BONES AND THEIR MARKINGS

BONES AND MARKINGS	DESCRIPTION
HYOID	U-shaped bone in the neck between the mandible and upper part of the larynx; distinctive as the only bone in the body not forming a joint with any other bone; suspended by ligaments from the styloid processes of the temporal bones
VERTEBRAL COLUMN	Not actually a column, but a flexible, segmented curved rod; forms the axis of the body; head balanced above, ribs and viscera suspended in front, and lower extremities attached below; encloses the spinal cord
	General features: Anterior part of each vertebra (except the first two cervical) consists of the body; posterior part of the vertebrae consists of the neural arch, which in turn consists of two pedicles, two laminae, and seven processes projecting from the laminae
Body	Main part; flat, round mass located anteriorly; supporting or weight-bearing part of the vertebra
Pedicles	Short projections extending posteriorly from the body
Lamina	Posterior part of the vertebra to which pedicles join and from which processes project
Neural arch	Formed by the pedicles and laminae; protects the spinal cord posteriorly; congenital absence of one or more neural arches is known as *spina bifida* (the cord may protrude right through the skin)
Spinous process	Sharp process projecting inferiorly from laminae in the midline
Transverse processes	Right and left lateral projections from laminae
Superior articulating processes	Project upward from laminae; have smooth *superior articular facets*
Inferior articulating processes	Project downward from laminae; articulate with the superior articulating processes of vertebrae below; have smooth *inferior articular facets*
Spinal foramen	Hole in the center of the vertebra formed by union of the body, pedicles, and laminae; spinal foramina, when vertebrae are superimposed on one another, form the spinal cavity that houses the spinal cord
Intervertebral foramina	Opening between the vertebrae through which the spinal nerves emerge

Continued

HYOID, VERTEBRAE, AND THORACIC BONES AND THEIR MARKINGS—cont'd

BONES AND MARKINGS	DESCRIPTION
CERVICAL VERTEBRAE	First or upper seven vertebrae; the foramen in each transverse process for transmission of the vertebral artery, vein, and plexus of nerves; short bifurcated spinous processes except on the seventh vertebra, where it is extra long and may be felt as a protrusion when head is bent forward; the bodies of these vertebrae are small, whereas spinal foramina are large and triangular
Atlas	First cervical vertebra; lacks a body and spinous process; superior articulating processes are concave ovals that act as rockerlike cradles for the condyles of the occipital bone; named *atlas* because it supports the head as Atlas supports the world in Greek mythology
Axis (epistropheus)	Second cervical vertebra, so named because the atlas rotates about this bone in rotating movements of the head; the *dens,* or odontoid process, is a peglike projection extending upward from the body of the axis that forms a pivot for rotation of the atlas
THORACIC VERTEBRAE	Next 12 vertebrae; 12 pairs of ribs attached to these vertebrae; stronger, with more massive bodies than the cervical vertebrae; no transverse foramina; two sets of facets for articulations with the corresponding rib: one on the body, the second on the transverse process; the upper thoracic vertebrae have elongated spinous processes
LUMBAR VERTEBRAE	Next five vertebrae; strong, massive; superior articulating processes directed medially instead of upward; inferior articulating processes, laterally instead of downward; short, blunt spinous processes
SACRUM	Five separate vertebrae until about 25 years of age; then fused to form one wedge-shaped bone
Sacral promontory	Protuberance from the anterior, upper border of the sacrum into the pelvis; of obstetrical importance because its size limits the anteroposterior diameter of the pelvic inlet
COCCYX	Four or five separate vertebrae in a child but fused into one in an adult

HYOID, VERTEBRAE, AND THORACIC BONES AND THEIR MARKINGS—cont'd

BONES AND MARKINGS	DESCRIPTION
CURVATURES	Curvatures have great structural importance because they increase the carrying strength of the vertebral column, make balance possible in an upright position (if the column was straight, the weight of the viscera would pull the body forward), absorb jolts from walking (a straight column would transmit jolts straight to the head), and protect the column from fracture
Primary curvatures Thoracic curvature Sacral curvature	Column curves at birth from the head to the sacrum with the convexity posteriorly; after the child stands, the convexity persists only in the *thoracic* and *sacral* regions, which are therefore called *primary curves*
Secondary curvatures Cervical curvature Lumbar curvature	Concavities in the *cervical* and *lumbar* regions; the cervical concavity results from the infant's attempts to hold the head erect (2 to 4 months); the lumbar concavity, from balancing efforts in learning to walk (10 to 18 months)
STERNUM	Breastbone; flat dagger-shaped bone; the sternum, ribs, and thoracic vertebrae together form a bony cage known as the *thorax*
Body	Main central part of the bone
Manubrium	Flaring, upper part
Xiphoid process	Projection of cartilage at the lower border of the bone
RIBS **Types**	
True ribs	Upper seven pairs; fasten to the sternum by costal cartilages
False ribs	False ribs do not attach to the sternum directly; the upper three pairs of false ribs attach by means of the costal cartilage of the seventh ribs
Floating ribs	The last two pairs of false ribs do not attach to the sternum at all and are therefore called *"floating" ribs*
Parts	
Head	Projection at the posterior end of a rib; articulates with the corresponding thoracic vertebra and one above, except the last three pairs, which join the corresponding vertebrae only
Neck	Constricted portion just below the head
Tubercle	Small knob just below the neck; articulates with the transverse process of the corresponding thoracic vertebra; missing in the lowest three ribs
Body or shaft	Main part of a rib
Costal cartilage	Cartilage at the sternal end of true ribs; attaches ribs (except floating ribs) to the sternum

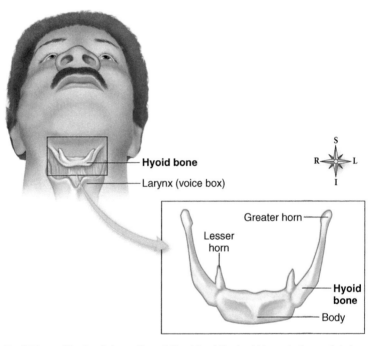

Hyoid Bone. The *inset* shows the relationship of the hyoid bone in the neck below the skull and above the voice box (larynx). Note that the hyoid does not articulate with any other bony structure.

Vertebral Column

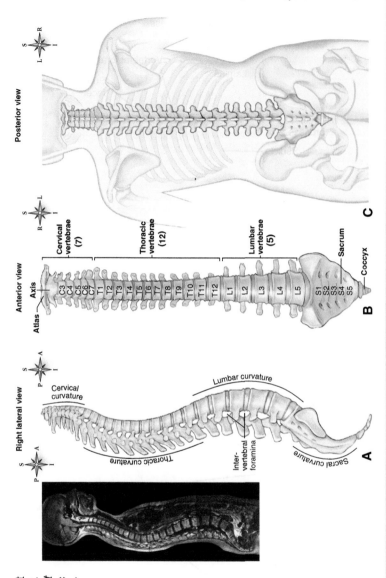

The Vertebral Column. A, Right lateral view. **B,** Anterior view. **C,** Posterior view. The *photo inset* shows a midline sagittal magnetic resonance image (MRI) of the vertebral column.

Right lateral view

Cervical curvature

Thoracic curvature

Lumbar curvature

Sacral curvature

Intervertebral foramina

A

Anterior view

Atlas

Axis

Cervical vertebrae (7)

C3
C4
C5
C6
C7

Thoracic vertebrae (12)

T1
T2
T3
T4
T5
T6
T7
T8
T9
T10
T11
T12

Lumbar vertebrae (5)

L1
L2
L3
L4
L5

Sacrum

S1
S2
S3
S4
S5

Coccyx

B

Posterior view

C

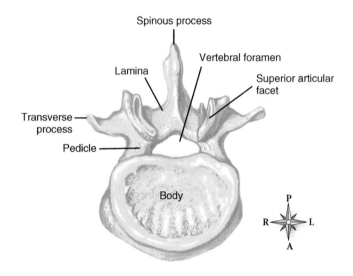

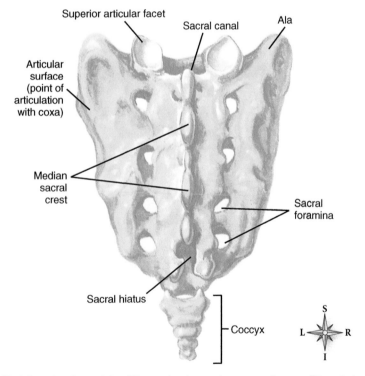

Vertebrae. Lumbar vertebra **(A)**, superior view, and sacrum and coccyx **(B)**, posterior view.

Thoracic Cage

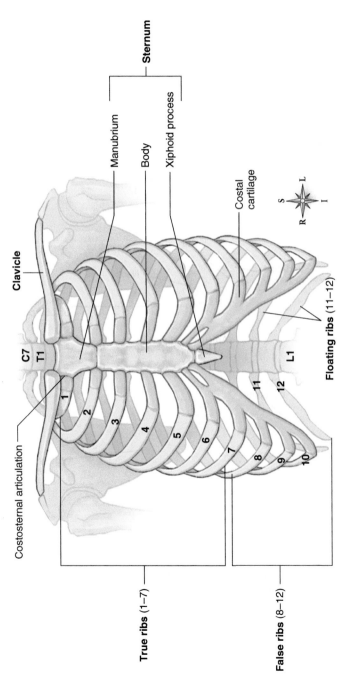

Thoracic Cage. Note the costal cartilages and their articulations with the body of the sternum.

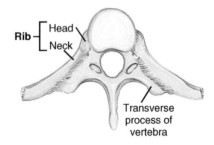

A

B

Rib. Articulation of the ribs with the thoracic vertebra **(A)** and a rib of the left side seen from behind (posterior view) **(B)**.

Upper Extremity

UPPER EXTERMITY BONES AND THEIR MARKINGS

BONES AND MARKINGS	DESCRIPTION
CLAVICLE	Collarbones; the shoulder girdle is joined to the axial skeleton by articulation of the clavicles with the sternum (the scapula does not form a joint with the axial skeleton)
SCAPULA	Shoulder blades; the scapulae and clavicles together make up the shoulder girdle
Borders	
Superior	Upper margin
Medial (vertebral)	Margin toward the vertebral column
Lateral (axillary)	Lateral margin, toward axilla
Spine	Sharp ridge running diagonally across the posterior surface of the shoulder blade
Acromion	Slightly flaring projection at the lateral end of the scapular spine; may be felt at the tip of the shoulder; articulates with the clavicle
Coracoid process	Projection on the anterior surface from the upper border of the bone; may be felt in the groove between the deltoid and pectoralis major muscles, about 1 inch below the clavicle
Glenoid cavity	Arm socket
HUMERUS	Long bone of the arm
Head	Smooth, hemispherical enlargement at the proximal end of the humerus
Anatomical neck	Oblique groove just below the head
Greater tubercle	Rounded projection lateral to the head on the anterior surface
Lesser tubercle	Prominent projection on the anterior surface just below the anatomical neck
Intertubercular groove	Deep groove between the greater and lesser tubercles; the long tendon of the biceps muscle lodges here
Surgical neck	Region just below the tubercles; so named because of its liability to fracture
Deltoid tuberosity	V-shaped, rough area about midway down the shaft where the deltoid muscle inserts
Radial groove	Groove running obliquely downward from the deltoid tuberosity; lodges the radial nerve

Continued

UPPER EXTERMITY BONES AND THEIR MARKINGS—cont'd

BONES AND MARKINGS	DESCRIPTION
Epicondyles (medial and lateral)	Rough projections at both sides of the distal end
Capitulum	Rounded knob below the lateral epicondyle; articulates with the radius; sometimes called the *radial head of the humerus*
Trochlea	Projection with a deep depression through the center similar to the shape of a pulley; articulates with the ulna
Olecranon fossa	Depression on the posterior surface just above the trochlea; receives the olecranon of the ulna when the forearm extends
Coronoid fossa	Depression on the anterior surface above the trochlea; receives the coronoid process of the ulna in flexion of the forearm
RADIUS	Bone of the thumb side of the forearm
Head	Disk-shaped process forming the proximal end of the radius; articulates with the capitulum of the humerus and with the radial notch of the ulna
Radial tuberosity	Roughened projection on the ulnar side, a short distance below the head; the biceps muscle inserts here
Styloid process	Protuberance at the distal end on the lateral surface (with the forearm in the anatomical position)
ULNA	Bone of the little finger side of the forearm; longer than the radius
Olecranon	Scooplike process that joins the trochlea of the humerus at the elbow
Coronoid process	Projection on the anterior surface of the proximal end of the ulna; the trochlea of the humerus fits snugly between the olecranon and coronoid processes
Trochlear notch	Curved notch between the olecranon and coronoid process into which the trochlea fits; also called *semilunar notch*

UPPER EXTERMITY BONES AND THEIR MARKINGS—cont'd

BONES AND MARKINGS	DESCRIPTION
Radial notch	Curved notch lateral and inferior to the trochlear notch; the head of the radius fits into this concavity
Head	Rounded process at the distal end; does not articulate with the wrist bones but with the fibrocartilaginous disk
Styloid process	Sharp protuberance at the distal end; can be seen from outside on the posterior surface
CARPAL BONES	Wrist bones; arranged in two rows at the proximal end of the hand; proximal row (from the little finger toward the thumb)—pisiform, triquetrum, lunate, and scaphoid; distal row—hamate, capitate, trapezoid, and trapezium
METACARPAL BONES	Long bones forming the framework of the palm of the hand; numbered (from lateral side) I, II, III, IV, V
PHALANGES	Miniature long bones of the fingers, three (proximal, middle, distal) in each finger, two (proximal, distal) in each thumb; numbered (from lateral side) I (except first middle), II, III, IV, V

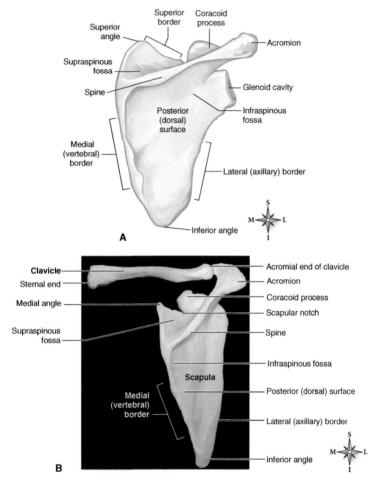

Right Scapula. A, Posterior view. **B,** Posterior view showing articulation of the right scapula with the clavicle.

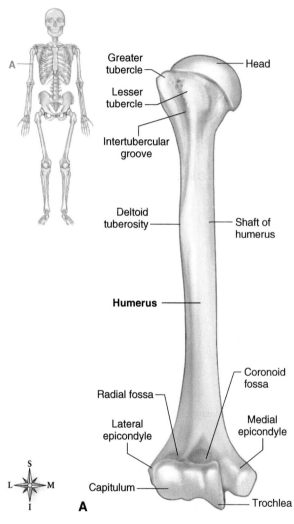

Bone of the Arm (right arm). Humerus. **A,** Anterior view.

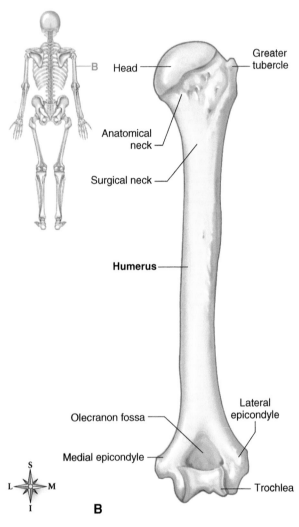

Head — Greater tubercle

Anatomical neck

Surgical neck

Humerus —

Olecranon fossa

Medial epicondyle

Lateral epicondyle

Trochlea

S
L — M
I

B

Bone of the Arm (right arm)—cont'd. B, Posterior view. (The *skeleton insets* show the relative position of these bones within the entire skeleton.)

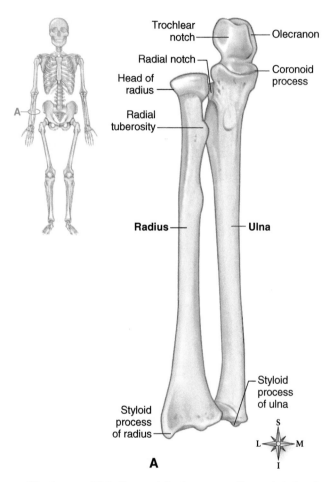

Bones of the Forearm (Right Forearm). Radius and ulna (forearm). **A,** Anterior view.

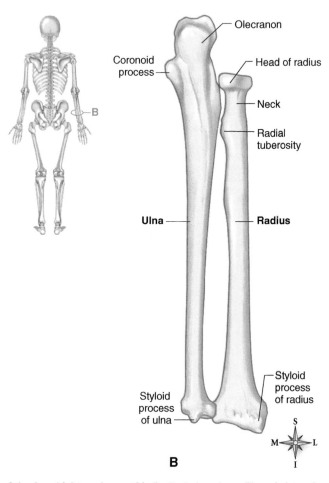

Bone of the Arm (right arm)—cont'd. B, Posterior view. (The *skeleton insets* show the relative position of these bones within the entire skeleton.)

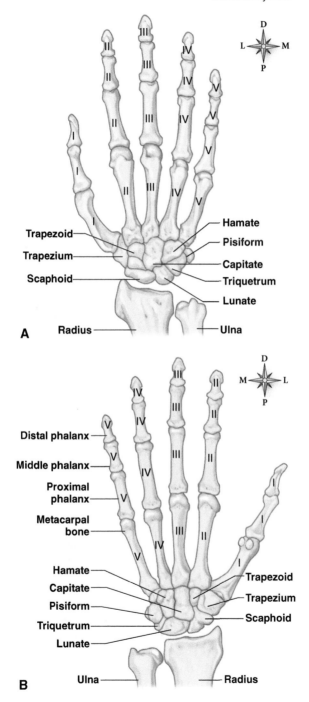

Bones of the Hand and Wrist. A, Dorsal view of the right hand and wrist. **B,** Palmar view of the right hand and wrist.

Lower Extremity

LOWER EXTREMITY BONES AND THEIR MARKINGS

BONES AND MARKINGS	DESCRIPTION
COXAL	Large hip bone (pelvic bone); with the sacrum and coccyx, forms the basinlike pelvic cavity; lower extremities attached to the axial skeleton by the coxal bones
Ilium	Upper, flaring portion
Ischium	Lower, posterior portion
Pubis	Medial, anterior section
Acetabulum	Hip socket; formed by union of the ilium, ischium, and pubis
Iliac crests	Upper, curving boundary of the ilium
Iliac spines	
Anterior superior	Prominent projection at the anterior end of the iliac crest; can be felt externally as the "point" of the hip
Anterior inferior	Less prominent projection short distance below anterior superior spine
Posterior superior	At the posterior end of the iliac crest
Posterior inferior	Just below the posterior superior spine
Greater sciatic notch	Large notch on the posterior surface of the ilium just below the posterior inferior spine
Ischial tuberosity	Large, rough, quadrilateral process forming the inferior part of the ischium; in an erect sitting position the body rests on these tuberosities
Ischial spine	Pointed projection just above the tuberosity
Pubic symphysis	Cartilaginous, amphiarthrotic joint between the pubic bones
Superior pubic ramus	Part of the pubis lying between the symphysis and acetabulum; forms the upper part of the obturator foramen
Inferior pubic ramus	Part extending down from the symphysis; unites with the ischium
Pubic arch	Curve formed by the two inferior rami
Subpubic angle	Angle formed under the inferior pubic rami; generally larger in women than in men
Pubic crest	Upper margin of the superior ramus
Pubic tubercle	Rounded process at the end of the crest

LOWER EXTREMITY BONES AND THEIR MARKINGS—cont'd

BONES AND MARKINGS	DESCRIPTION
Obturator foramen	Large hole in the anterior surface of the coxal bone; formed by the pubis and ischium; largest foramen in the body
Pelvic inlet (or brim)	Boundary of the aperture leading into the true pelvis; formed by the pubic crests, iliopectineal lines, and sacral promontory; the size and shape of this inlet have obstetrical importance because if any of its diameters are too small, the infant's skull cannot enter the true pelvis for natural birth (or lesser pelvis)
True pelvis (or greater pelvis)	Space below the pelvic brim; true "basin" with bone and muscle walls and a muscle floor; pelvic organs located in this space
False pelvis (or lesser pelvis)	Broad, shallow space above the pelvic brim, or the pelvic inlet; name *"false pelvis"* is misleading because this space is actually part of the abdominal cavity, not the pelvic cavity
Pelvic outlet	Irregular circumference marking the lower limits of the true pelvis; bounded by the tip of the coccyx and two ischial tuberosities
Pelvic girdle (or bony pelvis)	Complete bony ring; composed of two hip bones (ossa coxae), the sacrum, and the coccyx; forms a firm base by which the trunk rests on the thighs and for attachment of the lower extremities to the axial skeleton
FEMUR	Thigh bone; largest, strongest bone of the body
Head	Rounded upper end of the bone; fits into the acetabulum
Neck	Constricted portion just below the head
Greater trochanter	Protuberance located inferiorly and laterally to the head
Lesser trochanter	Small protuberance located inferiorly and medially to the greater trochanter
Intertrochanteric line	Line extending between the greater and lesser trochanter

Continued

LOWER EXTREMITY BONES AND THEIR MARKINGS—cont'd

BONES AND MARKINGS	DESCRIPTION
Linea aspera	Prominent ridge extending lengthwise along the concave posterior surface
Supracondylar ridges	Two ridges formed by division of the linea aspera at its lower end; the medial supracondylar ridge extends inward to the inner condyle, the lateral ridge to the outer condyle
Condyles	Large, rounded bulges at the distal end of the femur; one medial and one lateral
Epicondyles	Blunt projections from the sides of the condyles; one on the medial aspect and one on the lateral aspect
Adductor tubercle	Small projection just above the medial condyle; marks the termination of the medial supracondylar ridge
Trochlea	Smooth depression between the condyles on the anterior surface; articulates with the patella
Intercondylar fossa (notch)	Deep depression between the condyles on the posterior surface; the cruciate ligaments, which help bind the femur to the tibia, lodge in this notch
PATELLA	Kneecap; largest sesamoid bone of the body; embedded in the tendon of the quadriceps femoris muscle
TIBIA	Shin bone
Condyles	Bulging prominences at the proximal end of the tibia; upper surfaces concave for articulation with the femur
Intercondylar eminence	Upward projection on the articular surface between the condyles
Crest	Sharp ridge on the anterior surface
Tibial tuberosity	Projection in the midline on the anterior surface
Medial malleolus	Rounded downward projection at the distal end of the tibia; forms the prominence on the medial surface of the ankle

LOWER EXTREMITY BONES AND THEIR MARKINGS—cont'd

BONES AND MARKINGS	DESCRIPTION
FIBULA	Long, slender bone of the lateral side of the leg
Lateral malleolus	Rounded prominence at the distal end of the fibula; forms the prominence on the lateral surface of the ankle
TARSAL BONES	Bones that form the heel and proximal or posterior half of the foot; include calcaneus, talus, navicular, cuboid, medial cuneiform (I), intermediate cuneiform (II), and lateral cuneiform (III)
Calcaneus	Heel bone
Talus	Uppermost of the tarsal bones; articulates with the tibia and fibula; boxed in the medial and lateral malleoli
ARCHES OF FOOT	Curves of the bones of the foot and ankle that, along with muscles and other soft tissues, efficiently support the mass of the skeleton
Longitudinal arches	Tarsal and metatarsal bones so arranged as to form an arch from the front to the back of the foot
Medial	Formed by the calcaneus, talus, navicular, cuneiforms, and three medial metatarsal bones
Lateral	Formed by the calcaneus, cuboid, and two lateral metatarsal bones
Transverse (or metatarsal) arch	Metatarsal and distal row of tarsal bones (cuneiforms and cuboid) articulated so as to form an arch across the foot; bones kept in two arched positions by means of powerful ligaments in the sole of the foot and by muscles and tendons
METATARSAL BONES	Long bones of the feet; numbered (from medial side) I, II, III, IV, V
Phalanges	Miniature long bones of the toes; two in each great toe; three in the other toes; from metatarsal bone: proximal, middle (except first toe), distal; numbered (from medial side) I (except first toe), II, III, IV, V

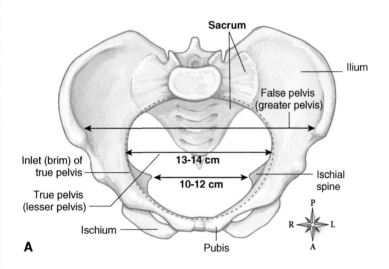

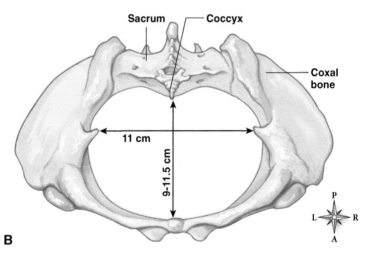

The Female Pelvis. A, Pelvis viewed from above. Note that the brim of the true pelvis *(dotted line)* marks the boundary between the superior false pelvis (pelvis major) and the inferior true pelvis (pelvis minor). **B,** Pelvis viewed from below.

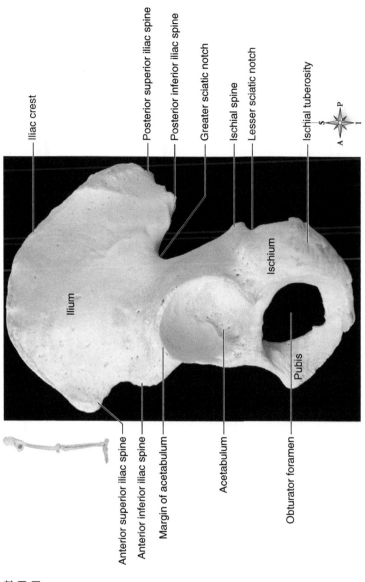

Iliac crest

Posterior superior iliac spine

Posterior inferior iliac spine

Greater sciatic notch

Ischial spine

Lesser sciatic notch

Ischial tuberosity

Ilium

Ischium

Pubis

Anterior superior iliac spine

Anterior inferior iliac spine

Margin of acetabulum

Acetabulum

Obturator foramen

Left Coxal (Hip) Bone. The left coxal bone is disarticulated from the bony pelvis and viewed from the side.

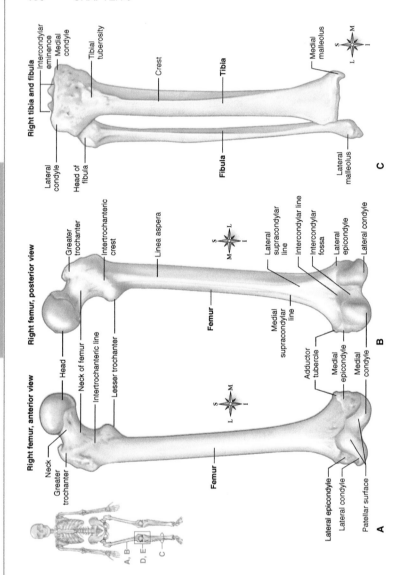

Bones of the Thigh and Leg.
A, Right femur, anterior surface.
B, Right femur, posterior view.
C, Right tibia and fibula, anterior surface. (The *skeleton inset* shows the relative position of the bones of the thigh and leg within the entire skeleton.)

Right tibia and fibula

Intercondylar eminence
Medial condyle
Tibial tuberosity
Crest
Tibia
Medial malleolus
Lateral condyle
Head of fibula
Fibula
Lateral malleolus

C

Right femur, posterior view

Greater trochanter
Intertrochanteric crest
Linea aspera
Lateral supracondylar line
Intercondylar fossa
Lateral epicondyle
Lateral condyle
Medial supracondylar line
Adductor tubercle
Medial epicondyle
Medial condyle
Head
Neck of femur
Intertrochanteric line
Lesser trochanter
Femur

B

Right femur, anterior view

Neck
Greater trochanter
Head
Lateral epicondyle
Lateral condyle
Patellar surface
Femur

A

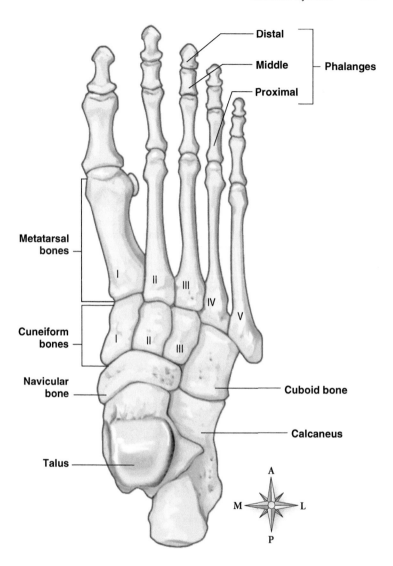

The Foot. Bones of the right foot viewed from above. The tarsal bones consist of the cuneiforms, navicular, talus, cuboid, and calcaneus.

Skeletal Differences Between Men and Women

COMPARISON OF MALE AND FEMALE SKELETONS

PORTION OF SKELETON	MALE	FEMALE
GENERAL FORM	Bones heavier and thicker Muscle attachment sites more massive Joint surfaces relatively large	Bones lighter and thinner Muscle attachment sites less distinct Joint surfaces relatively small
SKULL	Forehead shorter vertically Mandible and maxillae relatively smaller Facial area rounder, with less pronounced features Processes less pronounced	Forehead more elongated vertically Mandible and maxillae relatively larger Facial area more pronounced Processes more prominent
PELVIS		
Pelvic cavity	Narrower in all dimensions Deeper Pelvic outlet relatively small	Wider in all dimensions Shorter and roomier Pelvic outlet relatively large
Sacrum	Long, narrow, with a smooth concavity (sacral curvature); sacral promontory more pronounced	Short, wide, flat concavity more pronounced in a posterior direction; sacral promontory less pronounced
Coccyx	Less movable	More movable and follows the posterior direction of the sacral curvature
Pubic arch	60- to 90-degree angle	90- to 120-degree angle
Pubic symphysis	Relatively deep	Relatively shallow
Ischial spine, ischial tuberosity, and anterior superior iliac spine	Turned more inward	Turned more outward and further apart
Greater sciatic notch	Narrow	Wide

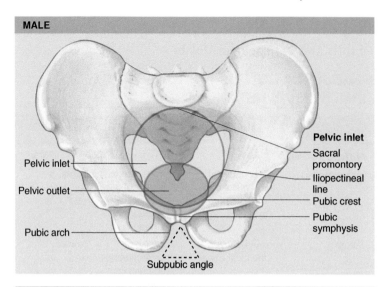

MALE

Pelvic inlet

Pelvic outlet

Pubic arch

Pelvic inlet

Sacral promontory

Iliopectineal line

Pubic crest

Pubic symphysis

Subpubic angle

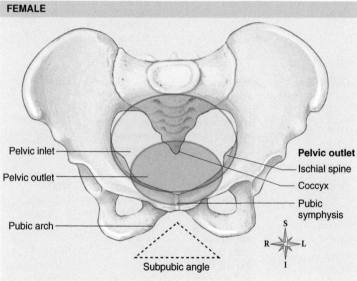

FEMALE

Pelvic inlet

Pelvic outlet

Pubic arch

Pelvic outlet

Ischial spine

Coccyx

Pubic symphysis

Subpubic angle

S
R — L
I

Comparison of the Bony Pelvises of the Male and Female Skeletons. The male pelvis is generally narrower than the female pelvis, with smaller pelvic openings and more prominent bone processes for muscle attachment.

ARTICULATIONS

Fibrous and Cartilaginous Joints

CLASSIFICATION OF FIBROUS AND CARTILAGINOUS JOINTS

TYPES	EXAMPLES	STRUCTURAL FEATURES	MOVEMENT
FIBROUS JOINTS			
Syndesmoses	Joints between the distal ends of the radius and ulna	Fibrous bands (ligaments) connect articulating bones	Slight
Sutures	Joints between the skull bones	Teethlike projections of articulating bones interlock with a thin layer of fibrous tissue connecting them	None
Gomphoses	Joints between the roots of the teeth and the jaw bones	Fibrous tissue connects the roots of the teeth to the alveolar processes	None
CARTILAGINOUS JOINTS			
Synchondroses	Costal cartilage attachments of the first rib to the sternum; epiphyseal plate between the diaphysis and epiphysis of a growing long bone	Hyaline cartilage connects articulating bones	Slight
Symphyses	Pubic symphysis; joints between bodies of vertebrae	Fibrocartilage between articulating bones	Slight

Synovial Joints

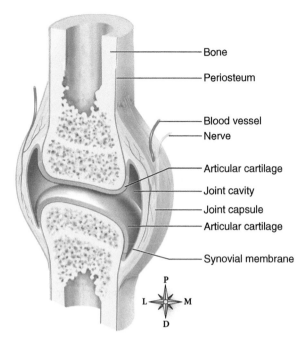

Bone

Periosteum

Blood vessel

Nerve

Articular cartilage

Joint cavity

Joint capsule

Articular cartilage

Synovial membrane

Structure of Synovial Joints. Artist's interpretation (composite drawing) of a typical synovial joint.

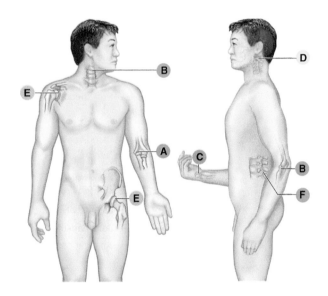

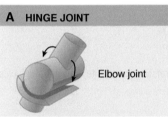

A HINGE JOINT

Elbow joint

B PIVOT JOINT

Dens of axis
rotating against
atlas

Head of radius
rotating against
ulna

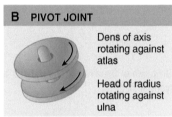

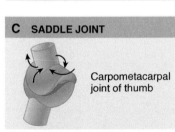

C SADDLE JOINT

Carpometacarpal
joint of thumb

D CONDYLOID JOINT

Atlantooccipital
joint

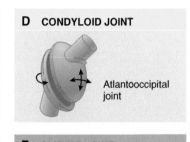

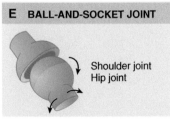

E BALL-AND-SOCKET JOINT

Shoulder joint
Hip joint

F GLIDING JOINT

Articular
processes
between
vertebrae

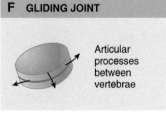

Types of Synovial Joints. Uniaxial: **A,** hinge, and **B,** pivot. Biaxial: **C,** saddle, and **D,** condyloid. Multiaxial: **E,** ball and socket, and **F,** gliding.

CLASSIFICATION OF SYNOVIAL JOINTS

TYPES	EXAMPLES	STRUCTURE	MOVEMENT
UNIAXIAL			*Around one axis; in one place*
Hinge	Elbow joint	Spool-shaped process fits into a concave socket	Flexion and extension only
Pivot	Joint between the first and second cervical vertebrae	Arch-shaped process fits around a peglike process	Rotation
BIAXIAL			*Around two axes, perpendicular to each other; in two planes*
Saddle	Thumb joint between the first metacarpal and carpal bone	Saddle-shaped bone fits into a socket that is concave-convex-concave	Flexion, extension in one plane; abduction, adduction in the other plane; opposing the thumb to the fingers
Condyloid (ellipsoidal)	Joint between the radius and carpal bones	Oval condyle fits into an elliptical socket	Flexion, extension in one plane; abduction, adduction in the other plane

Continued

CLASSIFICATION OF SYNOVIAL JOINTS—cont'd

TYPES	EXAMPLES	STRUCTURE	MOVEMENT
MULTIAXIAL			*Around many axes*
Ball and socket 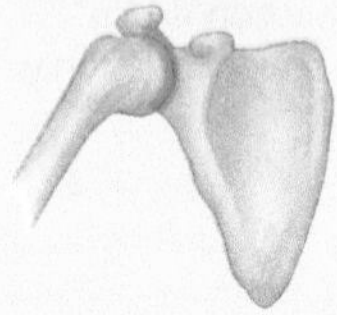	Shoulder joint and hip	Ball-shaped process fits into a concave socket	Widest range of movement: flexion, extension, abduction, adduction, rotation, circumduction
Gliding 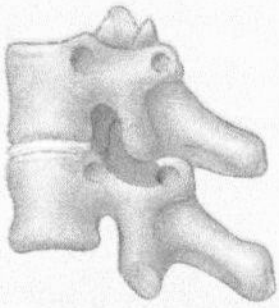	Joints between the articular facets of adjacent vertebrae; joints between the carpal and tarsal bones	Relatively flat articulating surfaces	Gliding movements without any angular or circular movements

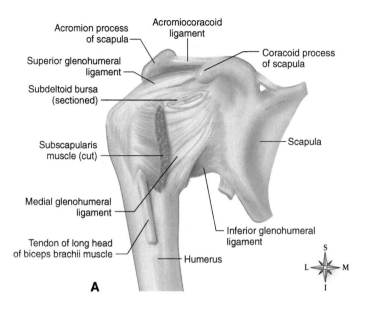

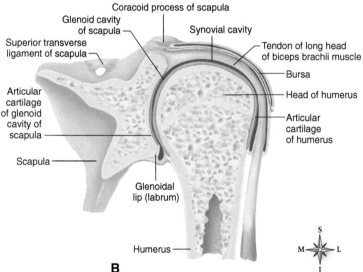

The Shoulder Joint. A, Artist's diagram, anterior view. **B,** Artist's diagram, viewed from behind through shoulder joint.

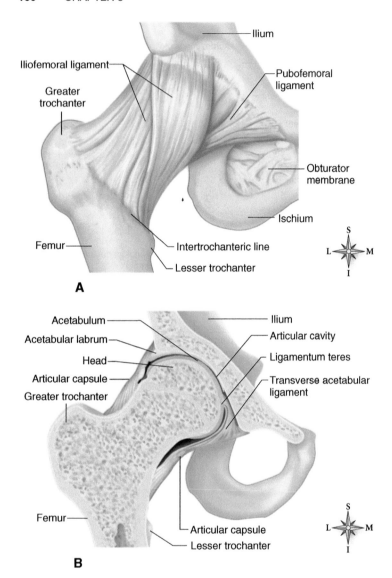

The Hip Joint. A, Artist's diagram, anterior view. **B,** Artist's diagram, frontal section.

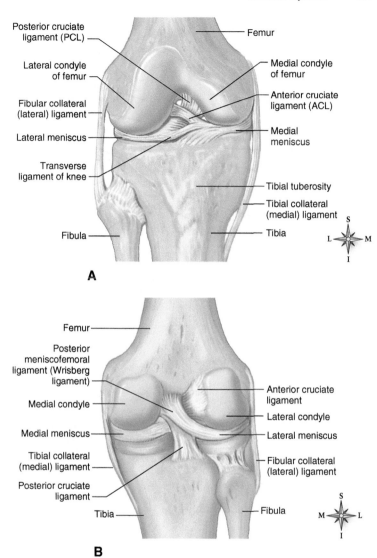

The Right Knee Joint. A, Labeled dissection of the right knee viewed from in front. **B,** Viewed from behind.

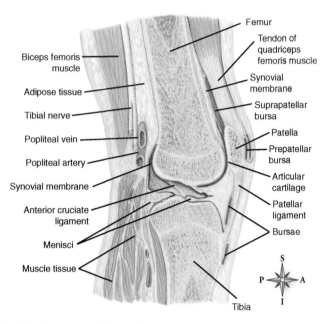

Femur

Tendon of quadriceps femoris muscle

Biceps femoris muscle

Synovial membrane

Adipose tissue

Suprapatellar bursa

Tibial nerve

Patella

Popliteal vein

Prepatellar bursa

Popliteal artery

Articular cartilage

Synovial membrane

Patellar ligament

Anterior cruciate ligament

Bursae

Menisci

Muscle tissue

Tibia

Sagittal Section through Knee Joint.

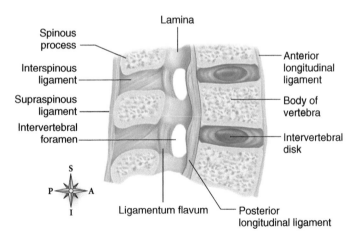

Lamina

Spinous process

Interspinous ligament

Anterior longitudinal ligament

Supraspinous ligament

Body of vertebra

Intervertebral foramen

Intervertebral disk

Ligamentum flavum

Posterior longitudinal ligament

Vertebrae and Their Ligaments. Sagittal section of two lumbar vertebrae and their ligaments.

MAJOR SYNOVIAL (DIARTHROTIC) & CARTILAGINOUS (AMPHIARTHROTIC) JOINTS

NAME	ARTICULATING BONES	TYPE	MOVEMENTS
Atlantoepistropheal	Anterior arch of the atlas rotates about the dens of the axis (epistropheus)	Synovial (pivot)	Pivoting or partial rotation of the head
Vertebral	Between bodies of vertebrae	Cartilaginous (symphyses)	Slight movement between any two vertebrae but considerable motility for the column as a whole
	Between articular processes	Synovial (gliding)	Gliding
Sternoclavicular	Medial end of the clavicle with the manubrium of the sternum	Synovial (gliding)	Gliding
Acromioclavicular	Distal end of the clavicle with the acromion of the scapula	Synovial (gliding)	Gliding; elevation, depression, protraction, and retraction
Thoracic	Heads of ribs with bodies of vertebrae	Synovial (gliding)	Gliding
	Tubercles of ribs with transverse processes of vertebrae	Synovial (gliding)	Gliding
Shoulder	Head of the humerus in the glenoid cavity of the scapula	Synovial (ball and socket)	Flexion, extension, abduction, adduction, rotation, and circumduction of the upper part of the arm
Elbow	Trochlea of the humerus with the semilunar notch of the ulna; head of the radius with the capitulum of the humerus	Synovial (hinge)	Flexion and extension
	Head of the radius in the radial notch of the ulna	Synovial (pivot)	Supination and pronation of the forearm and hand; rotation of the forearm on the upper extremity
Wrist	Scaphoid, lunate, and triquetral bones articulate with the radius and articular disk	Synovial (condyloid)	Flexion, extension, abduction, and adduction of the hand

Continued

MAJOR SYNOVIAL (DIARTHROTIC) & CARTILAGINOUS (AMPHIARTHROTIC) JOINTS—cont'd

NAME	ARTICULATING BONES	TYPE	MOVEMENTS
Carpal	Between various carpal bones	Synovial (gliding)	Gliding
Hand	Proximal end of the first metacarpal bone with the trapezium	Synovial (saddle)	Flexion, extension, abduction, adduction, and circumduction of the thumb and opposition to the fingers
	Distal end of the metacarpal bones with the proximal end of the phalanges	Synovial (hinge)	Flexion, extension, limited abduction, and adduction of the fingers
	Between phalanges	Synovial (hinge)	Flexion and extension of finger sections
Sacroiliac	Between the sacrum and two ilia	Synovial (gliding)	None or slight
Pubic symphysis	Between two pubic bones	Cartilaginous (symphysis)	Slight, particularly during pregnancy and delivery
Hip	Head of the femur in the acetabulum of the coxal bone	Synovial (ball and socket)	Flexion, extension, abduction, adduction, rotation, and circumduction
Knee	Between the distal end of the femur and proximal end of the tibia	Synovial (hinge)	Flexion and extension; slight rotation of the tibia
Tibiofibular (proximal)	Head of the fibula with the lateral condyle of the tibia	Synovial (gliding)	Gliding
Ankle	Distal end of the tibia and fibula with the talus	Synovial (hinge)	Flexion (dorsiflexion) and extension (plantar flexion)
Foot	Between tarsal bones	Synovial (gliding)	Gliding; inversion and eversion
	Between metatarsal bones and phalanges	Synovial (hinge)	Flexion, extension, slight abduction, and adduction
	Between phalanges	Synovial (hinge)	Flexion and extension

MAJOR TYPES OF JOINT MOVEMENTS

MOVEMENT	EXAMPLE	DESCRIPTION
Flexion (to flex a joint)	 Flexion	Reduces the angle of the joint, as in bending the elbow
Extension (to extend a joint)	 Extension	Increases the angle of a joint, as in straightening a bent elbow
Rotation (to rotate a joint)	 Rotation	Spin one bone relative to another, as in rotating the head at the neck joint

Continued

MAJOR TYPES OF JOINT MOVEMENTS—cont'd

MOVEMENT	EXAMPLE	DESCRIPTION
Circumduction (to circumduct a joint)	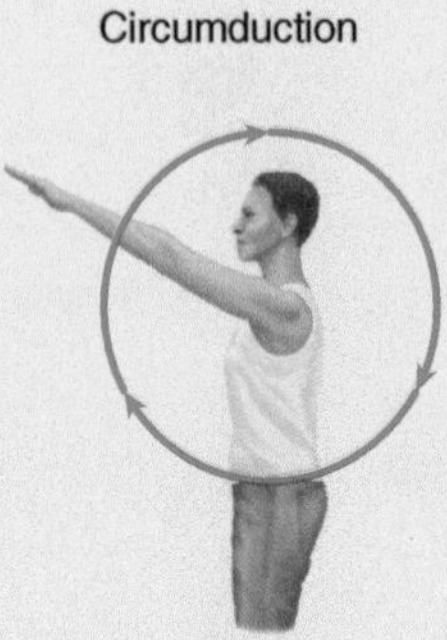 Circumduction	Moves the distal end of a bone in a circle, keeping the proximal end relatively stable, as in moving the arm in a circle and thus circumducting the shoulder joint
Abduction (to abduct a joint)	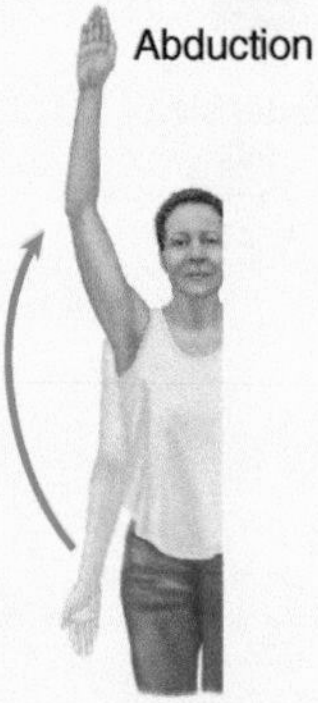 Abduction	Increases the angle of a joint to move a part away from the midline, as in moving the arm up and away from the side of the body
Adduction (to adduct a joint)	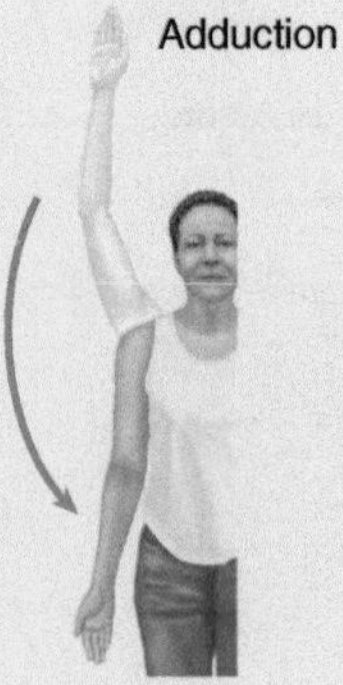 Adduction	Decreases the angle of a joint to move a part toward the midline, as in moving the arm in and down toward the side of the body

MAJOR TYPES OF JOINT MOVEMENTS—cont'd

MOVEMENT	EXAMPLE	DESCRIPTION
Hyperextension	Hyperextension	Increasing the angle of a joint beyond its usual anatomical position, as in tilting the neck backward; can also refer to abnormally extending a part, causing injury
Plantar flexion	Plantar flexion	Bending the ankle to point the toes and foot downward
Dorsiflexion	Dorsiflexion	Bending the ankle to point the toes and foot upward
Supination	Supination	Twists the forearm to move the hand to a thumb-outward (lateral) position; also applies to a similar twisting movement of the leg

Continued

MAJOR TYPES OF JOINT MOVEMENTS—cont'd

MOVEMENT	EXAMPLE	DESCRIPTION
Pronation	Pronation 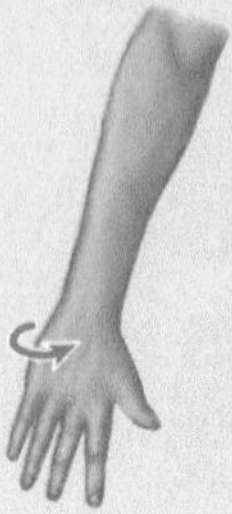	Twists the forearm to move the hand to a thumb-inward (medial) position; also applies to a similar twisting movement of the leg
Inversion	Inversion 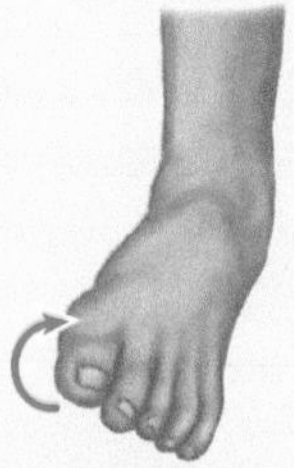	Bends the ankle to move the sole of the foot inward (medially)
Eversion	Eversion 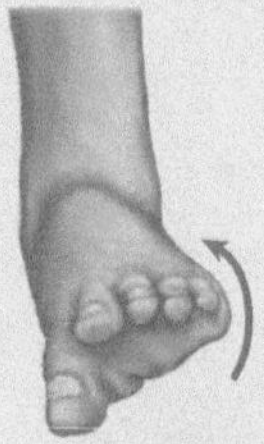	Bends the ankle to move the sole of the foot outward (laterally)
Protraction	Protraction 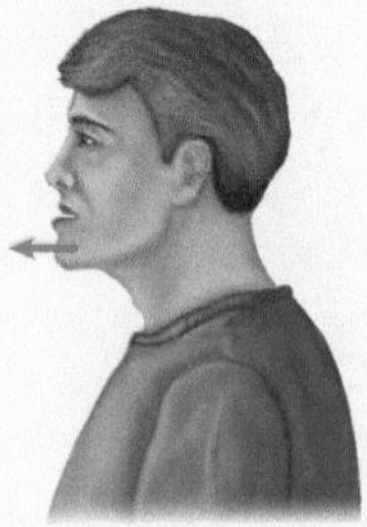	Moves a part forward, as in thrusting the mandible anteriorly

MAJOR TYPES OF JOINT MOVEMENTS—cont'd

MOVEMENT	EXAMPLE	DESCRIPTION
Retraction	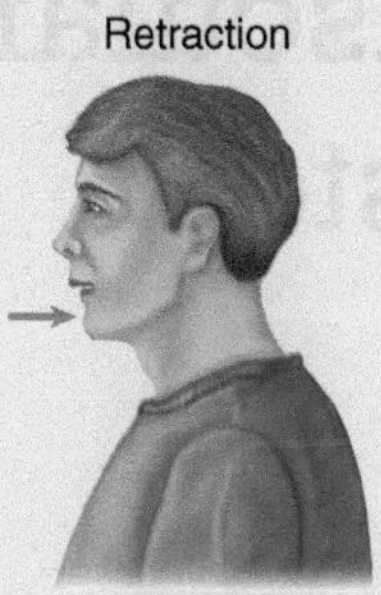 Retraction	Moves a part backward, as in pulling the mandible inward (posteriorly)
Elevation	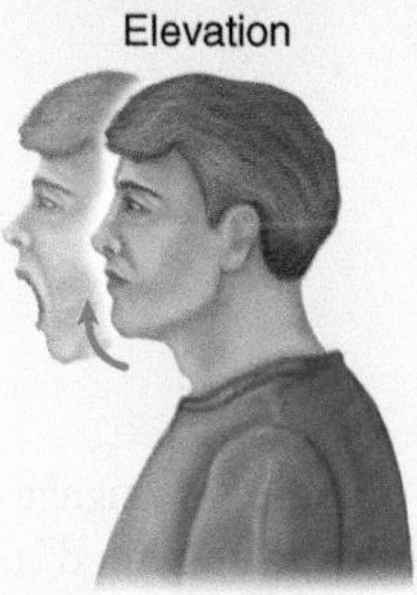 Elevation	Moves a part upward, as in raising the mandible to close the mouth
Depression	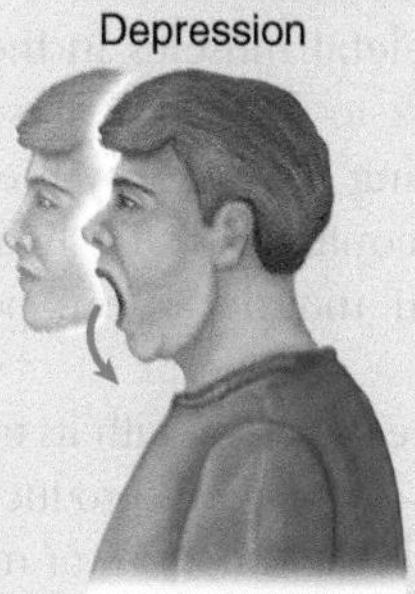 Depression	Moves a part downward, as in lowering the mandible to open the mouth

7

Muscular System

When we walk, talk, run, breathe, or engage in a multitude of other physical activities that are under the "willed" control of the individual, we do so by contraction of skeletal muscle.

There are over 600 skeletal muscles in the human body. Collectively, they constitute 40% to 50% of a person's body weight. And, together with the scaffolding provided by the skeleton, muscles also determine the form and contours of the body. Together with other body systems, the skeletal muscle system performs these essential functions:

1. **Movement.** Using the skeleton (with its moveable joints) as a scaffold, skeletal muscle contractions produce purposeful movement of the body as a whole (locomotion) or movement of its parts.
2. **Heat production.** Muscle cells, like all cells, produce heat by the metabolic process known as catabolism. The heat produced by just one cell is inconsequential, but because skeletal muscle cells are both highly active and numerous, together they produce a major share of total body heat. Skeletal muscle contractions therefore constitute one of the most important parts of the mechanism for maintaining homeostasis of temperature.
3. **Posture.** The continued partial contraction of many skeletal muscles makes possible standing, sitting, and maintaining a relatively stable position of the body while walking, running, or performing other movements.

SKELETAL MUSCLE STRUCTURE

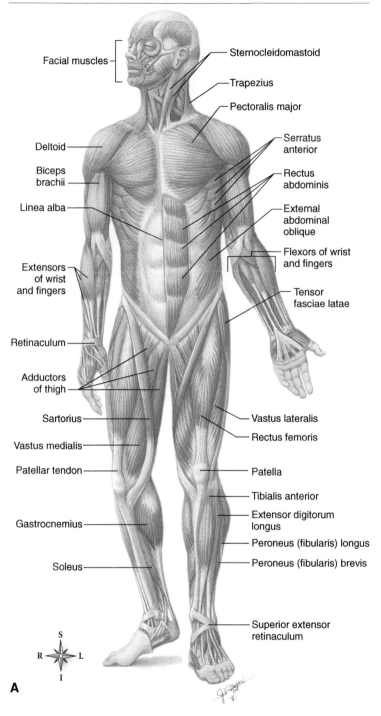

Facial muscles

Sternocleidomastoid

Trapezius

Pectoralis major

Deltoid

Serratus anterior

Biceps brachii

Rectus abdominis

Linea alba

External abdominal oblique

Flexors of wrist and fingers

Extensors of wrist and fingers

Tensor fasciae latae

Retinaculum

Adductors of thigh

Sartorius

Vastus lateralis

Rectus femoris

Vastus medialis

Patellar tendon

Patella

Tibialis anterior

Extensor digitorum longus

Gastrocnemius

Peroneus (fibularis) longus

Peroneus (fibularis) brevis

Soleus

Superior extensor retinaculum

S
R — L
I

A

General Overview of the Body's Musculature. **A,** Anterior view.

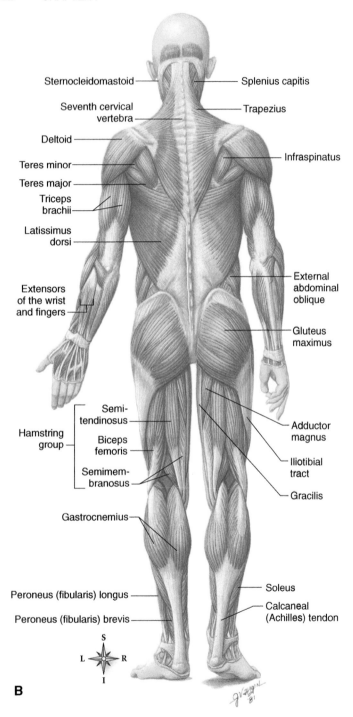

Sternocleidomastoid

Seventh cervical
vertebra

Deltoid

Teres minor

Teres major

Triceps
brachii

Latissimus
dorsi

Extensors
of the wrist
and fingers

Hamstring
group

Semi-
tendinosus

Biceps
femoris

Semimem-
branosus

Gastrocnemius

Peroneus (fibularis) longus

Peroneus (fibularis) brevis

Splenius capitis

Trapezius

Infraspinatus

External
abdominal
oblique

Gluteus
maximus

Adductor
magnus

Iliotibial
tract

Gracilis

Soleus

Calcaneal
(Achilles) tendon

S
L — R
I

B

General Overview of the Body's Musculature—cont'd. B, Posterior view.

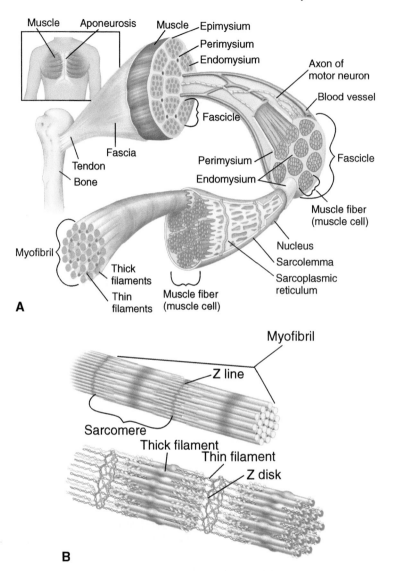

Structure of a Skeletal Muscle. Note in **A** that the connective tissue coverings, the epimysium, perimysium, and endomysium, are continuous with each other and with the tendon. The muscle fibers are held together by the perimysium in groups called *fascicles*. **B**, The magnification of the myofibril further shows sarcomere between successive Z lines (Z disks). Cross-striae are visible. The molecular structure of myofibril shows thick myofilaments and thin myofilaments.

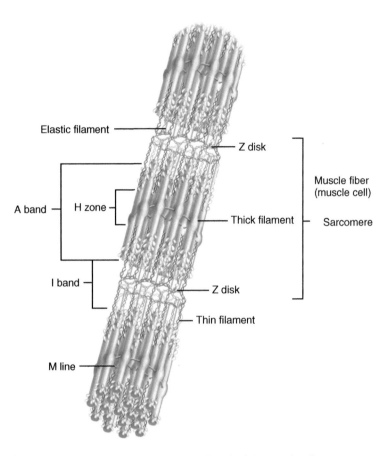

Sarcomere. Sarcomere is the basic contractile unit of the muscle cell.

Z disk: A dense plate or disk to which the thin filaments directly anchor; also called a *Z line*.

M line: Protein molecules that hold the thick (myosin) filaments together.

A band: The segment that runs the entire length of the thick filaments.

I band: The segment that includes the Z disk and the ends of the thin filaments, where they do not overlap the thick filaments.

H zone: The middle region of the thick filaments, where they do not overlap the thin filaments.

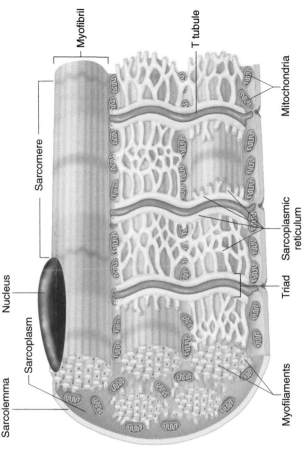

Unique Features of the Skeletal Muscle Cell. Notice especially the T tubules, which are extensions of the plasma membrane, or sarcolemma, and the sarcoplasmic reticulum (SR), a type of smooth endoplasmic reticulum that forms networks of tubular canals and sacs containing stored calcium ions. A triad is a triplet of adjacent tubules: a terminal (end) sac of the SR, a T tubule, and another terminal sac of the SR.

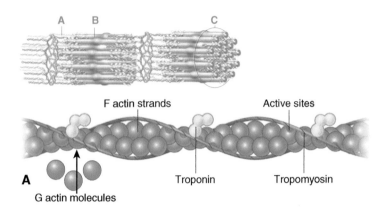

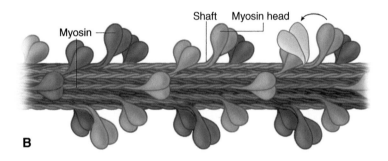

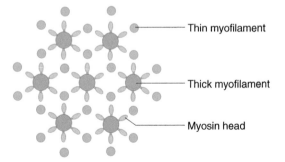

Structure of Myofilaments. A, Thin myofilament. **B,** Thick myofilament. **C,** Cross-section of several thick and thin myofilaments showing the relative positions of myofilaments and the myosin heads that will form cross-bridges between them.

MUSCLE CONTRACTION

MAJOR EVENTS OF MUSCLE CONTRACTION AND RELAXATION

Excitation and Contraction

1. A nerve impulse reaches the end of a motor neuron, triggering the release of the neurotransmitter acetylcholine (ACh).
2. Acetylcholine diffuses rapidly across the gap of the neuromuscular junction and binds to acetylcholine receptors on the motor end plate of the muscle fiber.
3. Stimulation of acetylcholine receptors initiates an impulse that travels along the sarcolemma, through the T tubules, to sacs of the sarcoplasmic reticulum.
4. Calcium (Ca^{++}) is released from the sarcoplasmic reticulum into the sarcoplasm, where it binds to troponin molecules in the thin myofilaments.
5. Tropomyosin molecules in the thin myofilaments shift, exposing actin's active sites.
6. Energized myosin cross-bridges of the thick myofilaments bind to actin and use their energy to pull the thin myofilaments toward the center of each sarcomere. This cycle repeats itself many times per second, as long as adenosine triphosphate (ATP) is available.
7. As the thin filaments slide past the thick myofilaments, the entire muscle fiber shortens.

Relaxation

1. After the impulse is over, the sarcoplasmic reticulum begins actively pumping Ca^{++} back into its sacs.
2. As Ca^{++} is stripped from troponin molecules in the thin myofilaments, tropomyosin returns to its position, blocking actin's active sites.
3. Myosin cross-bridges are prevented from binding to actin and thus can no longer sustain the contraction.
4. Since the thick and thin myofilaments are no longer connected, the muscle fiber may return to its longer, resting length.

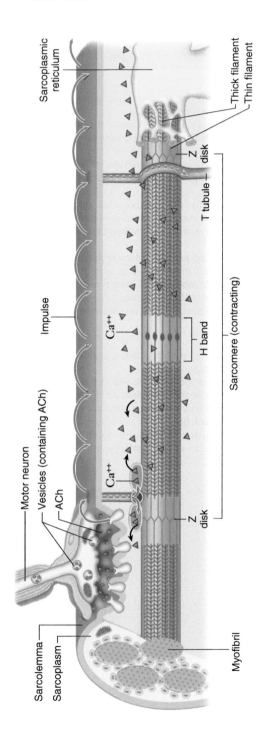

Effects of Excitation on a Muscle Fiber. Excitation of the sarcolemma by a nerve impulse initiates an impulse in the sarcolemma. The impulse travels across the sarcolemma and through the T tubules, where it triggers adjacent sacs of the sarcoplasmic reticulum to release a flood of calcium ions (Ca^{++}) into the sarcoplasm. Ca^{++} is then free to bind to troponin molecules in the thin filaments. This binding, in turn, initiates the chemical reactions that produce a contraction.

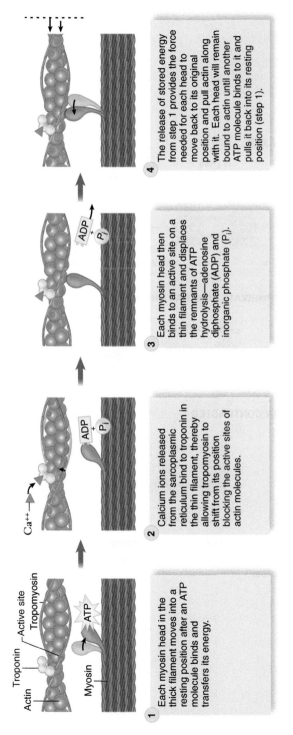

The Molecular Basis of Muscle Contraction.

1. Each myosin head in the thick filament moves into a resting position after an ATP molecule binds and transfers its energy.

2. Calcium ions released from the sarcoplasmic reticulum bind to troponin in the thin filament, thereby allowing tropomyosin to shift from its position blocking the active sites of actin molecules.

3. Each myosin head then binds to an active site on a thin filament and displaces the remnants of ATP hydrolysis—adenosine diphosphate (ADP) and inorganic phosphate (P_i).

4. The release of stored energy from step 1 provides the force needed for each head to move back to its original position and pull actin along with it. Each head will remain bound to actin until another ATP molecule binds to it and pulls it back into its resting position (step 1).

Actin
Troponin
Active site
Tropomyosin
Myosin
Ca^{++}
ATP
ADP + P_i
ADP + P_i

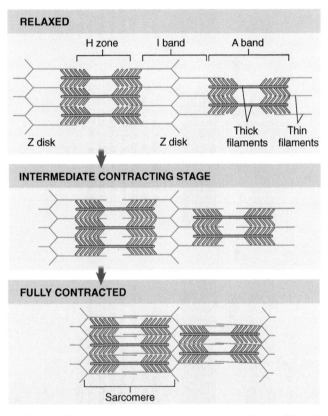

RELAXED

H zone   I band   A band

Z disk   Z disk   Thick filaments   Thin filaments

INTERMEDIATE CONTRACTING STAGE

FULLY CONTRACTED

Sarcomere

Sliding-Filament Model. During contraction, myosin cross-bridges pull the thin filaments toward the center of each sarcomere, thus shortening the myofibril and the entire muscle fiber.

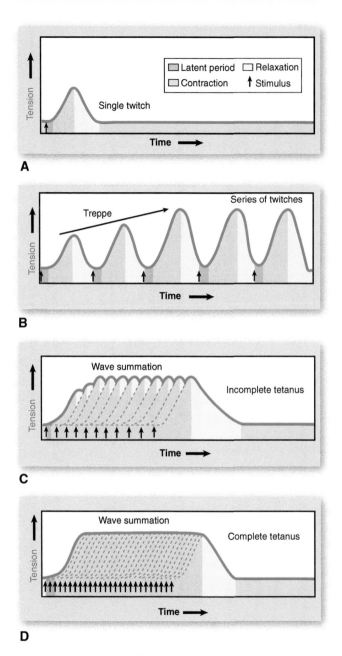

Myograms of Various Types of Muscle Contractions. A, A single twitch contraction. **B,** The treppe phenomenon, or "staircase effect," is a steplike increase in the force of contraction over the first few in a series of twitches. **C,** Incomplete tetanus occurs when a rapid succession of stimuli produces "twitches" that seem to add together (wave summation) to produce a rather sustained contraction. **D,** Complete tetanus is a smoother sustained contraction produced by the summation of "twitches" that occur so close together that the muscle cannot relax at all.

MUSCLE TISSUES

CHARACTERISTICS OF MUSCLE TISSUES

	SKELETAL	CARDIAC	SMOOTH
PRINCIPAL LOCATION	Skeletal muscle organs	Wall of heart	Walls of many hollow organs
PRINCIPAL FUNCTIONS	Movement of bones, heat production, posture	Pumping of blood	Movement in walls of hollow organs (peristalsis, mixing of fluids)
TYPE OF CONTROL	Voluntary	Involuntary	Involuntary
STRUCTURAL FEATURES			
Striations	Present	Present	Absent
Nucleus	Many near the sarcolemma	Single (sometimes double); near the center of the cell	Single; near the center of the cell
T tubules	Narrow; form triads with the SR	Large diameter; form dyads with the SR, regulate Ca^{++} entry into the sarcoplasm	Absent
Sarcoplasmic reticulum	Extensive; stores and releases Ca^{++}	Less extensive than in skeletal muscle	Very poorly developed
Cell junctions	No gap junctions	Intercalated disks	*Single-unit**: many gap junctions *Multiunit*: few gap junctions
CONTRACTION STYLE	Rapid twitch contractions of motor units usually summate to produce sustained tetanic contractions; must be stimulated by a neuron	Syncytium of fibers compress the heart chambers in slow, separate contractions (does not exhibit tetanus or fatigue); exhibits autorhythmicity	*Single-unit*: electrically coupled sheets of fibers contract autorhythmically and produce peristalsis or mixing movements *Multiunit*: individual fibers contract when stimulated by a neuron

*Also referred to as *visceral smooth muscle tissue*.

SR, Sarcoplasmic reticulum.

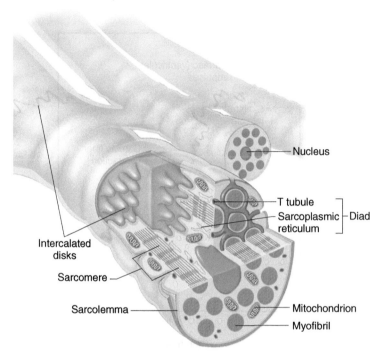

Cardiac Muscle Fiber. Unlike other types of muscle fibers, cardiac muscle fiber is typically branched and forms junctions, called **intercalated disks,** with adjacent cardiac muscle fibers. Like skeletal muscle fibers, cardiac muscle fibers contain sarcoplasmic reticula and T tubules—although these structures are not as highly organized as in skeletal muscle fibers.

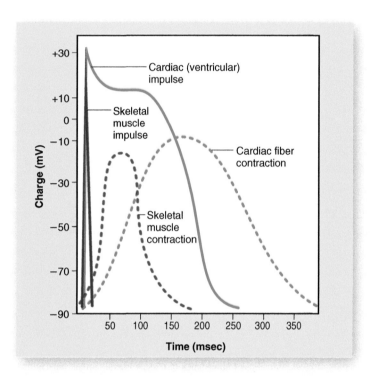

Cardiac and Skeletal Muscle Contractions Compared. A brief nerve impulse triggers a brief twitch contraction in skeletal muscle *(blue)*, but a prolonged impulse in the heart tissue produces a rather slow, drawn-out contraction in cardiac muscle *(red)*.

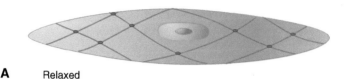

A   Relaxed

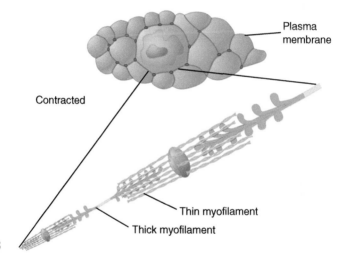

Plasma
membrane

Contracted

Thin myofilament

Thick myofilament

B

Smooth Muscle Fiber. A, Thin bundles of myofilaments span the diameter of a
relaxed fiber. **B,** During contraction, sliding of the myofilaments causes the fiber to
shorten by "balling up." The figure shows that the fiber becomes shorter and thicker,
exhibiting "dimples" where the myofilament bundles are pulling on the plasma
membrane.

ATTACHMENT OF MUSCLES

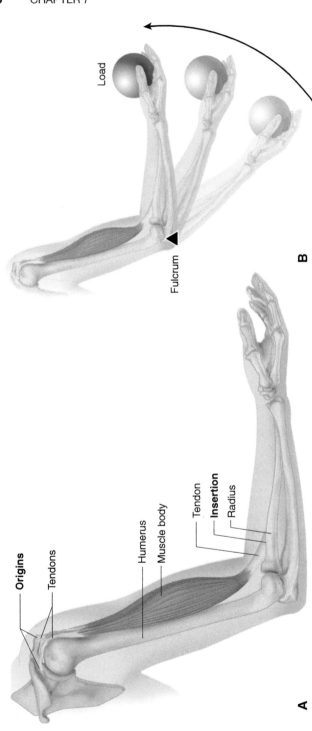

Attachments of a Skeletal Muscle. A, Origin and insertion of a skeletal muscle. A muscle originates at a relatively stable part of the skeleton (origin) and inserts at the skeletal part that is moved when the muscle contracts (insertion). **B,** Movement of the forearm during weightlifting. Muscle contraction moves bones, which serve as levers, and by acting on joints, which serve as fulcrums for those levers.

IMPORTANT MUSCLE GROUPINGS
SELECTED MUSCLES GROUPED BY LOCATION

LOCATION	MUSCLES
Neck	Sternocleidomastoid
Back	Trapezius Latissimus dorsi
Chest	Pectoralis major Serratus anterior
Abdominal wall	External oblique
Shoulder	Deltoid
Arm	Biceps brachii Triceps brachii Brachialis
Forearm	Brachioradialis Pronator teres
Buttocks	Gluteus maximus Gluteus minimus Gluteus medius Tensor fasciae latae
THIGH	
Anterior surface	Quadriceps femoris group Rectus femoris Vastus lateralis Vastus medialis Vastus intermedius
Medial surface	Gracilis Adductor group (brevis, longus, magnus)
Posterior surface	Hamstring group Biceps femoris Semitendinosus Semimembranosus
LEG	
Anterior surface	Tibialis anterior
Posterior surface	Gastrocnemius Soleus
Pelvic floor	Levator ani Coccygeus

SELECTED MUSCLES GROUPED BY FUNCTION

PART MOVED	EXAMPLE OF FLEXOR	EXAMPLE OF EXTENSOR	EXAMPLE OF ABDUCTOR	EXAMPLE OF ADDUCTOR
Head	Sternocleidomastoid	Semispinalis capitis		
Arm	Pectoralis major	Trapezius Latissimus dorsi	Deltoid	Pectoralis major with latissimus dorsi
Forearm	With forearm supinated: biceps brachii With forearm pronated: brachialis With semisupination or semipronation: brachioradialis	Triceps brachii		
Hand	Flexor carpi radialis and ulnaris Palmaris longus	Extensor carpi radialis, longus, and brevis Extensor carpi ulnaris	Flexor carpi radialis	Flexor carpi ulnaris
Thigh	Iliopsoas Rectus femoris (of quadriceps femoris group)	Gluteus maximus	Gluteus medius and minimus	Adductor group
Leg	Hamstrings	Quadriceps femoris group		
Foot	Tibialis anterior	Gastrocnemius Soleus	*Evertors* Fibularis longus Fibularis brevis	*Invertor* Tibialis anterior
Trunk	Iliopsoas Rectus abdominis	Erector spinae		

IMPORTANT SKELETAL MUSCLES

MUSCLES OF FACIAL EXPRESSION AND MASTICATION

MUSCLE	ORIGIN	INSERTION	FUNCTION	NERVE SUPPLY
MUSCLES OF FACIAL EXPRESSION				
Occipitofrontalis (Part of Epicranius)				
Frontal belly	Epicranial aponeurosis	Tissues of eyebrows and bridge of nose	Raises eyebrows, wrinkles forehead horizontally	Cranial nerve VII
Occipital belly	Occipital bone (highest nuchal line)	Epicranial aponeurosis	Draws scalp backward	Cranial nerve VII
Corrugator supercilii	Frontal bone (superciliary ridge)	Skin of eyebrow	Wrinkles forehead vertically	Cranial nerve VII
Orbicularis oculi	Encircles eyelid		Closes eye	Cranial nerve VII
Zygomaticus major	Zygomatic bone	Angle of mouth	Laughing (elevates angle of mouth)	Cranial nerve VII
Orbicularis oris	Encircles mouth		Draws lips together	Cranial nerve VII
Buccinator	Maxillae	Skin of sides of mouth	Facilitates smiling; blowing, as in playing trumpet	Cranial nerve VII
Depressor anguli oris	Mandible	Angle of mouth	Draws ends of mouth downward, as when frowning	Cranial nerve IV
MUSCLES OF MASTICATION				
Masseter	Zygomatic arch	Mandible (external surface)	Elevates mandible; closing jaw	Cranial nerve V
Temporalis	Temporal bone	Mandible	Elevates mandible; closing jaw	Cranial nerve V
Pterygoids (lateral and medial)	Undersurface of skull	Mandible (medial surface)	Grates teeth	Cranial nerve V

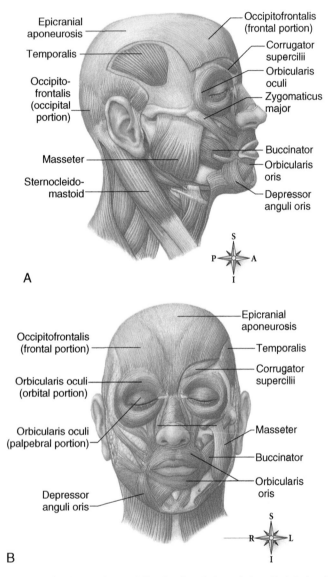

Muscles of Facial Expression and Mastication. A, Lateral view. **B,** Anterior view.

MUSCLES THAT MOVE THE HEAD

MUSCLE	ORIGIN	INSERTION	FUNCTION	NERVE SUPPLY
Sternocleidomastoid	Sternum	Temporal bone (mastoid process)	Flexes head and neck ("prayer muscle")	Accessory nerve
	Clavicle		One muscle alone rotates head toward opposite side; spasm of this muscle alone or associated with trapezius called *torticollis*, or *wryneck*	
Semispinalis capitis	Vertebrae (transverse processes of upper six thoracic, articular processes of lower four cervical)	Occipital bone (between superior and inferior nuchal lines)	Extends head and neck; bends it laterally	First five cervical nerves
Splenius capitis	Ligamentum nuchae	Temporal bone (mastoid process)	Extends head/neck	Second, third, and fourth cervical nerves
	Vertebrae (spinous processes of upper three or four thoracic)	Occipital bone	Bends and rotates head toward same side as contracting muscle	
Longissimus capitis	Vertebrae (transverse processes of upper six thoracic, articular processes of lower four cervical)	Temporal bone (mastoid process)	Extends head and neck. Bends and rotates head toward contracting side	Multiple innervation

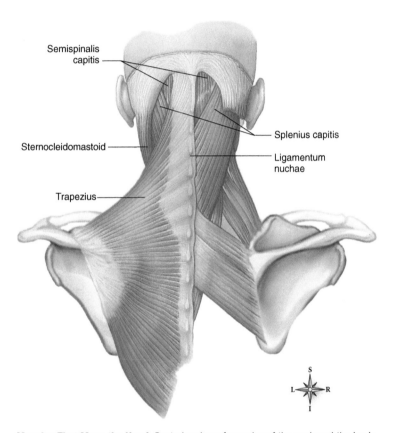

Muscles That Move the Head. Posterior view of muscles of the neck and the back.

MUSCLES OF THE THORAX

MUSCLE	ORIGIN	INSERTION	FUNCTION	NERVE SUPPLY
External intercostals	Rib (lower border; forward fibers)	Rib (upper border of rib below origin)	Elevate ribs	Intercostal nerves
Internal intercostals	Rib (inner surface, lower border; backward fibers)	Rib (upper border of rib below origin)	Depress ribs	Intercostal nerves
Diaphragm	Lower circumference of thorax (of rib cage)	Central tendon of diaphragm	Enlarges thorax, thereby causing inspiration	Phrenic nerves

MUSCLES OF THE ABDOMINAL WALL

MUSCLE	ORIGIN	INSERTION	FUNCTION	NERVE SUPPLY
External oblique	Ribs (lower eight)	Pelvis (iliac crest and pubis by way of the inguinal ligament)	Compresses abdomen	Lower seven intercostal nerves and iliohypogastric nerves
		Linea alba by way of an aponeurosis	Rotates trunk laterally	
Internal oblique	Pelvis (iliac crest and iliopsoas fascia)	Ribs (lower three)	Important postural function of all abdominal muscles is to pull the front of the pelvis upward, thereby flattening the lumbar curve of the spine; when these muscles lose their tone, common figure faults of protruding abdomen and lordosis develop	Last three intercostal nerves; iliohypogastric and ilioinguinal nerves
	Lumbodorsal fascia	Linea alba		
Transversus abdominis	Ribs (lower six)	Pubic bone	Same as external oblique	Last three intercostal nerves; iliohypogastric and ilioinguinal nerves
	Pelvis (iliac crest, iliopsoas fascia)	Linea alba		
	Lumbodorsal fascia	Ribs (costal cartilage of fifth, sixth, and seventh ribs)	Same as external oblique	Last five intercostal nerves; iliohypogastric and ilioinguinal nerves
Rectus abdominis	Pelvis (pubic bone and pubic symphysis)	Sternum (xiphoid process)	Same as external oblique; because abdominal muscles compress the abdominal cavity, they aid in straining, defecation, forced expiration, childbirth; abdominal muscles are antagonists of the diaphragm, relaxing as it contracts and vice versa	Last six intercostal nerves
			Flexes trunk	
Quadratus lumborum	Iliolumbar ligament; iliac crest	Last rib; transverse process of vertebrae (L1–L4)	Flexes vertebral column laterally; depresses last rib	Lumbar

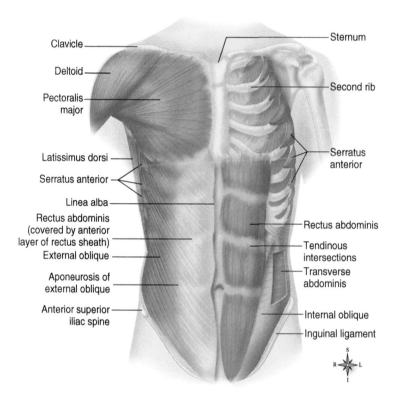

Clavicle

Deltoid

Pectoralis major

Latissimus dorsi

Serratus anterior

Linea alba

Rectus abdominis (covered by anterior layer of rectus sheath)

External oblique

Aponeurosis of external oblique

Anterior superior iliac spine

Sternum

Second rib

Serratus anterior

Rectus abdominis

Tendinous intersections

Transverse abdominis

Internal oblique

Inguinal ligament

Muscles of the Trunk and Abdominal Wall. Superficial muscles are visible on the right side of the body and deeper muscles on the left side of the body.

MUSCLES OF THE BACK

MUSCLE	ORIGIN	INSERTION	FUNCTION	NERVE SUPPLY
ERECTOR SPINAE GROUP				
Iliocostalis group	Various regions of the pelvis and ribs	Ribs and vertebra (superior to the origin)	Extends, laterally flexes the vertebral column	Spinal, thoracic, or lumbar nerves
Longissimus group	Cervical and thoracic vertebrae, ribs	Mastoid process, upper cervical vertebrae, or upper lumbar vertebrae	Extends head, neck, or vertebral column	Cervical or thoracic and lumbar nerves
Spinalis group	Lower cervical or lower thoracic/upper lumbar vertebrae	Upper cervical or middle/upper thoracic vertebrae (superior to the origin)	Extends the neck or vertebral column	Cervical or thoracic nerves
TRANSVERSOSPINALIS GROUP				
Semispinalis group	Transverse processes of vertebrae (T2–T11)	Spinous processes of vertebrae (C2–T4)	Extends neck or vertebral column	Cervical or thoracic nerves
Multifidus group	Transverse processes of vertebrae; sacrum, and ilium	Spinous processes of (next superior) vertebrae	Extends, rotates vertebral column	Spinal nerves
Rotatores group	Transverse processes of vertebrae	Spinous processes of (next superior) vertebrae	Extends, rotates vertebral column	Spinal nerves
Splenius	Spinous processes of vertebrae (C7–T1 or T3–T6)	Lateral occipital/mastoid or transverse processes of vertebrae (C1–C4)	Rotates, extends neck, and flexes neck laterally	Cervical nerves
Interspinales group	Spinous processes of vertebra	Spinous processes (of next superior vertebra)	Extends back and neck	Spinal nerves

Superficial muscles   **Intermediate muscles**

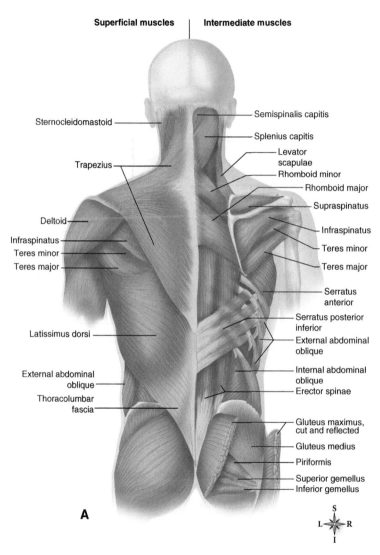

Sternocleidomastoid

Trapezius

Deltoid

Infraspinatus

Teres minor

Teres major

Latissimus dorsi

External abdominal
oblique

Thoracolumbar
fascia

Semispinalis capitis

Splenius capitis

Levator
scapulae

Rhomboid minor

Rhomboid major

Supraspinatus

Infraspinatus

Teres minor

Teres major

Serratus
anterior

Serratus posterior
inferior

External abdominal
oblique

Internal abdominal
oblique

Erector spinae

Gluteus maximus,
cut and reflected

Gluteus medius

Piriformis

Superior gemellus

Inferior gemellus

A

Muscles of the Back. A, Superficial *(left)* and intermediate *(right)* muscle dissection
of the neck and back, posterior view. The illustration shows a two-stage dissection.

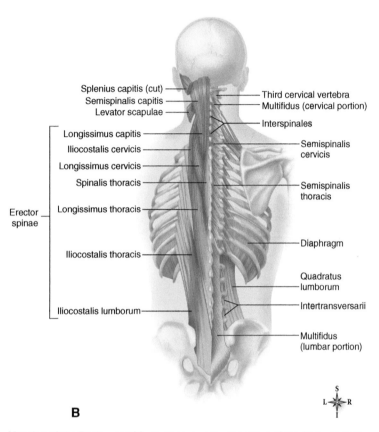

Splenius capitis (cut)
Semispinalis capitis
Levator scapulae
Third cervical vertebra
Multifidus (cervical portion)
Interspinales
Longissimus capitis
Iliocostalis cervicis
Longissimus cervicis
Spinalis thoracis
Longissimus thoracis
Iliocostalis thoracis
Iliocostalis lumborum
Erector spinae
Semispinalis cervicis
Semispinalis thoracis
Diaphragm
Quadratus lumborum
Intertransversarii
Multifidus (lumbar portion)

B

Muscles of the Back—cont'd. B, Deep muscle dissection of the back, posterior view. The superficial and intermediate muscles have been removed. The muscles in the gluteal region have been removed to expose the pelvic insertion of the multifidus.

MUSCLES OF THE PELVIC FLOOR

MUSCLE	ORIGIN	INSERTION	FUNCTION	NERVE SUPPLY
Levator ani	Pubis and spine of the ischium	Coccyx	Together with the coccygeus muscles form the floor of the pelvic cavity and support the pelvic organs	Pudendal nerve
Ischiocavernosus	Ischium	Penis or clitoris	Compress the base of the penis or clitoris	Perineal nerve
Bulbospongiosus				
Male	Bulb of the penis	Perineum and bulb of the penis	Constricts the urethra and erects the penis	Pudendal nerve
Female	Perineum	Base of the clitoris	Erects the clitoris	Pudendal nerve
Deep transverse perineal	Ischium	Central tendon (median raphe)	Supports the pelvic floor	Pudendal nerve
Urethral sphincter	Pubic ramus	Central tendon (median raphe)	Constricts the urethra	Pudendal nerve
External anal sphincter	Coccyx	Central tendon (median raphe)	Closes the anal canal	Pudendal and S4

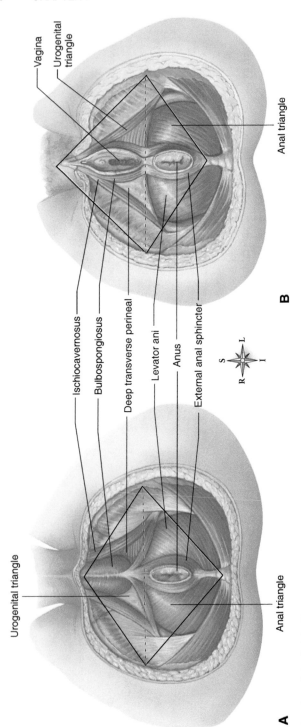

Muscles of the Pelvic Floor. A, Male, inferior view. **B,** Female, inferior view. Note the diamond-shaped outline of the perineum formed by the urogenital and anal triangles.

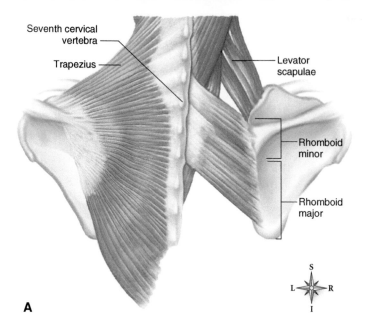

A

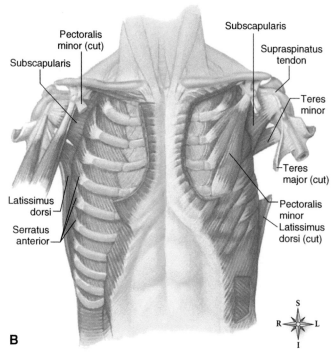

B

Muscles Acting on the Shoulder Girdle. A, Posterior view. The trapezius has been removed on the right to reveal the deeper muscles. **B,** Anterior view. The pectoralis major has been removed on both sides. The pectoralis minor has also been removed on the right side.

MUSCLES ACTING ON THE SHOULDER GIRDLE

MUSCLE	ORIGIN	INSERTION	FUNCTION	NERVE SUPPLY
Trapezius	Occipital bone (protuberance)	Clavicle	Raises or lowers the shoulders and shrugs them	Spinal accessory; second, third, and fourth cervical nerves
	Vertebrae (cervical and thoracic)	Scapula (spine and acromion)	Extends the head and neck when the occiput acts as the insertion	
Pectoralis minor	Ribs (second to fifth)	Scapula (coracoid)	Pulls the shoulder girdle down and forward	Medial and lateral anterior thoracic nerve
Serratus anterior	Ribs (upper eight or nine)	Scapula (anterior surface, vertebral border)	Pulls the shoulder down and forward; abducts and rotates it upward	Long thoracic nerve
Levator scapulae	C1–C4 (transverse processes)	Scapula (superior angle)	Elevates and retracts the scapula and abducts the neck	Dorsal scapular nerve
Rhomboid				
Major	T1–T4	Scapula (medial border)	Retracts, rotates, and fixes the scapula	Dorsal scapular nerve
Minor	C6–C7	Scapula (medial border)	Retracts, rotates, elevates, and fixes the scapula	Dorsal scapular nerve

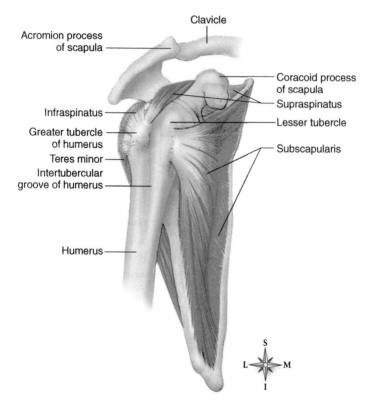

Rotator Cuff Muscles. Anterior view of the right shoulder showing the tendons of the teres minor, infraspinatus, supraspinatus, and subscapularis muscles surrounding the head of the humerus. These four muscles make up the *SITS muscles* that form the **rotator cuff** of the shoulder joint.

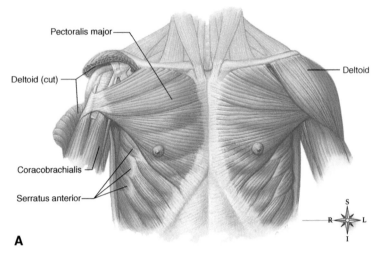

Pectoralis major

Deltoid (cut)

Deltoid

Coracobrachialis

Serratus anterior

A

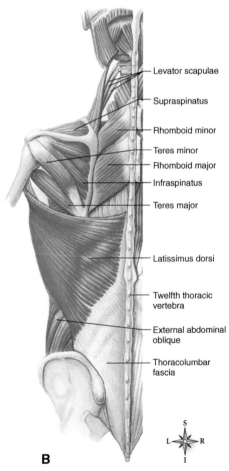

Levator scapulae

Supraspinatus

Rhomboid minor

Teres minor

Rhomboid major

Infraspinatus

Teres major

Latissimus dorsi

Twelfth thoracic vertebra

External abdominal oblique

Thoracolumbar fascia

B

Muscles That Move the Arm. A, Anterior view. **B,** Posterior view.

MUSCLES THAT MOVE THE ARM

MUSCLE	ORIGIN	INSERTION	FUNCTION	NERVE SUPPLY
AXIAL*				
Pectoralis major	Clavicle (medial half) Sternum Costal cartilages of the true ribs	Humerus (greater tubercle)	Flexes the arm Adducts the arm anteriorly; draws it across the chest	Medial and lateral anterior thoracic nerves
Latissimus dorsi	Vertebrae (spines of the lower thoracic, lumbar, and sacral) Ilium (crest) Lumbodorsal fascia	Humerus (intertubercular groove)	Extends the arm Adducts the arm posteriorly	Thoracodorsal nerve
SCAPULAR*				
Deltoid	Clavicle Scapula (spine and acromion)	Humerus (lateral side about halfway down—deltoid tubercle)	Abducts the arm Assists in flexion and extension of the arm	Axillary nerve
Coracobrachialis	Scapula (coracoid process)	Humerus (middle third, medial surface)	Adduction; assists in flexion and medial rotation of the arm	Musculocutaneous nerve
Supraspinatus†	Scapula (supraspinous fossa)	Humerus (greater tubercle)	Assists in abducting the arm	Suprascapular nerve
Teres minor†	Scapula (axillary border)	Humerus (greater tubercle)	Rotates the arm outward	Axillary nerve
Teres major	Scapula (lower part, axillary border)	Humerus (upper part, anterior surface)	Assists in extension, adduction, and medial rotation of the arm	Lower subscapular nerve
Infraspinatus†	Scapula (infraspinatus border)	Humerus (greater tubercle)	Rotates the arm outward	Suprascapular nerve
Subscapularis†	Scapula (subscapular fossa)	Humerus (lesser tubercle)	Medial rotation	Suprascapular nerve

*Axial muscles originate on the axial skeleton. Scapular muscles originate on the scapula.
†Muscles of the rotator cuff (SITS muscles).

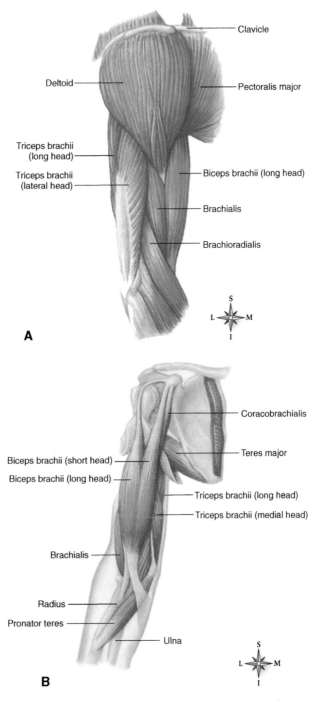

Muscles Acting on the Forearm. A, Lateral view of the right shoulder and arm. **B,** Anterior view of the right shoulder and arm (deep). The deltoid and pectoralis major muscles have been removed to reveal deeper structures.

MUSCLES THAT MOVE THE FOREARM

MUSCLE	ORIGIN	INSERTION	FUNCTION	NERVE SUPPLY
FLEXORS				
Biceps brachii	Scapula (supraglenoid tuberosity) Scapula (coracoid)	Radius (tuberosity at the proximal end)	Flexes the supinated forearm Supinates the forearm and hand	Musculocutaneous nerve
Brachialis	Humerus (distal half, anterior surface)	Ulna (front of the coronoid process)	Flexes the pronated forearm	Musculocutaneous nerve
Brachioradialis	Humerus (above the lateral epicondyle)	Radius (styloid process)	Flexes the semipronated or semisupinated forearm; supinates the forearm and hand	Radial nerve
EXTENSOR				
Triceps brachii	Scapula (infraglenoid tuberosity) Humerus (posterior surface—lateral head above the radial groove; medial head, below)	Ulna (olecranon)	Extends the lower arm	Radial nerve
PRONATORS				
Pronator teres	Humerus (medial epicondyle) Ulna (coronoid process)	Radius (middle third of the lateral surface)	Pronates and flexes the forearm	Median nerve
Pronator quadratus	Ulna (distal fourth, anterior surface)	Radius (distal fourth, anterior surface)	Pronates the forearm	Median nerve
SUPINATOR				
Supinator	Humerus (lateral epicondyle) Ulna (proximal fifth)	Radius (proximal third)	Supinates the forearm	Radial nerve

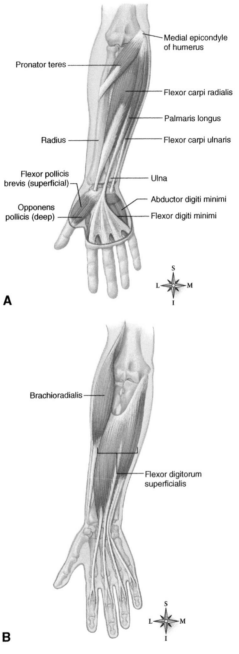

Muscles of the Forearm. A, Anterior view showing the right forearm (superficial). The brachioradialis muscle has been removed. **B,** Anterior view showing the right forearm (deeper than **A**). The pronator teres, flexor carpi radialis and ulnaris, and palmaris longus muscles have been removed.

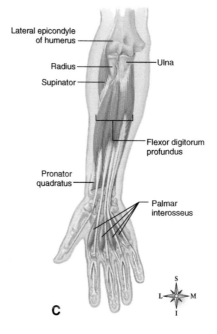

C

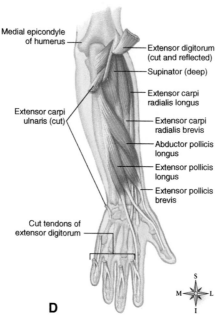

D

Muscles of the Forearm—cont'd. **C,** Anterior view showing the right forearm (deeper than **A** or **B**). The brachioradialis, pronator teres, flexor carpi radialis and ulnaris, palmaris longus, and flexor digitorum superficialis muscles have been removed. **D,** Posterior view showing the deep muscles of the right forearm. The extensor digitorum, extensor digiti minimi, and extensor carpi ulnaris muscles have been cut to reveal deeper muscles.

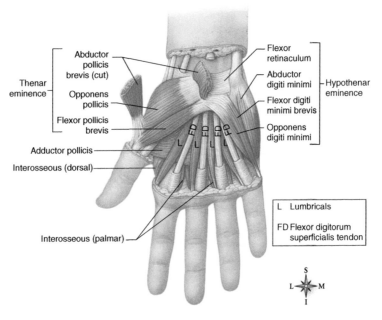

Thenar eminence

Abductor pollicis brevis (cut)

Opponens pollicis

Flexor pollicis brevis

Adductor pollicis

Interosseous (dorsal)

Interosseous (palmar)

Flexor retinaculum

Abductor digiti minimi

Flexor digiti minimi brevis

Opponens digiti minimi

Hypothenar eminence

L Lumbricals

FD Flexor digitorum superficialis tendon

S
L M
I

Intrinsic Muscles of the Hand, Anterior (Palmar) View.

CARPAL TUNNEL SYNDROME

Some epidemiologists specialize in the field of occupational health, the study of health matters related to work or the workplace. Many problems seen by occupational health experts are caused by repetitive motions of the wrists or other joints. Meat cutters and workers who use word processors, for example, are at risk for conditions caused by repetitive motion injuries.

One common problem often caused by such repetitive motion is **tenosynovitis** (ten-oh-sin-oh-VYE-tis)—inflammation of a tendon sheath. Tenosynovitis can be painful, and the swelling characteristic of this condition can limit movement in affected parts of the body. For example, swelling of the tendon sheath around tendons in an area of the wrist known as the **carpal tunnel** can limit movement of the wrist, hand, and fingers.

The figure shows the relative positions of the tendon sheath and median nerve within the carpal tunnel. The carpal tunnel is formed as a fibrous band called the **flexor retinaculum** wraps over the tendons of the flexor muscles that lie within an arch formed by the carpal bones. If swelling, or any other lesion within the carpal tunnel, presses on the **median nerve,** a condition called **carpal tunnel syndrome** may result. Because the median nerve connects to the palm and radial side (thumb side) of the hand, carpal tunnel syndrome is characterized by weakness, pain, and tingling in this part of the hand. The pain and tingling may also radiate to the forearm and shoulder. Prolonged or severe cases of carpal tunnel syndrome may be relieved by injection of anti-inflammatory agents. A permanent cure is sometimes accomplished by surgically cutting the flexor retinaculum to relieve the pressure on the median nerve.

The procedure called **carpal tunnel release** is the most common hand operation in the United States. Such operations are performed more than 200,000 times every year. When the procedure was first introduced in 1933, it was performed as an "open" procedure. A less invasive endoscopic approach was introduced in 1989; that and many other innovative surgical techniques and advances are now being used.

Continued

CARPAL TUNNEL SYNDROME—cont'd

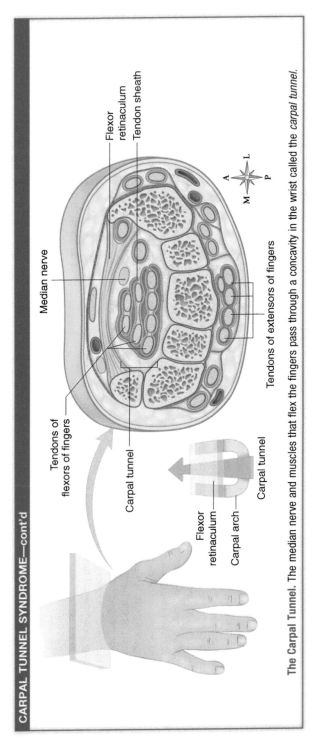

Median nerve

Tendons of
flexors of fingers

Carpal tunnel

Flexor retinaculum

Carpal arch

Carpal tunnel

Flexor
retinaculum

Tendon sheath

Tendons of extensors of fingers

M
A
L
P

The Carpal Tunnel. The median nerve and muscles that flex the fingers pass through a concavity in the wrist called the *carpal tunnel*.

MUSCLES THAT MOVE THE WRIST, HAND, AND FINGERS

MUSCLE	ORIGIN	INSERTION	FUNCTION	NERVE SUPPLY
EXTRINSIC				
Flexor carpi radialis	Humerus (medial epicondyle)	Second metacarpal (base of)	Flexes the hand Flexes the forearm	Median nerve
Palmaris longus	Humerus (medial epicondyle)	Fascia of the palm	Flexes the hand	Median nerve
Flexor carpi ulnaris	Humerus (medial epicondyle) Ulna (proximal two thirds)	Pisiform bone Third, fourth, and fifth metacarpals	Flexes the hand Adducts the hand	Ulnar nerve
Extensor carpi radialis longus	Humerus (ridge above the lateral epicondyle)	Second metacarpal (base of)	Extends the hand Abducts the hand (moves toward the thumb side when the hand is supinated)	Radial nerve
Extensor carpi radialis brevis	Humerus (lateral epicondyle)	Second, third metacarpals (bases of)	Extends the hand	Radial nerve
Extensor carpi ulnaris	Humerus (lateral epicondyle) Ulna (proximal three fourths)	Fifth metacarpal (base of)	Extends the hand Adducts the hand (moves toward the little finger side when the hand is supinated)	Radial nerve
Flexor digitorum profundus	Ulna (anterior surface)	Distal phalanges (fingers 2 to 5)	Flexes the distal interphalangeal joints	Median and ulnar nerves
Flexor digitorum superficialis	Humerus (medial epicondyle) Radius Ulna (coronoid process)	Tendons of the fingers	Flexes the fingers	Median nerve
Extensor digitorum	Humerus (lateral epicondyle)	Phalanges (fingers 2 to 5)	Extends the fingers	Radial nerve

Continued

MUSCLES THAT MOVE THE WRIST, HAND, AND FINGERS—cont'd

MUSCLE	ORIGIN	INSERTION	FUNCTION	NERVE SUPPLY
INTRINSIC				
Opponens pollicis	Trapezium	Thumb metacarpal	Opposes the thumb to the fingers	Median nerve
Abductor pollicis brevis	Trapezium	Proximal phalanx of the thumb	Abducts the thumb	Median nerve
Adductor pollicis	Second and third metacarpals Trapezoid Capitate	Proximal phalanx of the thumb	Adducts the thumb	Ulnar nerve
Flexor pollicis brevis	Flexor retinaculum	Proximal phalanx of the thumb	Flexes the thumb	Median and ulnar nerves
Abductor digiti minimi	Pisiform	Proximal phalanx of the fifth finger (base of)	Abducts the fifth finger Flexes the fifth finger	Ulnar nerve
Flexor digiti minimi brevis	Hamate	Proximal and middle phalanx of the fifth finger	Flexes the fifth finger	Ulnar nerve
Opponens digiti minimi	Hamate Flexor retinaculum	Fifth metacarpal	Opposes the fifth finger slightly	Ulnar nerve
Interosseous (palmar and dorsal)	Metacarpals	Proximal phalanges	Adducts the second, fourth, and fifth fingers (palmar) Abducts the second, third, and fourth fingers (dorsal)	Ulnar nerve
Lumbricals	Tendons of the flexor digitorum profundus	Phalanges (2 to 5)	Flexes the proximal phalanges (2 to 5) Extends the middle and distal phalanges (2 to 5)	Median nerve (phalanges 2 and 3) Ulnar nerve (phalanges 4 and 5)

MUSCLES THAT MOVE THE THIGH

MUSCLE	ORIGIN	INSERTION	FUNCTION	NERVE SUPPLY
Iliopsoas (iliacus, psoas major, and psoas minor)	Ilium (iliac fossa)	Femur (lesser trochanter)	Flexes the thigh	Femoral and second to fourth lumbar nerves
	Vertebrae (bodies of twelfth thoracic to fifth lumbar)		Flexes the trunk (when the femur acts as the origin)	
Rectus femoris	Ilium (anterior, inferior spine)	Tibia (by way of the patellar tendon)	Flexes the thigh Extends the leg	Femoral nerve
GLUTEAL GROUP				
Maximus	Ilium (crest and posterior surface) Sacrum and coccyx (posterior surface) Sacrotuberous ligament	Femur (gluteal tuberosity) Iliotibial tract	Extends the thigh—rotates outward	Inferior gluteal nerve
Medius	Ilium (lateral surface)	Femur (greater trochanter)	Abducts the thigh—rotates outward; stabilizes the pelvis on the femur	Superior gluteal nerve
Minimus	Ilium (lateral surface)	Femur (greater trochanter)	Abducts the thigh; stabilizes the pelvis on the femur Rotates the thigh medially	Superior gluteal nerve
Tensor fasciae latae	Ilium (anterior part of the crest)	Tibia (by way of the iliotibial tract)	Abducts the thigh Tightens the iliotibial tract	Superior gluteal nerve
ADDUCTOR GROUP				
Brevis	Pubic bone	Femur (linea aspera)	Adducts the thigh	Obturator nerve
Longus	Pubic bone	Femur (linea aspera)	Adducts the thigh	Obturator nerve
Magnus	Pubic bone	Femur (linea aspera)	Adducts the thigh	Obturator nerve
Gracilis	Pubic bone (just below the symphysis)	Tibia (medial surface behind the sartorius)	Adducts the thigh and flexes and adducts the leg	Obturator nerve

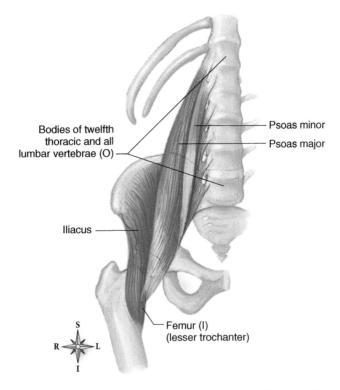

Psoas minor

Psoas major

Bodies of twelfth thoracic and all lumbar vertebrae (O)

Iliacus

Femur (I) (lesser trochanter)

S

R — L

I

Iliopsoas Muscle (Iliacus, Psoas Major, and Psoas Minor Muscles). *O,* Origin; *I,* insertion.

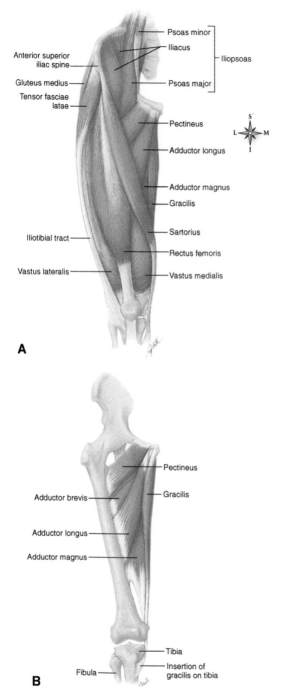

Muscles of the Anterior Aspect of the Thigh. A, Anterior view of the right thigh. **B,** Adductor region of the right thigh. The tensor fasciae latae, sartorius, and quadriceps muscles have been removed.

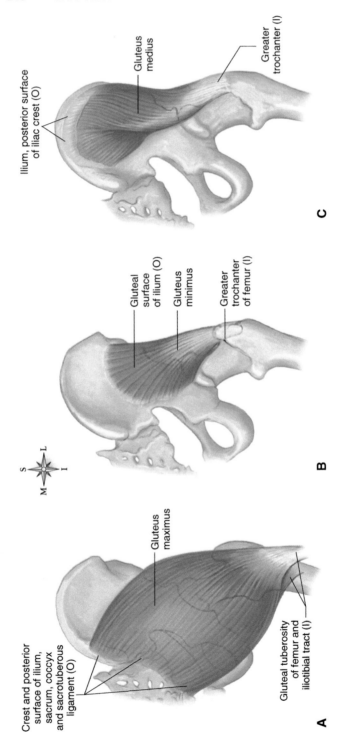

Ilium, posterior surface of iliac crest (O)

Gluteus medius

Greater trochanter (I)

C

Gluteal surface of ilium (O)

Gluteus minimus

Greater trochanter of femur (I)

B

Gluteus maximus

Crest and posterior surface of ilium, sacrum, coccyx and sacrotuberous ligament (O)

Gluteal tuberosity of femur and iliotibial tract (I)

A

Gluteal Muscles. **A,** Gluteus maximus. **B,** Gluteus minimus. **C,** Gluteus medius. *O,* Origin; *I,* insertion.

MUSCLES THAT MOVE THE LEG

MUSCLE	ORIGIN	INSERTION	FUNCTION	NERVE SUPPLY
QUADRICEPS FEMORIS GROUP				
Rectus femoris	Ilium (anterior inferior spine)	Tibia (by way of patellar tendon)	Flexes the thigh and extends the leg	Femoral nerve
Vastus lateralis	Femur (linea aspera)	Tibia (by way of the patellar tendon)	Extends the leg	Femoral nerve
Vastus medialis	Femur	Tibia (by way of the patellar tendon)	Extends the leg	Femoral nerve
Vastus intermedius	Femur (anterior surface)	Tibia (by way of the patellar tendon)	Extends the leg	Femoral nerve
Sartorius	Coxal (anterior superior iliac spines)	Tibia (medial surface of the upper end of the shaft)	Adducts and flexes the leg Permits crossing of the legs tailor fashion	Femoral nerve
HAMSTRING GROUP				
Biceps femoris	Ischium (tuberosity)	Fibula (head of)	Extends the thigh; flexes the leg	Common fibular nerve (branch of the sciatic nerve)
	Femur (linea aspera)	Tibia (lateral condyle)	Flexes the leg	Tibial nerve
Semitendinosus	Ischium (tuberosity)	Tibia (proximal end, medial surface)	Extends the thigh; flexes the leg	Tibial nerve
Semimembranosus	Ischium (tuberosity)	Tibia (medial condyle)	Extends the thigh; flexes the leg	Tibial nerve

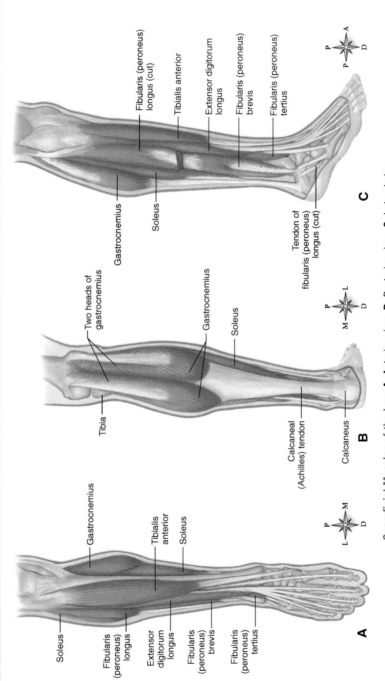

Superficial Muscles of the Leg. A, Anterior view. **B,** Posterior view. **C,** Lateral view.

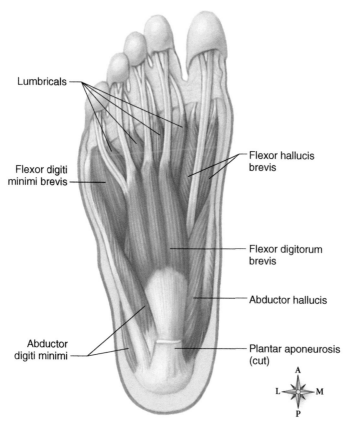

Intrinsic Muscles of the Foot. Inferior (plantar) view.

Lumbricals

Flexor digiti minimi brevis

Flexor hallucis brevis

Flexor digitorum brevis

Abductor hallucis

Abductor digiti minimi

Plantar aponeurosis (cut)

A
L — M
P

MUSCLES THAT MOVE THE FOOT

MUSCLE	ORIGIN	INSERTION	FUNCTION	NERVE SUPPLY
EXTRINSIC				
Tibialis anterior	Tibia (lateral condyle of the upper body)	Tarsal (first cuneiform)	Flexes the foot	Common and deep peroneal nerves
		Metatarsal (base of first)	Inverts the foot	
Gastrocnemius	Femur (condyles)	Tarsal (calcaneus by way of the Achilles tendon)	Extends the foot Flexes leg	Tibial nerve (branch of the sciatic nerve)
Soleus	Tibia (underneath the gastrocnemius) Fibula	Tarsal (calcaneus by way of the Achilles tendon)	Extends the foot (plantar flexion)	Tibial nerve
Fibularis longus (peroneus longus)	Tibia (lateral condyle) Fibula (head and shaft)	First cuneiform	Extends the foot (plantar flexion)	Common peroneal nerve
		Base of the first metatarsal	Everts the foot	
Fibularis brevis (peroneus brevis)	Fibula (lower two thirds of the lateral surface of the shaft)	Fifth metatarsal (tubercle, dorsal surface)	Everts the foot Flexes the foot	Superficial peroneal nerve
Fibularis tertius (peroneus tertius)	Fibula (distal third)	Fourth and fifth metatarsals (bases of)	Flexes the foot Everts the foot	Deep peroneal nerve
Extensor digitorum longus	Tibia (lateral condyle) Fibula (anterior surface)	Second and third phalanges (four lateral toes)	Dorsiflexion of the foot; extension of the toes	Deep peroneal nerve

INTRINSIC				
Lumbricals	Tendons of the flexor digitorum longus	Phalanges (2 to 5)	Flex the proximal phalanges; Extend the middle and distal phalanges	Lateral and medial plantar nerve
Flexor digiti minimi brevis	Fifth metatarsal	Proximal phalanx of the fifth toe	Flexes the fifth (small) toe	Lateral plantar nerve
Flexor hallucis brevis	Cuboid; Medial and lateral cuneiform	Proximal phalanx of the first (great) toe	Flexes the first (great) toe	Medial and lateral plantar nerve
Flexor digitorum brevis	Calcaneus; Plantar fascia	Middle phalanges of the toes (2 to 5)	Flexes toes 2 through 5	Medial plantar nerve
Abductor digiti minimi	Calcaneus	Proximal phalanx of the fifth (small) toe	Abducts the fifth (small) toe; Flexes the fifth toe	Lateral plantar nerve
Abductor hallucis	Calcaneus	First (great) toe	Abducts the first (great) toe	Medial plantar nerve

8

Nervous System

The nervous system is organized to detect changes (stimuli) in the internal and external environments, evaluate that information, and possibly respond by initiating changes in muscles or glands. To make this complex network of information lines and processing circuits easier to understand, biologists have subdivided the nervous system into smaller "systems" and "divisions." The nervous system can be divided in various ways:

1. According to structure (Central Nervous System and Peripheral Nervous System)
2. Direction of information flow (Afferent [Sensory] Division and Efferent [Motor] Division)
3. Control of effectors (Somatic Nervous System and Autonomic Nervous System)

The diagram on the facing page summarizes a common scheme used to understand the organization of the nervous system.

Two main types of cells compose the nervous system, namely, *neurons* and *glia*. **Neurons** are excitable cells that conduct the impulses that make possible all nervous system functions. In other words, they form the "wiring" of the nervous system's information circuits. **Glia**, or *glial cells*, on the other hand, do not usually conduct information themselves but support the function of neurons in various ways. Some of the major types of glia and neurons are described in the following sections.

NERVOUS SYSTEM CELLS

Organizational Plan of the Nervous System. Diagram summarizes the scheme used by most neurobiologists in studying the nervous system. Both the somatic nervous system (SNS) and the autonomic nervous system (ANS) include components in the central nervous system (CNS) and peripheral nervous system (PNS). Somatic sensory pathways conduct information toward integrators in the CNS, and somatic motor pathways conduct information toward somatic effectors. In the ANS, visceral sensory pathways conduct information toward CNS integrators, whereas the sympathetic and parasympathetic pathways conduct information toward autonomic effectors.

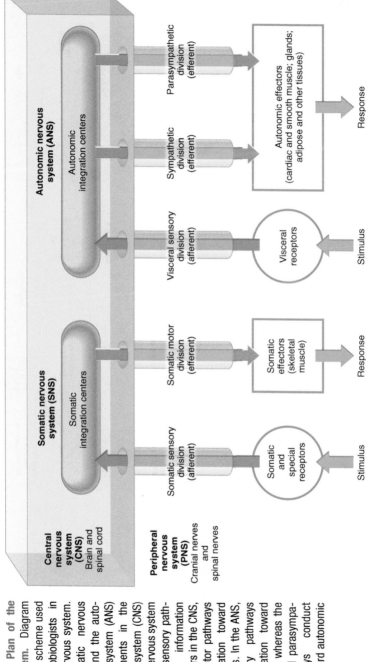

Central nervous system (CNS)
Brain and spinal cord

Peripheral nervous system (PNS)
Cranial nerves and spinal nerves

Somatic nervous system (SNS)
Somatic integration centers

Autonomic nervous system (ANS)
Autonomic integration centers

Somatic sensory division (afferent)

Somatic motor division (efferent)

Visceral sensory division (afferent)

Sympathetic division (efferent)

Parasympathetic division (efferent)

Somatic and special receptors

Somatic effectors (skeletal muscle)

Visceral receptors

Autonomic effectors (cardiac and smooth muscle; glands; adipose and other tissues)

Stimulus

Response

Stimulus

Response

Types of Neuroglia. *Neuroglia of the central nervous system (CNS):* **A,** Astrocytes attached to the outside of a capillary blood vessel in the brain. **B,** A phagocytic microglial cell. **C,** Ciliated ependymal cells forming a sheet that usually lines fluid cavities in the brain. **D,** An oligodendrocyte with processes that wrap around nerve fibers in the CNS to form myelin sheaths. *Neuroglia of the peripheral nervous system (PNS):* **E,** A Schwann cell supporting a bundle of nerve fibers in the PNS. **F,** Another type of Schwann cell wrapping around a peripheral nerve fiber to form a thick myelin sheath. **G,** Satellite cells, another type of Schwann cell, surround and support cell bodies of neurons in the PNS.

CENTRAL NERVOUS SYSTEM NEUROGLIA

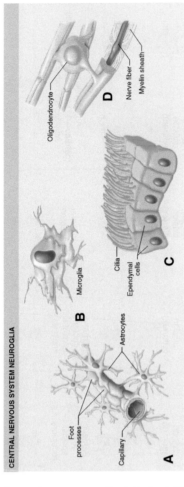

PERIPHERAL NERVOUS SYSTEM NEUROGLIA

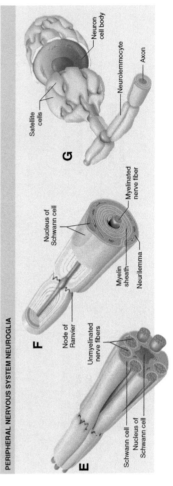

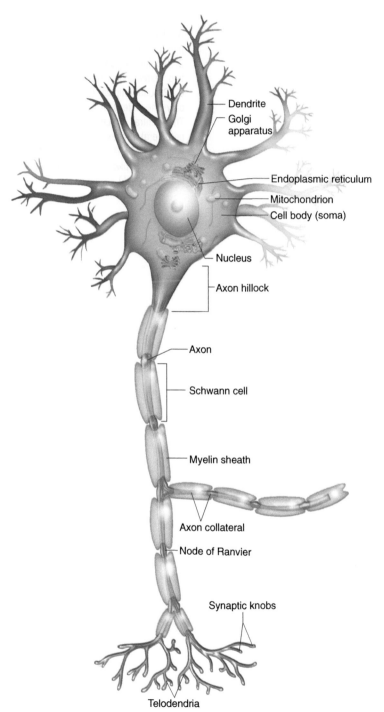

Structure of a Typical Neuron.

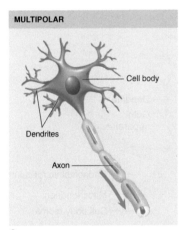

A

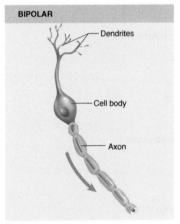

B

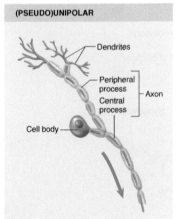

C

Structural Classification of Neurons.
A, Multipolar neuron: neuron with multiple extensions from the cell body. **B,** Bipolar neuron: neuron with exactly two extensions from the cell body. **C,** (Pseudo) unipolar neuron: neuron with only one extension from the cell body. The central process is an axon; the peripheral process is a modified axon with branched dendrites at its extremity. (The *red arrows* show the direction of impulse travel.)

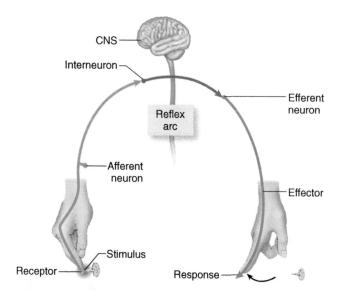

Functional Classification of Neurons in a Reflex Arc. Neurons can be classified according to the direction in which they conduct impulses. Notice that the most basic route of signal conduction follows a pattern called the *reflex arc*.

Nerves and Nerve Impulses

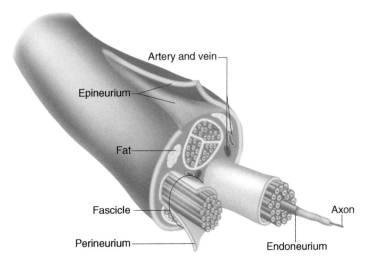

The Nerve. Each nerve contains axons bundled into fascicles. A fibrous endoneurium surrounds each axon and its Schwann cells within a fascicle. A perineurium surrounds each fascicle. A connective tissue epineurium wraps the entire nerve. The superficial epineurium is shown in blue and the deep epineurium (collagen fibers, adipose tissue, and blood vessels) is shown in brown.

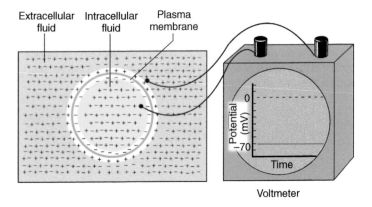

Membrane Potential. The diagram on the *left* represents a cell maintaining a very slight difference in the concentration of oppositely charged ions across its plasma membrane. The voltmeter records the magnitude of electrical difference over time, which, in this case, does not fluctuate from −70 mV (voltage recorded over time as a *red line*).

Action Potential

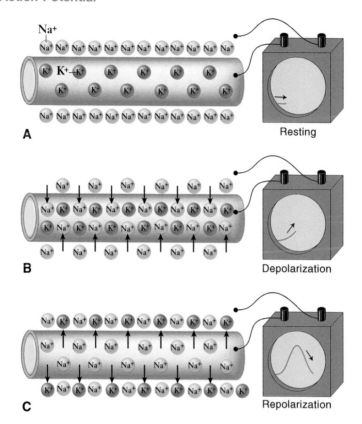

Depolarization and Repolarization. A, Resting membrane potential (RMP) results from an excess of positive ions on the outer surface of the plasma membrane. More Na$^+$ ions are on the outside of the membrane than K$^+$ ions are on the inside of the membrane. **B,** Depolarization of a membrane occurs when Na$^+$ channels open, allowing Na$^+$ to move to an area of lower concentration (and more negative charge) *inside* the cell—reversing the polarity to an inside-positive state. **C,** Repolarization of a membrane occurs when K$^+$ channels then open, allowing K$^+$ to move to an area of lower concentration (and more negative charge) *outside* the cell—reversing the polarity back to an inside-negative state. Each voltmeter records the changing membrane potential as a *red line*.

TYPES OF MEMBRANE POTENTIALS

MEMBRANE POTENTIAL	POLARIZATION	TYPICAL VOLTAGE*	SUMMATION	CONDUCTION	DESCRIPTION
Resting membrane potential (RMP)	Polarized	−70 mV	Not applicable	Not applicable	Membrane voltage when the neuron is not excited and not conducting an impulse
Local potential	Depolarized (excitatory; EPSP)	Graded; varies greater than −70 mV	Yes	Decremental	Temporary fluctuation in a local region of the membrane in response to a sensory or nerve stimulus; may be an upward or downward fluctuation in voltage; loses amplitude as it spreads along membrane
	Hyperpolarized (inhibitory; IPSP)	Graded; varies at levels less than −70 mV	Yes	Decremental	
Threshold potential	Depolarized	−59 mV	Yes	Triggers action potential	Minimum local depolarization needed to trigger voltage-gated channels that produce the action potential
Action potential	Depolarized	+30 mV	No	Nondecremental	Temporary maximum depolarization of membrane voltage that travels to end of axon without losing amplitude

*Example used in this chapter; actual values in body vary depending on many diverse factors.
EPSP, Excitatory postsynaptic potential; *IPSP,* inhibitory postsynaptic potential.

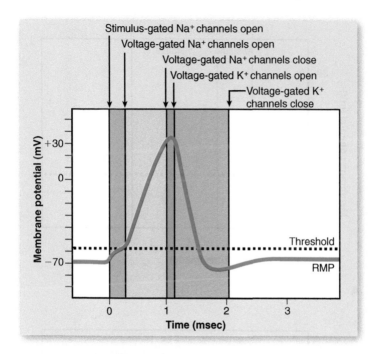

The Action Potential. Changes in membrane potential in a local area of a neuron's membrane result from changes in membrane permeability.

STEPS OF THE MECHANISM THAT PRODUCES AN ACTION POTENTIAL

STEP	DESCRIPTION
1	A stimulus triggers stimulus-gated Na^+ channels to open and allow inward Na^+ diffusion. This causes the membrane to depolarize.
2	As the threshold potential is reached, voltage-gated Na^+ channels open.
3	As more Na^+ enters the cell through voltage-gated Na^+ channels, the membrane depolarizes even further.
4	The magnitude of the action potential peaks (at +30 mV) when voltage-gated Na^+ channels close.
5	Repolarization begins when voltage-gated K^+ channels open, allowing outward diffusion of K^+.
6	After a brief period of hyperpolarization, the resting potential is restored by the sodium-potassium pump and the return of ion channels to their resting state.

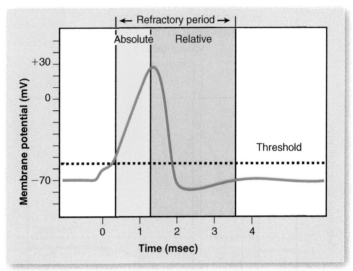

A

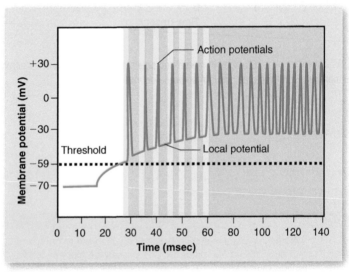

B

Refractory Period. A, During the absolute refractory period, the membrane will not respond to any stimulus. During the relative refractory period, however, a very strong stimulus may elicit a response in the membrane. **B,** As the local potential increases, a new action potential may begin during the relative refractory period. The higher the local potential, the sooner a new action potential can be generated. As the graph shows, high local potentials produce a higher frequency of action potentials than lower local potentials.

Synaptic Transmission

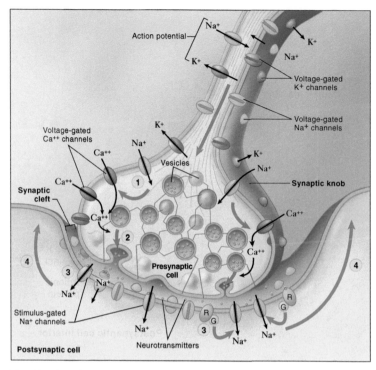

The Chemical Synapse. Diagram shows detail of synaptic knob, or axon terminal, of presynaptic neuron, the plasma membrane of a postsynaptic neuron, and a synaptic cleft. On the arrival of an action potential at a synaptic knob, voltage-gated Ca^{++} channels open and allow extracellular Ca^{++} to diffuse into the presynaptic cell *(step 1)*. In step 2, the Ca^{++} triggers the rapid exocytosis of neurotransmitter molecules from vesicles in the knob. In step 3, neurotransmitter diffuses into the synaptic cleft and binds to receptor molecules in the plasma membrane of the postsynaptic neuron. The postsynaptic receptors directly or indirectly trigger the opening of stimulus-gated ion channels, initiating a local potential in the postsynaptic neuron. In step 4, the local potential may move toward the axon, where an action potential may begin.

Neurotransmitters

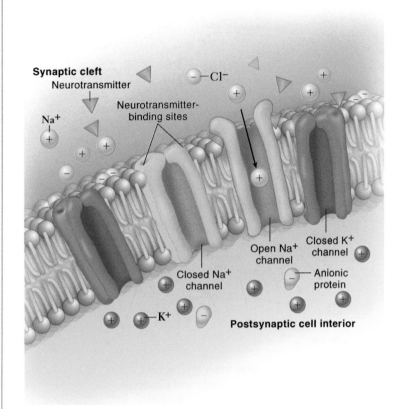

Direct Stimulation of a Postsynaptic Receptor. Some neurotransmitters, such as acetylcholine, initiate nerve signals by binding directly to one or both neurotransmitter-binding sites on the stimulus-gated ion channel. Such binding causes the channel to change its shape to an open position. When the neurotransmitter is removed, the channel again closes.

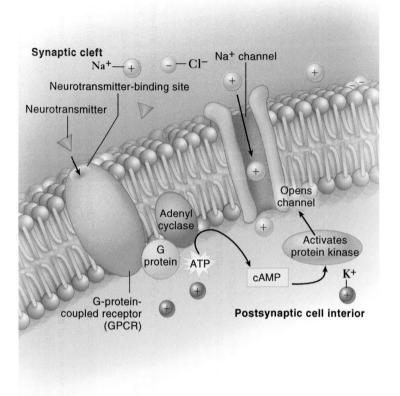

Second Messenger Stimulation of a Postsynaptic Receptor. Norepinephrine and many other neurotransmitters initiate nerve signals indirectly by binding to a G-protein–coupled receptor (GPCR) that changes shape to activate the enzyme adenylate cyclase, which in turn catalyzes the conversion of ATP to cyclic AMP (cAMP). cAMP is a "second messenger" that induces a change in the shape of a stimulus-gated channel.

EXAMPLES OF NEUROTRANSMITTERS

NEUROTRANSMITTER	LOCATION*	FUNCTION*
SMALL-MOLECULE TRANSMITTERS		
Class I		
Acetylcholine (ACh)	Junctions with motor effectors (muscles, glands); many parts of brain	Excitatory or inhibitory; involved in memory
Class II: Amines		
Monoamines		
Serotonin (5-HT†)	Several regions of the CNS	Mostly inhibitory; involved in moods and emotions, sleep
Histamine	Brain	Mostly excitatory; involved in emotions and regulation of body temperature and water balance
Catecholamines		
Dopamine (DA)	Brain; autonomic system	Mostly inhibitory; involved in emotions/moods and in regulating motor control
Epinephrine	Several areas of the CNS and in the sympathetic division of the ANS	Excitatory or inhibitory; acts as a hormone when secreted by sympathetic neurosecretory cells of the adrenal gland
Norepinephrine (NE)	Several areas of the CNS and in the sympathetic division of the ANS	Excitatory or inhibitory; regulates sympathetic effectors; in brain, involved in emotional responses

Class III: Amino Acids		
Glutamate (glutamic acid, Glu)	CNS	Excitatory; most common excitatory neurotransmitter in CNS
Gamma-aminobutyric acid (GABA)	Brain	Inhibitory; common inhibitory neurotransmitter in brain
Glycine (Gly)	Spinal cord	Inhibitory; common inhibitory neurotransmitter in brain
Class IV: Other Small Molecules		
Nitric oxide (NO)	Several regions of the nervous system	May be a signal from postsynaptic to presynaptic neuron
LARGE-MOLECULE TRANSMITTERS		
Neuropeptides		
Vasoactive intestinal peptide (VIP)	Brain; some ANS and sensory fibers; retina; gastrointestinal tract	Function in nervous system uncertain
Cholecystokinin (CCK)	Brain; retina	Function in nervous system uncertain
Substance P	Brain, spinal cord, sensory pain pathways; gastrointestinal tract	Mostly excitatory; transmits pain information
Enkephalins	Several regions of CNS; retina; intestinal tract	Mostly inhibitory; act like opiates to block pain
Endorphins	Several regions of CNS; retina; intestinal tract	Mostly inhibitory; act like opiates to block pain
Neuropeptide Y (NPY)	Brain, some ANS fibers	Variety of functions including enhancing blood vessel constriction by ANS, regulation of energy balance, learning, and memory

*These are examples only; most of these neurotransmitters are also found in other locations, and many have additional functions.
†5-hydroxytryptamine (synonym for serotonin).
ANS, Autonomic nervous system; *CNS*, central nervous system.

NEURAL NETWORKS

Nervous pathways, **or neural networks,** conduct information along complex series of neurons joined together by synapses.

Research shows that such networks develop during a person's early life and are influenced by the various sensory learning experiences that we have as our nerve tissue develops. One process that facilitates the formation of connections involves *neurotrophic factors* or **neurotrophins**—nerve growth factors that are released by various cells of the body. The axons of several developing neurons grow toward the cell that releases neurotrophins. However, only those axons that can be supported by the amount of available neurotrophin will remain—the rest of the neurons will degenerate. Many other factors, such as repeated stimulation of a pathway, influence this process. Once neural networks become mature in adulthood, they are less likely to accept the addition of new neurons—even though neural stem cells do exist in the adult nervous system.

Something that makes the pathways of neural networks complex is that they often *converge* and *diverge.*

Convergence occurs when more than one presynaptic axon synapses with a single postsynaptic neuron (part *A* of the figure). Convergence allows information from several different pathways to be funneled into a single pathway. For example, the pathways that innervate the skeletal muscles may originate in several different areas of the central nervous system. Because pathways from each of these motor control areas converge on a single motor neuron, each area has an opportunity to control the same muscle.

Divergence occurs when a single presynaptic axon synapses with many different postsynaptic neurons (part *B* of the figure). Divergence allows information from one pathway to be "split" or "copied" and sent to different destinations in the nervous system. For example, a single bit of visual information may be sent to many different areas of the brain for processing.

NEURAL NETWORKS—cont'd

CONVERGENCE

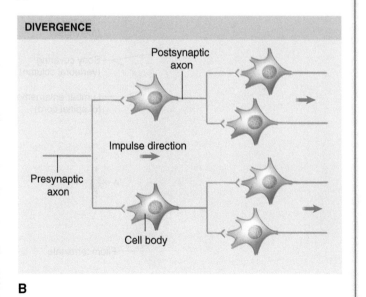

Cell body

Postsynaptic axon

Presynaptic axon

Impulse direction

A

DIVERGENCE

Postsynaptic axon

Impulse direction

Presynaptic axon

Cell body

B

CENTRAL NERVOUS SYSTEM

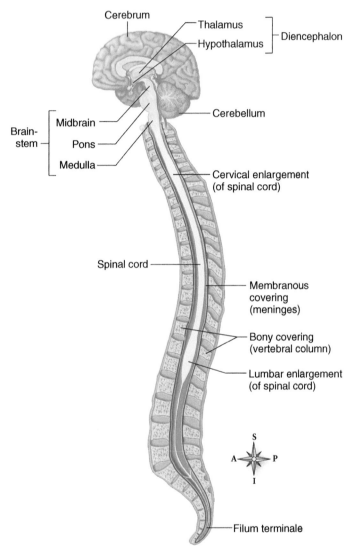

The Central Nervous System. Details of both the brain and the spinal cord are easily seen in this figure.

Coverings of the Brain and Spinal Cord

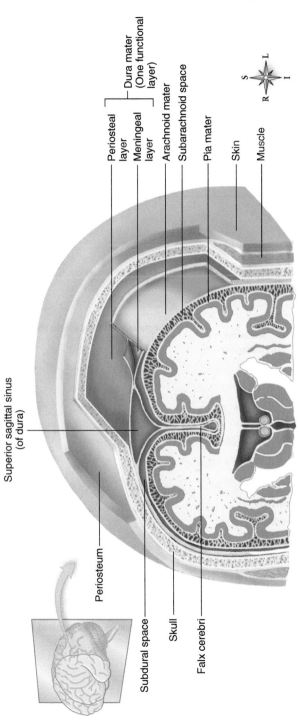

Coverings of the Brain. Frontal section of the superior portion of the head, as viewed from the front. Both the bony and the membranous coverings of the brain can be seen.

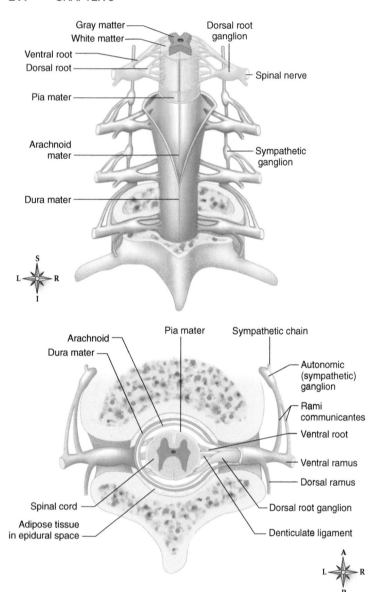

Coverings of the Spinal Cord. The dura mater is shown in purple. Note how it extends to cover the spinal nerve roots and nerves. The arachnoid is highlighted in pink, and the pia mater is shown in orange.

Cerebrospinal Fluid

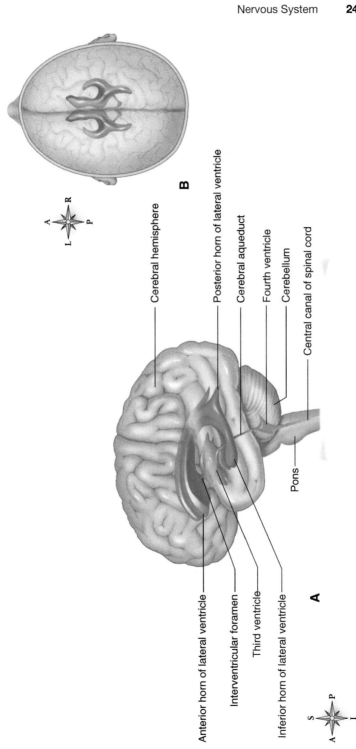

Anterior horn of lateral ventricle

Interventricular foramen

Third ventricle

Inferior horn of lateral ventricle

Cerebral hemisphere

Posterior horn of lateral ventricle

Cerebral aqueduct

Fourth ventricle

Cerebellum

Central canal of spinal cord

Pons

A

B

Fluid Spaces of the Brain. A, Ventricles highlighted in blue within a translucent brain in a left lateral view. **B,** Ventricles as seen from above.

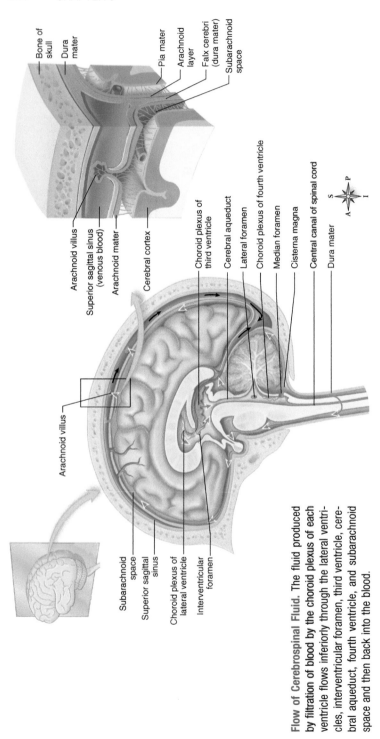

Flow of Cerebrospinal Fluid. The fluid produced by filtration of blood by the choroid plexus of each ventricle flows inferiorly through the lateral ventricles, interventricular foramen, third ventricle, cerebral aqueduct, fourth ventricle, and subarachnoid space and then back into the blood.

Spinal Cord

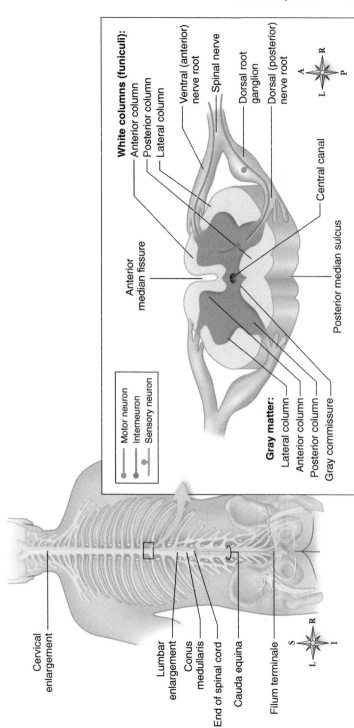

White columns (funiculi):
Anterior column
Posterior column
Lateral column

Ventral (anterior) nerve root

Spinal nerve

Dorsal root ganglion

Dorsal (posterior) nerve root

Central canal

Anterior median fissure

Posterior median sulcus

Motor neuron
Interneuron
Sensory neuron

Gray matter:
Lateral column
Anterior column
Posterior column
Gray commissure

Cervical enlargement

Lumbar enlargement
Conus medullaris
End of spinal cord
Cauda equina

Filum terminale

Spinal Cord. The *inset* illustrates a transverse section of the spinal cord shown in the broader view.

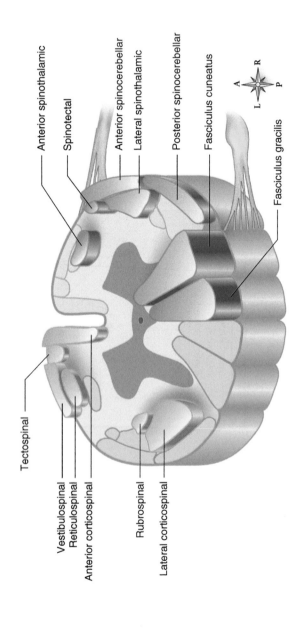

Anterior spinothalamic

Spinotectal

Anterior spinocerebellar

Lateral spinothalamic

Posterior spinocerebellar

Fasciculus cuneatus

Fasciculus gracilis

Tectospinal

Vestibulospinal
Reticulospinal
Anterior corticospinal

Rubrospinal

Lateral corticospinal

Major Tracts of the Spinal Cord. The major ascending (sensory) tracts are highlighted in blue. The major descending (motor) tracts are highlighted in red.

MAJOR ASCENDING TRACTS OF THE SPINAL CORD

NAME	FUNCTION	LOCATION	ORIGIN*	TERMINATION†
Lateral spinothalamic	Pain, temperature, and crude touch on opposite side	Lateral white columns	Posterior gray column on opposite side	Thalamus
Anterior spinothalamic	Crude touch and pressure	Anterior white columns	Posterior gray column on opposite side	Thalamus
Fasciculi gracilis and cuneatus	Discriminating touch and pressure sensations, including vibration, stereognosis, and two-point discrimination; also conscious kinesthesia	Posterior white columns	Spinal ganglia on same side	Medulla
Anterior and posterior spinocerebellar	Unconscious kinesthesia	Lateral white columns	Anterior or posterior gray column	Cerebellum
Spinotectal	Touch related to visual reflexes	Lateral white columns	Posterior gray columns	Superior colliculus (midbrain)

*Location of cell bodies of neurons from which axons of tract arise.
†Structure in which axons of tract terminate.

MAJOR DESCENDING TRACTS OF THE SPINAL CORD

NAME	FUNCTION	LOCATION	ORIGIN*	TERMINATION†
Lateral corticospinal (or crossed pyramidal)	Voluntary movement, contraction of individual or small groups of muscles, particularly those moving hands, fingers, feet, and toes of opposite side	Lateral white columns	Motor areas or cerebral cortex of opposite side from tract location in cord	Lateral or anterior gray columns
Anterior corticospinal (direct pyramidal)	Same as lateral corticospinal except mainly muscles of same side	Anterior white columns	Motor cortex but on same side as location in cord	Lateral or anterior gray columns
Reticulospinal	Maintain posture during movement	Anterior white columns	Reticular formation (midbrain, pons, medulla)	Anterior gray columns
Rubrospinal	Coordination of body movement and posture	Lateral white columns	Red nucleus (of midbrain)	Anterior gray columns
Tectospinal	Head and neck movement during visual reflexes	Anterior white columns	Superior colliculus (midbrain)	Medulla and anterior gray columns
Vestibulospinal	Coordination of posture/balance	Anterior white columns	Vestibular nucleus (pons, medulla)	Anterior gray columns

*Location of the cell bodies of neurons from which the axons of the tract arise.
†Structure in which the axons of the tract terminate.

Brain

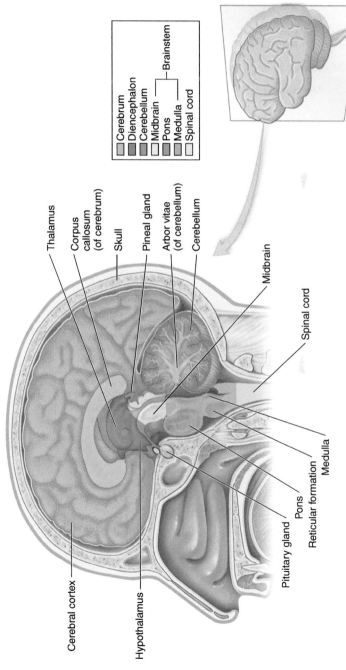

Cerebral cortex

Hypothalamus

Thalamus

Corpus callosum (of cerebrum)

Skull

Pineal gland

Arbor vitae (of cerebellum)

Cerebellum

Midbrain

Spinal cord

Medulla

Reticular formation

Pons

Pituitary gland

Cerebrum
Diencephalon
Cerebellum
Midbrain
Pons   Brainstem
Medulla
Spinal cord

Major Regions of the Central Nervous System. Sagittal section of the brain and spinal cord.

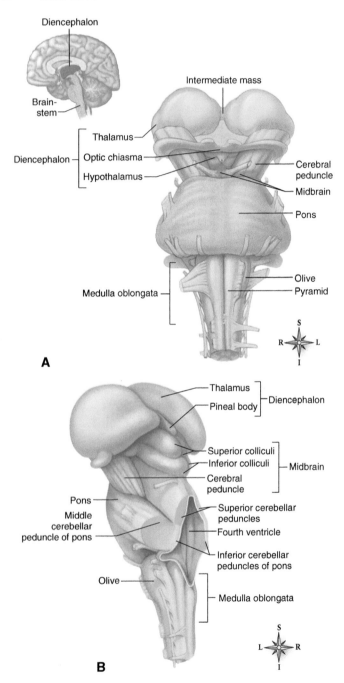

The Brainstem and the Diencephalon. A, Anterior aspect. **B,** Posterior aspect (shifted slightly to lateral).

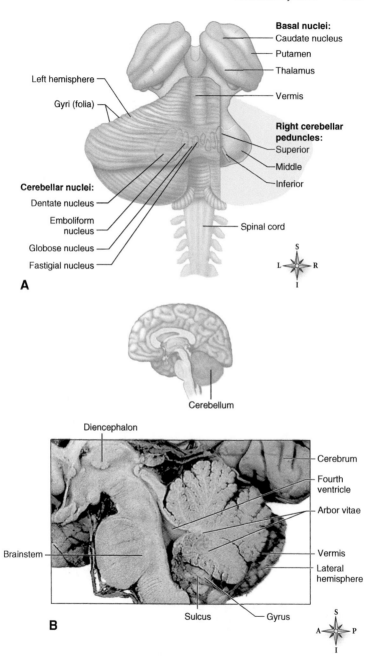

Basal nuclei:
Caudate nucleus
Putamen
Thalamus

Left hemisphere

Gyri (folia)

Vermis

Right cerebellar
peduncles:
Superior
Middle
Inferior

Cerebellar nuclei:
Dentate nucleus

Emboliform
nucleus

Globose nucleus

Fastigial nucleus

Spinal cord

A

Cerebellum

Diencephalon

Cerebrum

Fourth
ventricle

Arbor vitae

Brainstem

Vermis

Lateral
hemisphere

Sulcus   Gyrus

B

Cerebellum. A, Posterior view of the surface of the cerebellum. **B,** Photograph of midsagittal brain section shows internal features of the cerebellum and surrounding structures of the brain.

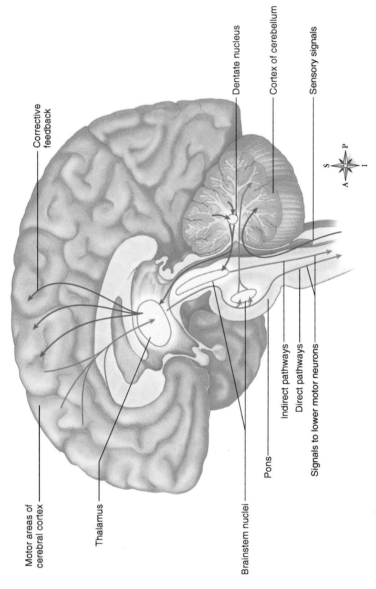

Coordinating Function of the Cerebellum. Impulses from the motor control areas of the cerebrum travel down to skeletal muscle tissue and to the cerebellum at the same time. The cerebellum, which also receives and evaluates sensory information, compares the intended movement with the actual movement. It then sends impulses to both the cerebrum and the muscles, thus coordinating and "smoothing" muscle activity.

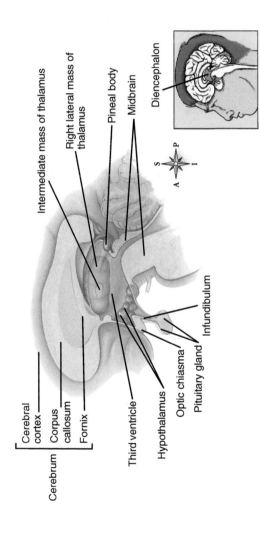

Cerebral cortex
Corpus callosum
Fornix
Cerebrum

Intermediate mass of thalamus

Right lateral mass of thalamus

Pineal body

Midbrain

Diencephalon

S
A   P
I

Third ventricle

Hypothalamus

Optic chiasma

Pituitary gland   Infundibulum

Diencephalon and Surrounding Structures. This midsagittal section highlights the largest regions of the diencephalon, the thalamus and hypothalamus, but also shows the smaller optic chiasma and pineal body. Note the position of the diencephalon between the midbrain and the cerebrum.

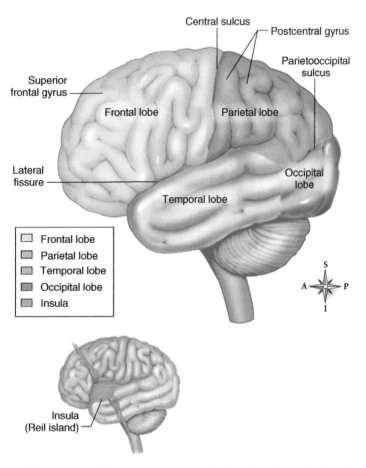

Left Hemisphere of the Cerebrum, Lateral Surface. Note the highlighted lobes of the cerebrum.

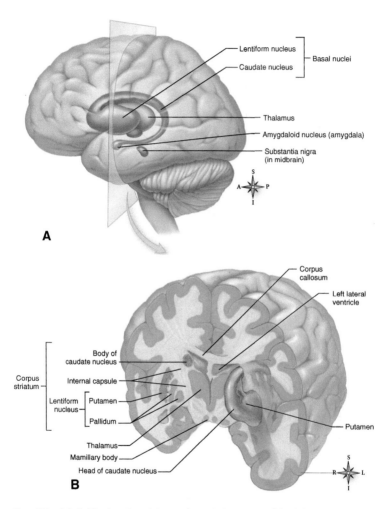

Basal Nuclei. A, The basal nuclei seen through the cortex of the left cerebral hemisphere. **B,** The basal nuclei seen in a frontal (coronal) section of the brain.

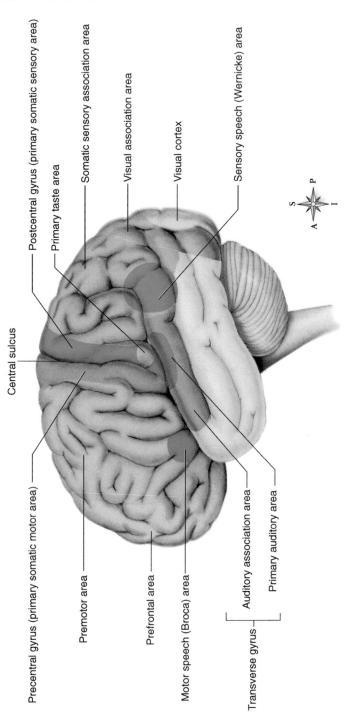

Precentral gyrus (primary somatic motor area)

Central sulcus

Premotor area

Prefrontal area

Motor speech (Broca) area

Transverse gyrus { Auditory association area

Primary auditory area

Postcentral gyrus (primary somatic sensory area)

Primary taste area

Somatic sensory association area

Visual association area

Visual cortex

Sensory speech (Wernicke) area

Functional Areas of the Cerebral Cortex.

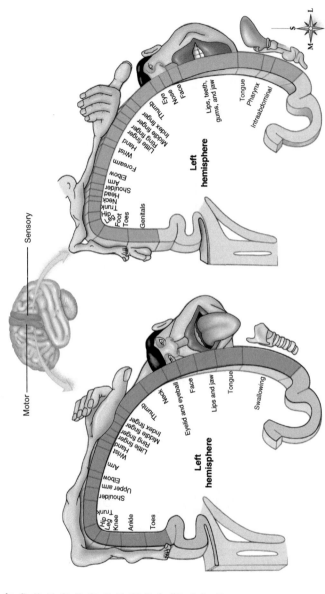

Primary Somatic Motor and Sensory Areas of the Cortex. The body parts illustrated here show which parts of the body are "mapped" to specific areas of each cortical area. The exaggerated face indicates that more cortical area is devoted to processing information to and from the many receptors and motor units of the face than for of the leg or arm, for example. **A,** Primary somatic motor area. **B,** Primary somatic sensory area.

Motor ——— Sensory

A   Primary somatic motor area

Left hemisphere

Trunk
Hip
Leg
Knee
Ankle
Toes
Shoulder
Upper arm
Elbow
Arm
Wrist
Hand
Little finger
Ring finger
Middle finger
Index finger
Thumb
Neck
Eyelid and eyeball
Face
Lips and jaw
Tongue
Swallowing

B   Primary somatic sensory area

Left hemisphere

Genitals
Toes
Foot
Leg
Hip
Trunk
Neck
Head
Shoulder
Arm
Elbow
Forearm
Wrist
Hand
Little finger
Ring finger
Middle finger
Index finger
Thumb
Eye
Nose
Face
Lips, teeth, gums, and jaw
Tongue
Pharynx
Intraabdominal

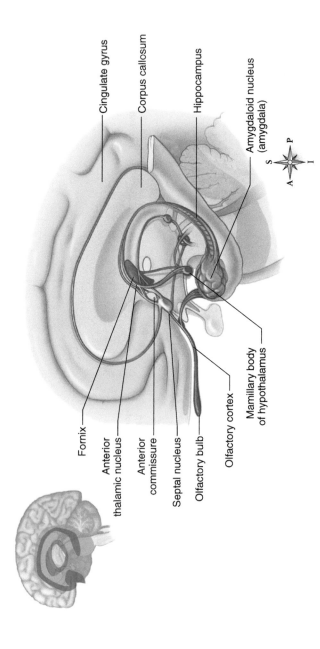

Cingulate gyrus

Corpus callosum

Hippocampus

Amygdaloid nucleus (amygdala)

Fornix

Anterior thalamic nucleus

Anterior commissure

Septal nucleus

Olfactory bulb

Olfactory cortex

Mamillary body of hypothalamus

Structures of the Limbic System. Sometimes referred to as "the emotional brain," this network of brain structures functions as we experience emotions.

THE ELECTROENCEPHALOGRAM (EEG)

Cerebral activity goes on as long as life itself. Only when life ceases (or moments before) does the cerebrum cease its functioning. Only then do all its neurons stop conducting impulses. Proof of this has come from records of brain electrical potentials known as **electroencephalograms,** or *EEGs*. These records are usually made from data detected by a number of electrodes placed on different regions of the scalp; they are records of wave activity—brainwaves (parts *A* and *B* of the figure).

Four types of brainwaves are recognized based on frequency and amplitude of the waves. *Frequency,* or the number of wave cycles per second, is usually referred to as *hertz (Hz,* from Hertz, a German physicist). *Amplitude* means voltage. Listed in order of frequency from fastest to slowest, brainwaves are designated as *beta, alpha, theta,* and *delta.* **Beta waves** have a frequency of more than 13 Hz and a relatively low voltage. **Alpha waves** have a frequency of 8 to 13 Hz and a relatively high voltage. **Theta waves** have both a relatively low frequency—4 to 7 Hz—and a low voltage. **Delta waves** have the slowest frequency (<4 Hz) but a high voltage. Brainwaves vary in different regions of the brain, in different states of awareness, and in abnormal conditions of the cerebrum.

Fast, low-voltage beta waves characterize EEGs recorded from the frontal and central regions of the cerebrum when an individual is awake, alert, and attentive, with eyes open. Beta waves predominate when the cerebrum is busiest, that is, when it is engaged with sensory stimulation or mental activities. In short, beta waves are "busy waves." Alpha waves, in contrast, are "relaxed waves." They are moderately fast, relatively high-voltage waves that dominate EEGs recorded from the parietal lobe, occipital lobe, and posterior parts of the temporal lobes when the cerebrum is idling, so to speak. The individual is awake but has eyes closed and is in a relaxed, nonattentive state. This state is sometimes called the "alpha state." When drowsiness descends, moderately slow, low-voltage theta waves appear. Theta waves are "drowsy waves." "Deep sleep waves," on the other hand, are known as delta waves. These slowest brainwaves characterize the deep sleep from which one is not easily aroused. For this reason, deep sleep is referred to as slow-wave sleep.

Physicians use electroencephalograms (EEGs) to help localize areas of brain dysfunction, to identify altered states of consciousness, and often to establish death. Two flat EEG recordings (no brainwaves) taken 24 hours apart in conjunction with no spontaneous respiration and total absence of somatic reflexes are criteria accepted as evidence of brain death.

Continued

THE ELECTROENCEPHALOGRAM (EEG)—cont'd

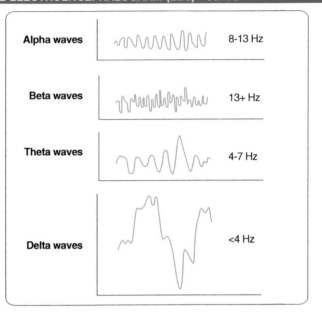

Alpha waves		8-13 Hz
Beta waves		13+ Hz
Theta waves		4-7 Hz
Delta waves		<4 Hz

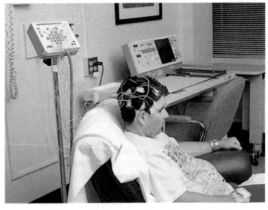

The Electroencephalogram. Diagnosis and evaluation of epilepsy or any seizure disorder often rely on electroencephalography. This illustration shows examples of alpha, beta, theta, and delta waves seen on an EEG.

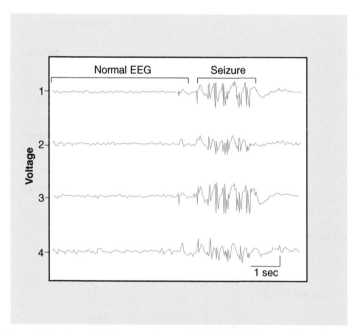

Abnormal Electroencephalogram. A normal electroencephalogram shows the moderate rise and fall of voltage in various parts of the brain, but a seizure manifests as an explosive increase in the size and frequency of voltage fluctuations. Different classifications of seizure disorders are based on the location(s) and durations of these changes in brain activity.

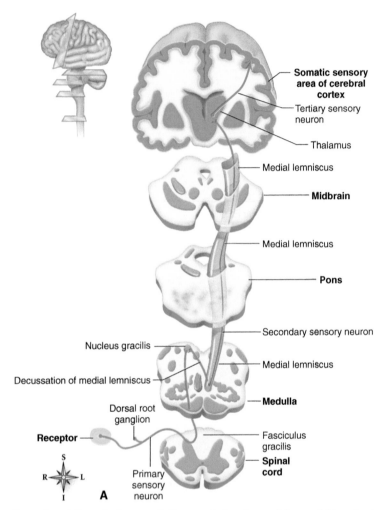

Examples of Somatic Sensory Pathways. A, A pathway of the medial lemniscal system that conducts information about discriminating touch and kinesthesia.

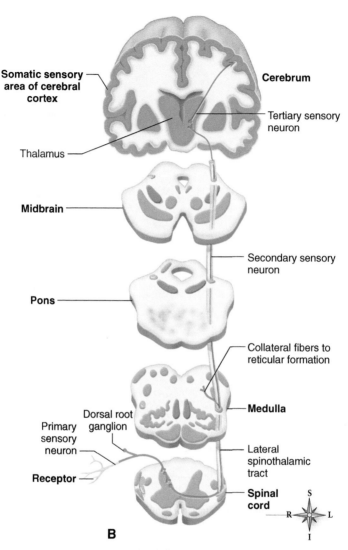

Examples of Somatic Sensory Pathways—cont'd. B, A spinothalamic pathway that conducts information about pain and temperature.

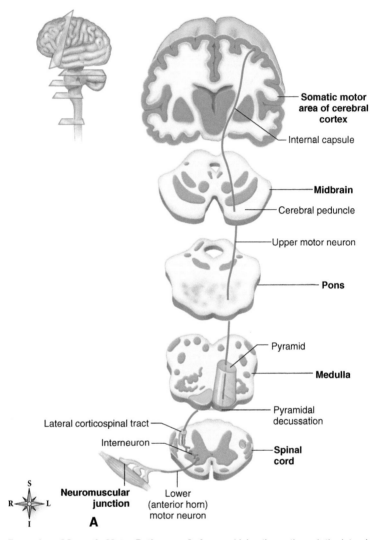

Somatic motor area of cerebral cortex

Internal capsule

Midbrain

Cerebral peduncle

Upper motor neuron

Pons

Pyramid

Medulla

Pyramidal decussation

Lateral corticospinal tract

Interneuron

Spinal cord

Neuromuscular junction

Lower (anterior horn) motor neuron

A

Examples of Somatic Motor Pathways. A, A pyramidal pathway through the lateral corticospinal tract.

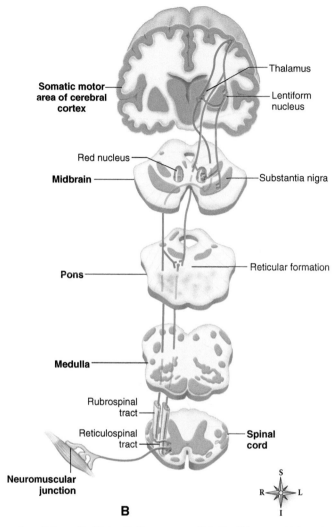

Thalamus

Somatic motor area of cerebral cortex

Lentiform nucleus

Red nucleus

Midbrain

Substantia nigra

Pons

Reticular formation

Medulla

Rubrospinal tract

Reticulospinal tract

Spinal cord

Neuromuscular junction

B

S
R — L
I

Examples of Somatic Motor Pathways—cont'd. B, Extrapyramidal pathways through the rubrospinal and reticulospinal tracts.

PERIPHERAL NERVOUS SYSTEM

Spinal Nerves

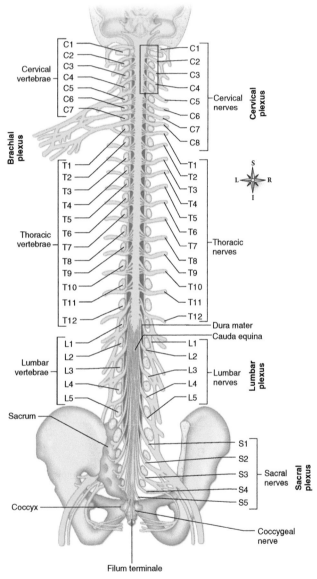

Spinal Nerves. Each of 31 pairs of spinal nerves exits the spinal cavity from the intervertebral foramina. The names of the vertebrae are given on the *left,* and the names of the corresponding spinal nerves on the *right*. Note that, after leaving the spinal cavity, many of the spinal nerves interconnect to form networks called *plexuses*.

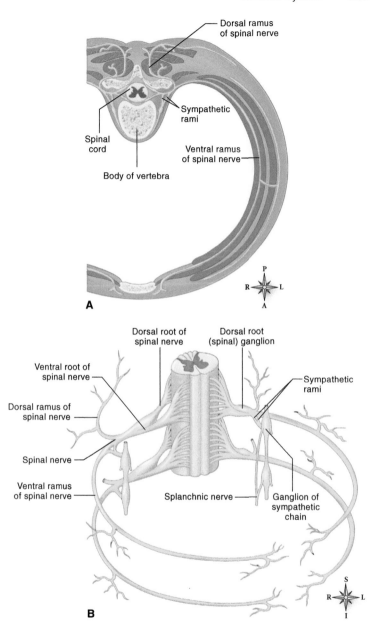

Rami of the Spinal Nerves. Note that ventral and dorsal roots join to form a spinal nerve. The spinal nerve then splits into a *dorsal ramus* (pl., *rami*) and *ventral ramus.* The ventral ramus communicates with a chain of sympathetic (autonomic) ganglia by way of a pair of thin sympathetic rami. **A,** Superior view of a pair of thoracic spinal nerves. **B,** Anterior view of several pairs of thoracic spinal nerves.

SPINAL NERVES AND PERIPHERAL BRANCHES

SPINAL NERVES	PLEXUSES FORMED FROM ANTERIOR RAMI	SPINAL NERVE BRANCHES FROM PLEXUSES	PARTS SUPPLIED
Cervical 1 2 3 4	Cervical plexus	Lesser occipital Greater auricular Cutaneous nerve of neck Supraclavicular nerves Branches to muscles Phrenic nerve	Sensory to back of head, front of neck, and upper part of shoulder; motor to numerous neck muscles Diaphragm
Cervical 5 6 7 8	Brachial plexus	Suprascapular and dorsoscapular Thoracic nerves, medial and lateral branches	Superficial muscles* of scapula Pectoralis major and minor
Thoracic (or Dorsal) 1 2 3		Long thoracic nerve Thoracodorsal Subscapular Axillary (circumflex) Musculocutaneous	Serratus anterior Latissimus dorsi Subscapular and teres major muscles Deltoid and teres minor muscles and skin over deltoid Muscles of front of arm (biceps brachii, coracobrachialis, brachialis) and skin on outer side of forearm

			Description
No plexus formed; branches run directly to intercostal muscles and skin of thorax			
4			
5			
6			
7	Ulnar		Flexor carpi ulnaris and part of flexor digitorum profundus; some muscles of hand; sensory to medial side of hand, little finger, and medial half of fourth finger
8	Median		Rest of muscles of front of forearm and hand; sensory to skin of palmar surface of thumb, index, and middle fingers
9	Radial		Triceps muscle and muscles of back of forearm; sensory to skin of back of forearm and hand
10	Medial cutaneous		Sensory to inner surface of arm and forearm
11			
12			
Lumbar	Iliohypogastric	Sometimes fused	Sensory to anterior abdominal wall
1	Ilioinguinal		Sensory to anterior abdominal wall and external genitalia; motor to muscles of abdominal wall
2	Genitofemoral		Sensory to skin of external genitalia and inguinal region
3	Lateral femoral cutaneous		Sensory to outer side of thigh
4			
5			

*Although nerves to muscles are considered motor nerves, they do contain some sensory fibers that transmit proprioceptive impulses.

†Sensory fibers from the tibial and peroneal nerves unite to form the medial cutaneous (or sural) nerve that supplies the calf of the leg and the lateral surface of the foot. In the thigh the tibial and common peroneal nerves are usually enclosed in a single sheath to form the sciatic nerve, the largest nerve in the body with a width of approximately ¾ inch (2 cm). About two thirds of the way down the posterior part of the thigh, the sciatic nerve divides into its component parts. Branches of the sciatic nerve extend into the hamstring muscles.

Continued

SPINAL NERVES AND PERIPHERAL BRANCHES—cont'd

SPINAL NERVES	PLEXUSES FORMED FROM ANTERIOR RAMI	SPINAL NERVE BRANCHES FROM PLEXUSES	PARTS SUPPLIED
Sacral 1 2 3 4 5	Lumbosacral plexus	Femoral	Motor to quadriceps, sartorius, and iliacus muscles; sensory to front of thigh and medial side of leg (saphenous nerve)
		Obturator	Motor to adductor muscles of thigh
		Tibial† (medial popliteal)	Motor to muscles of calf of leg; sensory to skin of calf of leg and sole of foot
		Common peroneal (lateral popliteal)	Motor to evertors and dorsiflexors of foot; sensory to lateral surface of leg and dorsal surface of foot
		Nerves to hamstring muscles	Motor to muscles of back of thigh
		Gluteal nerves	Motor to buttock muscles and tensor fasciae latae
		Posterior femoral cutaneous	Sensory to skin of buttocks, posterior surface of thigh, and leg
		Pudendal nerve	Motor to perineal muscles; sensory to skin of perineum
Coccygeal 1	Coccygeal plexus	Anococcygeal nerves	Sensory to skin overlying coccyx

Cervical plexus

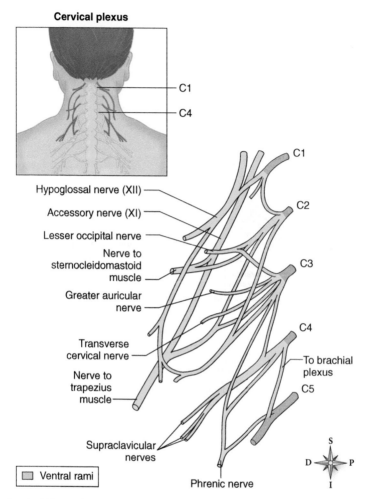

Cervical Plexus. Ventral rami of the first four cervical spinal nerves (C1 through C4) exchange fibers in this plexus found deep within the neck. Notice that some fibers from C5 also enter this plexus to form a portion of the phrenic nerve.

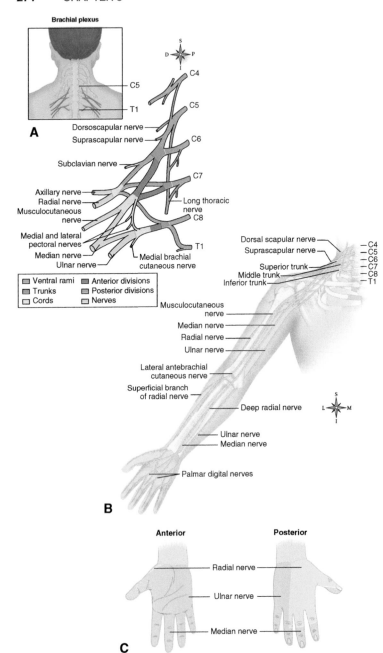

Brachial plexus

A

C5
T1

C4
C5
Dorsoscapular nerve —
Suprascapular nerve —
C6
Subclavian nerve —
C7
Axillary nerve —
Radial nerve —
Musculocutaneous nerve —
Long thoracic nerve
C8
Medial and lateral pectoral nerves —
T1
Median nerve —
Ulnar nerve —
Medial brachial cutaneous nerve

☐ Ventral rami   ☐ Anterior divisions
☐ Trunks   ☐ Posterior divisions
☐ Cords   ☐ Nerves

B

Dorsal scapular nerve — C4
Suprascapular nerve — C5, C6
Superior trunk — C7
Middle trunk — C8
Inferior trunk — T1

Musculocutaneous nerve —
Median nerve —
Radial nerve —
Ulnar nerve —
Lateral antebrachial cutaneous nerve —
Superficial branch of radial nerve —
Deep radial nerve —
Ulnar nerve —
Median nerve —
Palmar digital nerves —

C

Anterior   Posterior
Radial nerve
Ulnar nerve
Median nerve

Brachial Plexus. A, From the five rami (C5 through T1), the plexus forms three "trunks." Each trunk in turn subdivides into an anterior and posterior "division." The divisional branches then reorganize into three "cords." The cords then give rise to the individual nerves that exit this plexus. **B,** Nerves of the brachial plexus. **C,** Innervation of the hand.

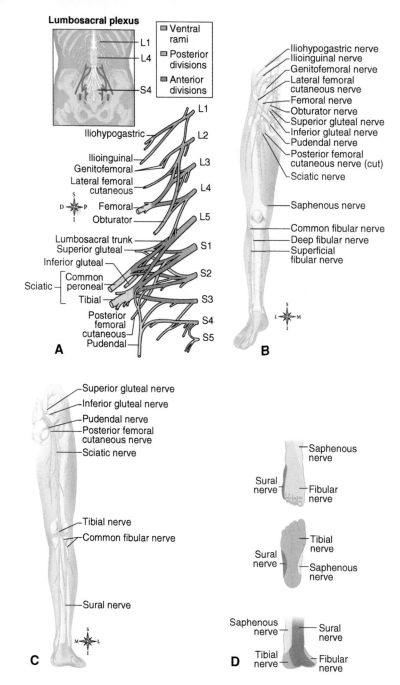

Lumbosacral Plexus. A, This plexus is formed by the combination of the lumbar plexus with the sacral plexus, as shown in the *inset*. Notice that the ventral rami split into anterior and posterior "divisions" before reorganizing into the various individual nerves that exit this plexus. **B,** Anterior view of lumbosacral plexus nerves. **C,** Posterior view of lumbosacral plexus nerves. **D,** Innervation of the foot and ankle.

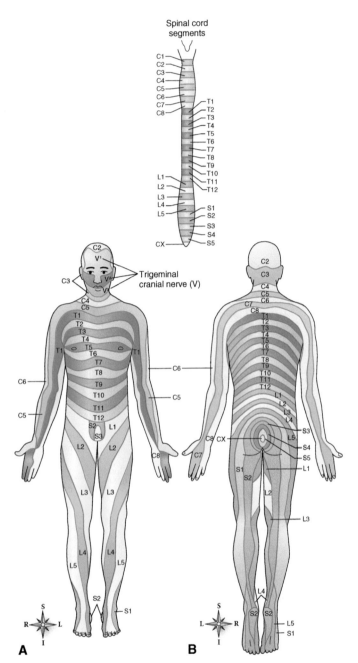

Dermatome Distribution of the Spinal Nerves. A, The front of the body's surface. **B,** The back of the body's surface. The *inset* shows the segments of the spinal cord connected with each of the spinal nerves associated with the sensory dermatomes shown. *C,* Cervical segments and spinal nerves; *T,* thoracic segments and spinal nerves; *L,* lumbar segments and spinal nerves; *S,* sacral segments and spinal nerves; *CX,* coccygeal segment and spinal nerves.

Cranial Nerves

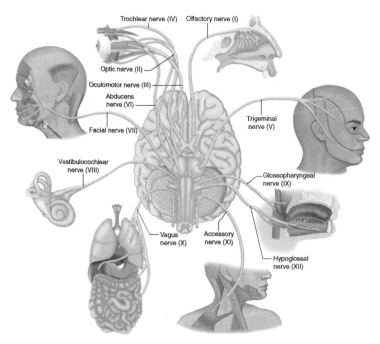

Cranial Nerves. Ventral surface of the brain showing attachment of the cranial nerves.

STRUCTURE AND FUNCTION OF THE CRANIAL NERVES

sensory (afferent)
motor (efferent)

| NERVE | | SENSORY FIBERS | | | MOTOR FIBERS | | |
		RECEPTORS	CELL BODIES	TERMINATION	CELL BODIES	TERMINATION	FUNCTIONS
I OLFACTORY 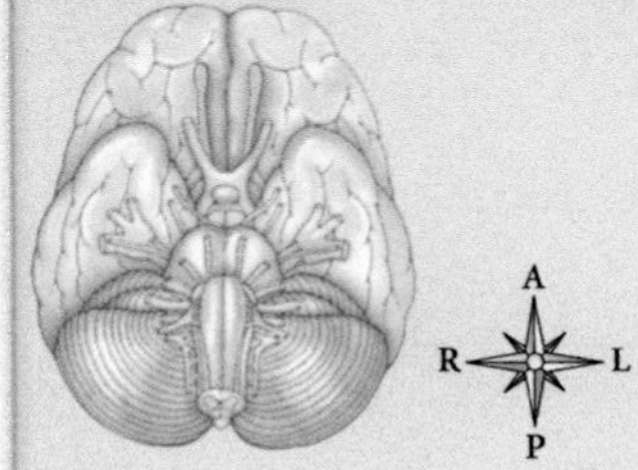		Nasal mucosa	Nasal mucosa	Olfactory bulbs (new relay of neurons to olfactory cortex)			Sense of smell
II OPTIC 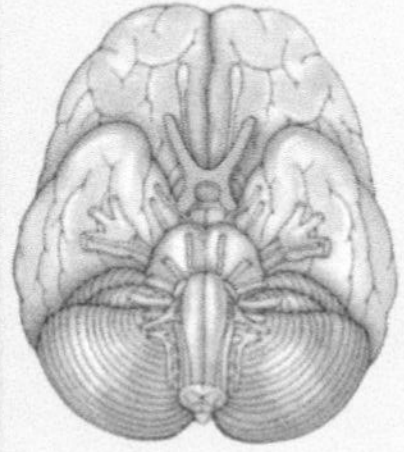		Retina (proprioceptive)	Retina	Nucleus in thalamus (lateral geniculate); some fibers terminate in superior colliculus of midbrain			Vision

Nerve					
III OCULOMOTOR 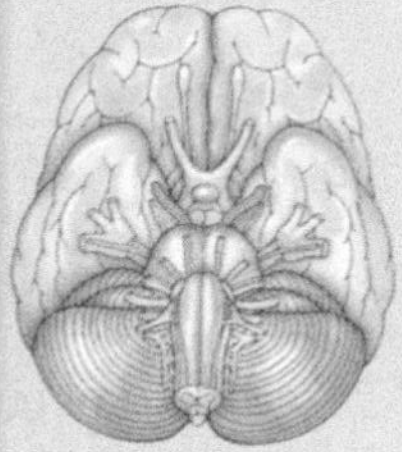	External eye muscles except superior oblique and lateral rectus	Trigeminal ganglion	Midbrain (oculomotor nucleus)	Midbrain (oculomotor nucleus)	External eye muscles except superior oblique and lateral rectus; autonomic fibers terminate in ciliary ganglion and then to ciliary and iris muscles	Eye movements, regulation of size of pupil, accommodation (for near vision), proprioception (muscle sense)
	Superior oblique (proprioceptive)					
IV TROCHLEAR 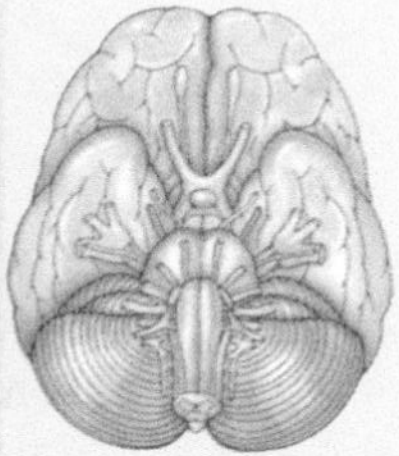	Superior oblique (proprioceptive)	Trigeminal ganglion	Midbrain	Midbrain	Superior oblique muscle of eye	Eye movements, proprioception

Continued

STRUCTURE AND FUNCTION OF THE CRANIAL NERVES—cont'd

■ sensory (afferent)
■ motor (efferent)

| NERVE | SENSORY FIBERS | | | MOTOR FIBERS | | |
	RECEPTORS	CELL BODIES	TERMINATION	CELL BODIES	TERMINATION	FUNCTIONS
V TRIGEMINAL 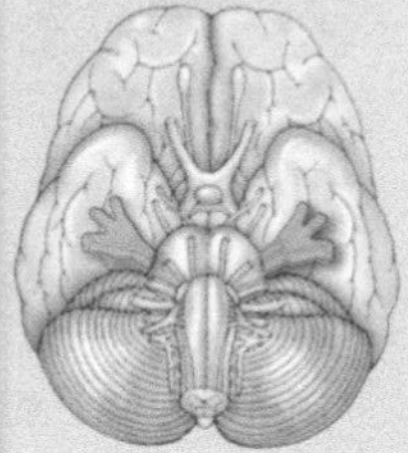	Skin and mucosa of head, teeth	Trigeminal ganglion	Pons (sensory nucleus)	Pons (motor nucleus)	Muscles of mastication	Sensations of head and face, chewing movements, proprioception
VI ABDUCENS 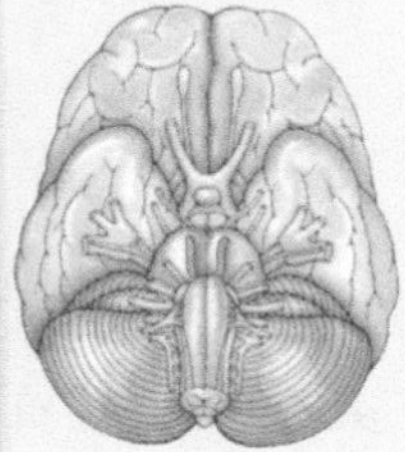	Lateral rectus (proprioceptive)	Trigeminal ganglion	Pons	Pons	Lateral rectus muscle of eye	Abduction of eye, proprioception

VII FACIAL 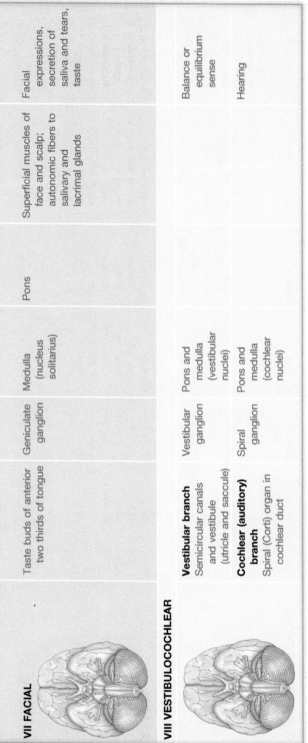	Taste buds of anterior two thirds of tongue	Geniculate ganglion	Medulla (nucleus solitarius)	Pons	Superficial muscles of face and scalp; autonomic fibers to salivary and lacrimal glands	Facial expressions, secretion of saliva and tears, taste
VIII VESTIBULOCOCHLEAR						
Vestibular branch Semicircular canals and vestibule (utricle and saccule)		Vestibular ganglion	Pons and medulla (vestibular nuclei)			Balance or equilibrium sense
Cochlear (auditory) branch Spiral (Corti) organ in cochlear duct		Spiral ganglion	Pons and medulla (cochlear nuclei)			Hearing

Continued

STRUCTURE AND FUNCTION OF THE CRANIAL NERVES—cont'd

■ sensory (afferent)
■ motor (efferent)

NERVE	SENSORY FIBERS				MOTOR FIBERS		
	RECEPTORS	CELL BODIES	TERMINATION	CELL BODIES	TERMINATION		FUNCTIONS
IX GLOSSOPHARYNGEAL	Pharynx; taste buds and other receptors of posterior third of tongue	Jugular and petrous ganglia	Medulla (nucleus solitarius)	Medulla (nucleus ambiguus)	Muscles of pharynx		Sensations of tongue, swallowing movements, secretion of saliva, aid in reflex control of blood pressure and respiration
	Carotid sinus and carotid body	Jugular and petrous ganglia	Medulla (respiratory and vasomotor centers)	Medulla at junction of pons (nucleus salivatorius)	Otic ganglion and then to parotid salivary gland		
X VAGUS	Pharynx, larynx, carotid body, thoracic and abdominal viscera	Jugular and nodose ganglia	Medulla (nucleus solitarius), pons (nucleus of fifth cranial nerve)	Medulla (dorsal motor nucleus)	Ganglia of vagal plexus and then to muscles of pharynx, larynx, and autonomic fibers to thoracic and abdominal viscera		Sensations and movements of organs supplied; e.g., slows heart, increases peristalsis, contracts muscles for voice production

XI ACCESSORY 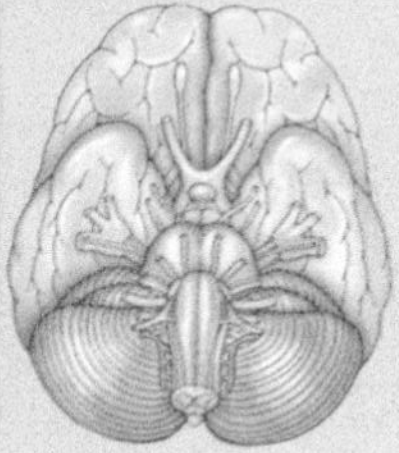	Trapezius and sternocleidomastoid (proprioceptive)	Upper cervical ganglia	Spinal cord	Anterior gray column of first five or six cervical segments of spinal cord	Trapezius and sternocleidomastoid muscle	Shoulder movements, turning movements of head, proprioception
XII HYPOGLOSSAL 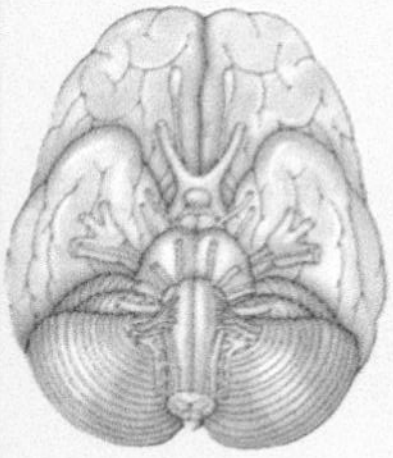	Tongue muscles (proprioceptive)	Trigeminal ganglion	Medulla (hypoglossal nucleus)	Medulla (hypoglossal nucleus)	Muscles of tongue and throat	Tongue movements, proprioception

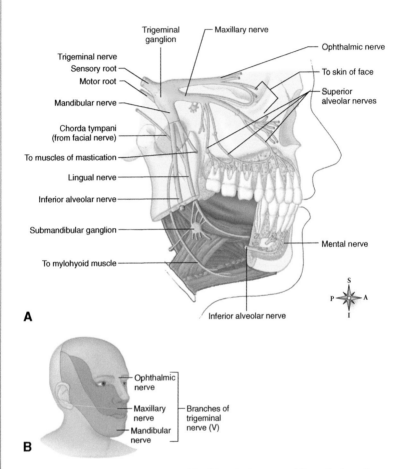

Trigeminal Nerve (V). A, The route of the trigeminal nerve and its major branches. **B,** Sensory fibers of the trigeminal nerve form three branch nerves (ophthalmic, maxillary, and mandibular nerves), each of which conducts information from a different region of the face.

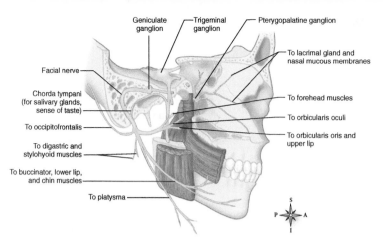

Facial Nerve (VII). Artist's interpretation of the location of the various branches of the facial nerve.

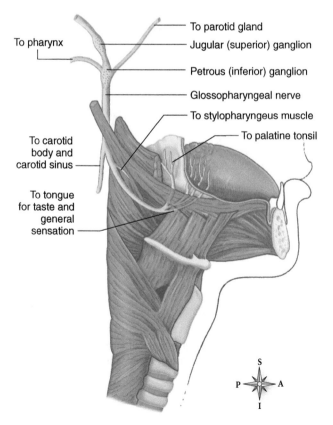

Glossopharyngeal Nerve (IX). As its name implies (*glosso-*, "tongue"; -*pharyng-*, "throat"), the ninth cranial nerve supplies fibers to the tongue and throat. It is a mixed nerve that carries both sensory and motor fibers.

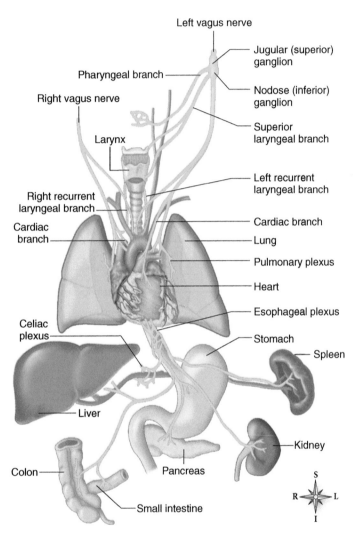

Vagus Nerve (X). The vagus nerve is a mixed cranial nerve with many widely distributed branches—hence the name *vagus*, which is the Latin word for "wanderer."

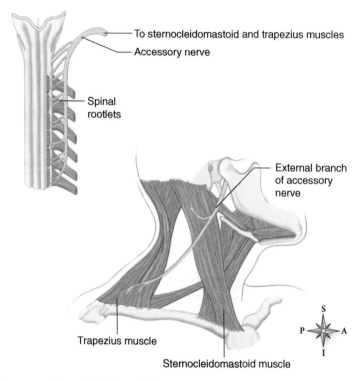

To sternocleidomastoid and trapezius muscles

Accessory nerve

Spinal rootlets

External branch of accessory nerve

Trapezius muscle

Sternocleidomastoid muscle

Accessory Nerve (XI). This cranial nerve is an "accessory" to the vagus nerve because some of its fibers join the vagus nerve before traveling on to the viscera, pharynx, and larynx. Fibers that originate in the cervical spinal segments travel through an external nerve branch to the trapezius and sternocleidomastoid muscles of the neck.

AUTONOMIC NERVOUS SYSTEM

Structure of the Autonomic Nervous System

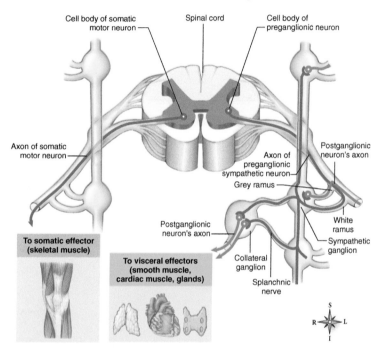

Diagram of Autonomic Conduction Paths. The *left side* of the diagram shows that one somatic motor neuron conducts impulses all the way from the spinal cord to a somatic effector. Conduction from the spinal cord to any visceral effector, however, requires a relay of at least two autonomic motor neurons—a preganglionic and a postganglionic neuron, shown on the *right side* of the diagram.

COMPARISON OF SOMATIC AND AUTONOMIC PATHWAYS

FEATURE	SOMATIC MOTOR PATHWAYS	AUTONOMIC EFFERENT PATHWAYS
Direction of information flow	Efferent	Efferent
Number of neurons between CNS and effector	One (somatic motor neuron)	Two (preganglionic and postganglionic)
Myelin sheath present	Yes	Preganglionic: yes Postganglionic: no
Location of peripheral fibers	Most cranial nerves and all spinal nerves	Most cranial nerves and all spinal nerves
Effector innervated	Skeletal muscle (voluntary)	Smooth and cardiac muscle, glands, and adipose and other tissues (involuntary)
Neurotransmitter	Acetylcholine	Acetylcholine or norepinephrine

CNS, Central nervous system.

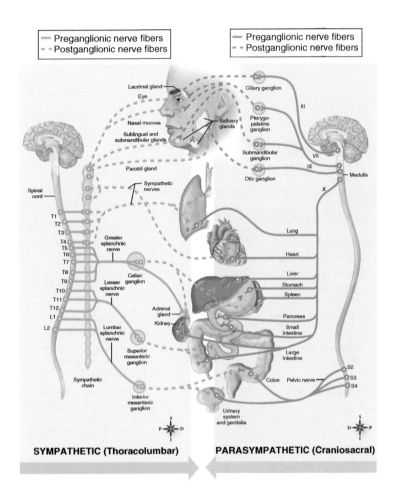

Major Autonomic Pathways.

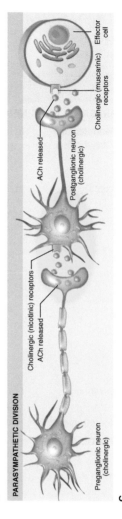

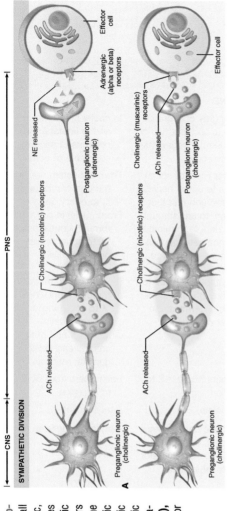

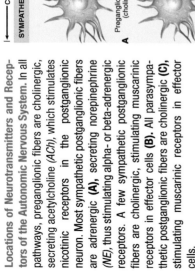

Locations of Neurotransmitters and Receptors of the Autonomic Nervous System. In all pathways, preganglionic fibers are cholinergic, secreting acetylcholine *(ACh)*, which stimulates nicotinic receptors in the postganglionic neuron. Most sympathetic postganglionic fibers are adrenergic **(A)**, secreting norepinephrine *(NE)*, thus stimulating alpha- or beta-adrenergic receptors. A few sympathetic postganglionic fibers are cholinergic, stimulating muscarinic receptors in effector cells **(B)**. All parasympathetic postganglionic fibers are cholinergic **(C)**, stimulating muscarinic receptors in effector cells.

COMPARISON OF STRUCTURAL FEATURES OF THE SYMPATHETIC AND PARASYMPATHETIC PATHWAYS

NEURONS	SYMPATHETIC PATHWAYS	PARASYMPATHETIC PATHWAYS
PREGANGLIONIC NEURONS		
Dendrites and cell bodies	In lateral gray columns of thoracic and first two or three lumbar segments of spinal cord	In nuclei of brainstem and in lateral gray columns of sacral segments of cord
Axons	In anterior roots of spinal nerves to spinal nerves (thoracic and first four lumbar), to and through white rami to terminate in sympathetic ganglia at various levels or to extend through sympathetic ganglia, to and through splanchnic nerves to terminate in collateral ganglia	From brainstem nuclei through cranial nerve III to ciliary ganglion From nuclei in pons through cranial nerve VII to sphenopalatine or submaxillary ganglion From nuclei in medulla through cranial nerve IX to otic ganglion or through cranial nerves X and XI to cardiac and celiac ganglia, respectively
Distribution	Short fibers from CNS to ganglion	Long fibers from CNS to ganglion
Neurotransmitter	Acetylcholine	Acetylcholine
GANGLIA	Sympathetic chain ganglia (22 pairs); collateral ganglia (celiac, superior, inferior mesenteric)	Terminal ganglia (in or near effector)

COMPARISON OF STRUCTURAL FEATURES OF THE SYMPATHETIC AND PARASYMPATHETIC PATHWAYS—cont'd

NEURONS	SYMPATHETIC PATHWAYS	PARASYMPATHETIC PATHWAYS
POSTGANGLIONIC NEURONS		
Dendrites and cell bodies	In sympathetic and collateral ganglia	In parasympathetic ganglia (e.g., ciliary, sphenopalatine, submaxillary, otic, cardiac, celiac) located in or near visceral effector organs
Receptors	Cholinergic (nicotinic)	Cholinergic (nicotinic)
Axons	In autonomic nerves and plexuses that innervate thoracic and abdominal viscera and blood vessels in these cavities In gray rami to spinal nerves, to smooth muscle of skin, blood vessels, and hair follicles, and to sweat glands	In short nerves to various visceral effector organs
Distribution	Long fibers from ganglion to widespread effectors	Short fibers from ganglion to single effector
Neurotransmitter	Norepinephrine (many); acetylcholine (few)	Acetylcholine

CNS, Central nervous system.

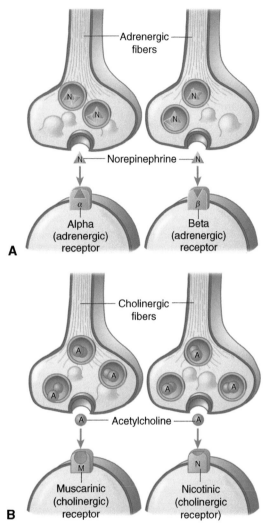

Functions of Autonomic Neurotransmitters and Receptors. A, Norepinephrine released from adrenergic fibers binds to alpha- or beta-adrenergic receptors according to the lock-and-key model to produce regulatory effects in the postsynaptic cell. **B,** Acetylcholine released from cholinergic fibers similarly binds to muscarinic or nicotinic cholinergic receptors to produce postsynaptic regulatory effects.

Neurotransmitters

- N Norepinephrine
- A Acetylcholine

Receptors

- α Alpha (adrenergic) receptor
- β Beta (adrenergic) receptor
- M Muscarinic (cholinergic) receptor
- N Nicotinic (cholinergic) receptor

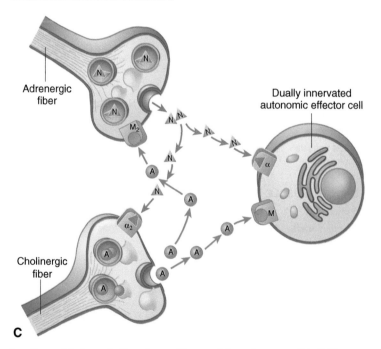

C

Functions of Autonomic Neurotransmitters and Receptors—cont'd. **C,** The complex manner in which neurotransmitters and receptors regulate dually innervated effector cells shows that a summation of effects on receptors at both presynaptic and postsynaptic locations may occur. For example, norepinephrine released by an adrenergic fiber may bind to postsynaptic alpha (or beta) receptors to influence the effector cell and may also bind to presynaptic alpha (α_2) receptors in a cholinergic fiber to inhibit the release of acetylcholine, a possible antagonist to norepinephrine.

Functions of the Autonomic Nervous System

AUTONOMIC FUNCTIONS

AUTONOMIC EFFECTOR	EFFECT OF SYMPATHETIC STIMULATION (NEUROTRANSMITTER: NOREPINEPHRINE UNLESS OTHERWISE STATED)	EFFECT OF PARASYMPATHETIC STIMULATION (NEUROTRANSMITTER: ACETYLCHOLINE)
CARDIAC MUSCLE	Increased rate and strength of contraction (beta receptors)	Decreased rate and strength of contraction
SMOOTH MUSCLE OF BLOOD VESSELS		
Skin blood vessels	Constriction (alpha receptors)	No effect
Skeletal muscle blood vessels	Dilation (beta receptors)	No effect
Coronary blood vessels	Constriction (alpha receptors) Dilation (beta receptors)	Dilation
Abdominal blood vessels	Constriction (alpha receptors)	No effect
Blood vessels of external genitalia	Constriction (alpha receptors)	Dilation of blood vessels causing erection
SMOOTH MUSCLE OF HOLLOW ORGANS AND SPHINCTERS		
Bronchioles	Relaxation (dilation)	Constriction
Digestive tract, except sphincters	Decreased peristalsis	Increased peristalsis
Sphincters of digestive tract	Contraction	Relaxation
Urinary bladder	Relaxation	Contraction
Urinary sphincters	Contraction	Relaxation
Reproductive ducts	Constriction	Relaxation

AUTONOMIC FUNCTIONS—cont'd

AUTONOMIC EFFECTOR	EFFECT OF SYMPATHETIC STIMULATION (NEUROTRANSMITTER: NOREPINEPHRINE UNLESS OTHERWISE STATED)	EFFECT OF PARASYMPATHETIC STIMULATION (NEUROTRANSMITTER: ACETYLCHOLINE)
EYE		
Iris	Contraction of radial muscle; dilated pupil	Contraction of circular muscle; constricted pupil
Ciliary	Relaxation; accommodates for far vision	Contraction; accommodates for near vision
Hairs (arrector pili muscles)	Contraction produces goose pimples or piloerection (alpha receptors)	No effect
GLANDS		
Sweat	Increased sweat (neurotransmitter, acetylcholine)	No effect
Lacrimal	No effect	Increased secretion of tears
Digestive (salivary, gastric, etc.)	Decreased secretion of saliva; not known for others	Increased secretion of saliva
Pancreas, including islets	Decreased secretion	Increased secretion of pancreatic juice and insulin
Liver	Increased glycogenolysis (beta receptors); increased blood sugar level	No effect
Adrenal medulla*	Increased epinephrine secretion	No effect
Adipose	Increased lipolysis	No effect
SKELETAL MUSCLE†	During intense exercise, regulates contractility to prevent fatigue (beta receptors)	No effect

*Sympathetic preganglionic axons terminate in contact with secreting cells of the adrenal medulla. Thus, the adrenal medulla functions, to quote someone's descriptive phrase, as a "giant sympathetic postganglionic neuron."

†Skeletal muscle is primarily a somatic effector but during intense exercise, subconscious autonomic stimulation also occurs.

SUMMARY OF THE SYMPATHETIC "FIGHT-OR-FLIGHT" REACTION

RESPONSE	ROLE IN PROMOTING ENERGY USE BY SKELETAL MUSCLES
Increased heart rate	Increased rate of blood flow, thus increased delivery of oxygen and glucose to skeletal muscles
Increased strength of cardiac muscle contractions	Increased rate of blood flow, thus increased delivery of oxygen and glucose to skeletal muscles
Dilation of coronary vessels of the heart	Increased delivery of oxygen and nutrients to cardiac muscle to sustain increased rate and strength of heart contractions
Dilation of blood vessels in skeletal muscles	Increased delivery of oxygen and nutrients to skeletal muscles
Increased stimulation at neuromuscular junctions and increased ion pump activity in skeletal muscles	Increased availability of ACh at the neuromuscular junction and more efficient restoration of resting ion balance in muscle fibers both reduce fatigue in skeletal muscles
Constriction of blood vessels in digestive and other organs	Shunting of blood to skeletal muscles to increase oxygen and glucose delivery
Contraction of spleen and other blood reservoirs	More blood discharged into general circulation, causing increased delivery of oxygen and glucose to skeletal muscles
Dilation of respiratory airways	Increased loading of oxygen into blood
Increased rate and depth of breathing	Increased loading of oxygen into blood (indirect effect)
Increased sweating	Increased dissipation of heat generated by skeletal muscle activity
Increased conversion of glycogen into glucose	Increased amount of glucose available to skeletal muscles
Increased breakdown of stored fats	Increased amount of fatty acids and glycerol available to skeletal muscles

SENSE ORGANS

Sensory Receptors

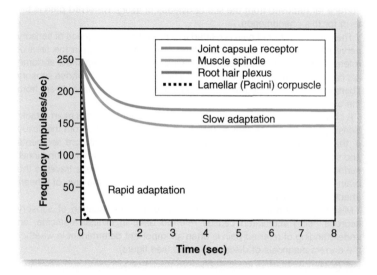

Adaptation of Sensory Receptors. In the presence of a continuous stimulus, the rate (frequency) of impulses declines quickly in rapidly adapting receptors of the skin. Here the initial stimulus, representing a change, is valuable information. However, continued sensation from the skin may be distracting. In slow-adapting joint and muscle receptors, the rate of impulses instead declines gradually and levels off to a constant, moderately high level. Thus information about body position is continually sent to the central nervous system.

REFERRED PAIN

The stimulation of pain receptors in deep structures may be felt as pain in the skin that lies over the affected organ or in an area of skin on the body surface far removed from the site of disease or injury. **Referred pain** is the term for this phenomenon.

The cause of referred pain is related to a mixing or convergence of sensory nerve impulses from both the diseased organ and the skin in the area of referred pain. For example, pain originating in an organ deep in the abdominal cavity is often interpreted as coming from an area of skin whose sensory fibers enter the same segment of the spinal cord as the sensory fibers from the deep structure.

A classic example is the referred pain often associated with a heart attack. Sensory fibers from the skin on the chest over the heart and from the tissue of the heart itself enter the first to the fifth thoracic spinal cord segments and so do sensory fibers from the skin areas over the left shoulder and inner surface of the left arm. Sensory impulses from all these areas travel to the brain over a common pathway. Thus the brain may feel the pain of a heart attack in the shoulder or arm.

Misinterpretation in the brain in regard to the true location of sensory neurons being stimulated causes referred pain. In clinical medicine, an understanding of referred pain is often an important determinant in whether the correct diagnosis of disease is made (see figure).

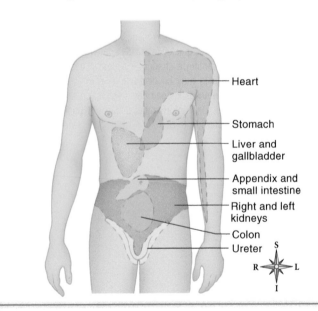

CLASSIFICATION OF SOMATIC SENSORY RECEPTORS

BY STRUCTURE	BY LOCATION AND TYPE	BY ACTIVATION STIMULUS	BY SENSATION OR FUNCTION
FREE NERVE ENDINGS			
Nociceptor Dendritic knobs	Either exteroceptor or visceroceptor—most body tissues	Almost any noxious stimulus; temperature change; mechanical	Pain; temperature; itch; tickle
Tactile (Merkel) disk (meniscus) Tactile epithelial cell — Tactile disk	Exteroceptor	Light pressure; mechanical	Discriminative touch

Continued

CLASSIFICATION OF SOMATIC SENSORY RECEPTORS—cont'd

BY STRUCTURE	BY LOCATION AND TYPE	BY ACTIVATION STIMULUS	BY SENSATION OR FUNCTION
Root hair plexus 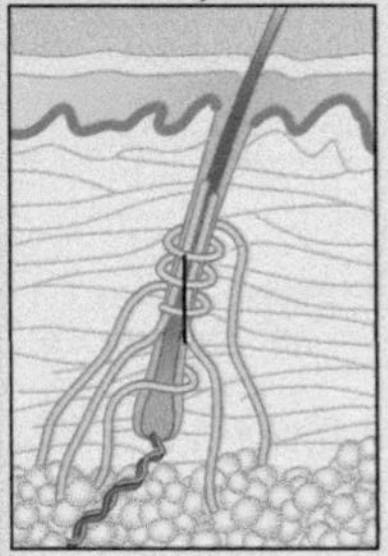	Exteroceptor	Hair movement; mechanical	Sense of "deflection" type of movement of hair
ENCAPSULATED NERVE ENDINGS **TOUCH AND PRESSURE RECEPTORS**			
Tactile (Meissner) corpuscle 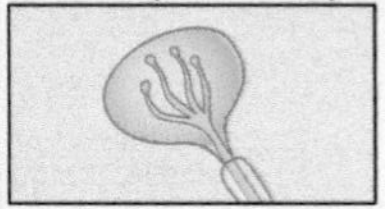	Exteroceptor; epidermis, hairless skin	Light pressure, mechanical	Touch; low-frequency vibration
Bulboid (Krause) corpuscle 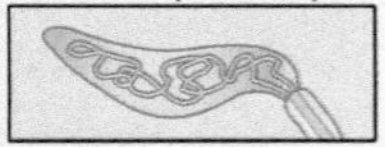	Exteroceptor; mucous membranes	Mechanical	Touch; low-frequency vibration; textural sensation
Bulbous (Ruffini) corpuscle 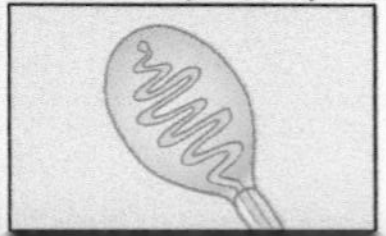	Exteroceptor; dermis of skin	Mechanical	Crude and persistent touch

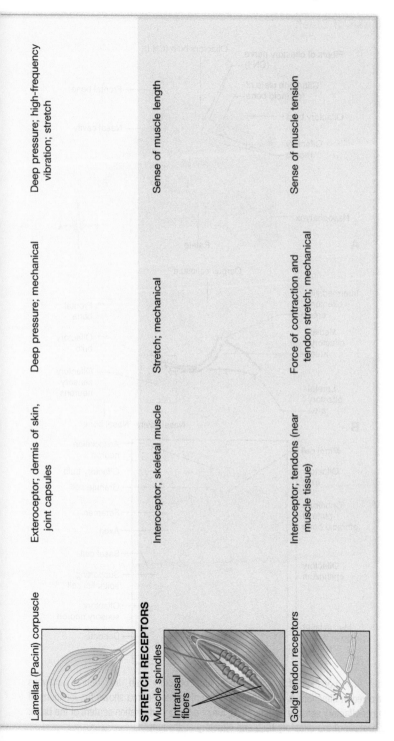

	Deep pressure; high-frequency vibration; stretch	Sense of muscle length	
	Deep pressure; mechanical	Stretch; mechanical	Sense of muscle tension
Exteroceptor; dermis of skin, joint capsules		Interoceptor; skeletal muscle	Force of contraction and tendon stretch; mechanical
			Interoceptor; tendons (near muscle tissue)

Lamellar (Pacini) corpuscle

STRETCH RECEPTORS

Muscle spindles

Intrafusal fibers

Golgi tendon receptors

Sense of Smell

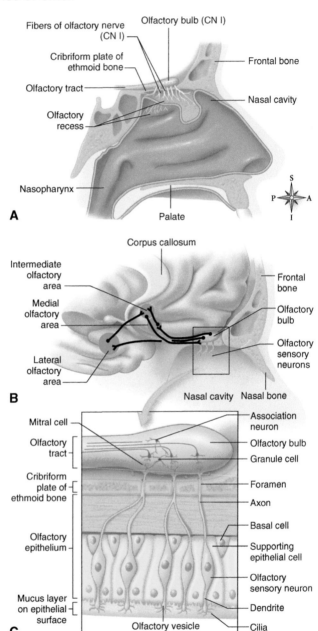

Olfaction. Location of olfactory epithelium, olfactory bulb, and neural pathways involved in olfaction. **A,** Midsagittal section of the nasal area shows the locations of major olfactory sensory structures. **B,** Major olfactory integration centers of the brain. **C,** Details of the olfactory bulb and olfactory epithelium.

Sense of Taste

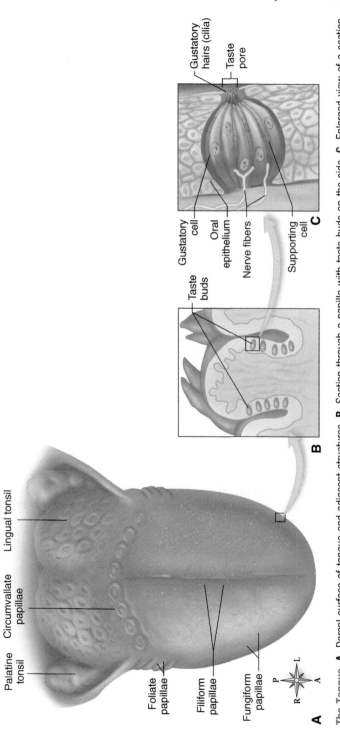

The Tongue. A, Dorsal surface of tongue and adjacent structures. **B,** Section through a papilla with taste buds on the side. **C,** Enlarged view of a section through a taste bud.

Labels in image A:
- Palatine tonsil
- Circumvallate papillae
- Lingual tonsil
- Foliate papillae
- Filiform papillae
- Fungiform papillae

Labels in image B:
- Taste buds

Labels in image C:
- Gustatory hairs (cilia)
- Taste pore
- Gustatory cell
- Oral epithelium
- Nerve fibers
- Supporting cell

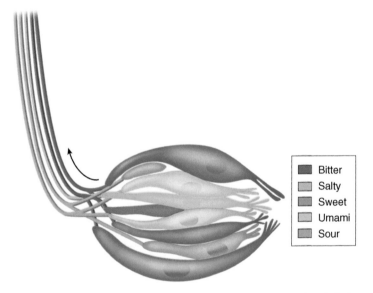

Taste Receptors. The labeled-line model of gustation (taste) holds that each distinct taste has a separate group of taste receptors, with each group sending its impulses along a distinct "line" or neural pathway.

Senses of Hearing and Balance: The Ear

External ear (not to scale)

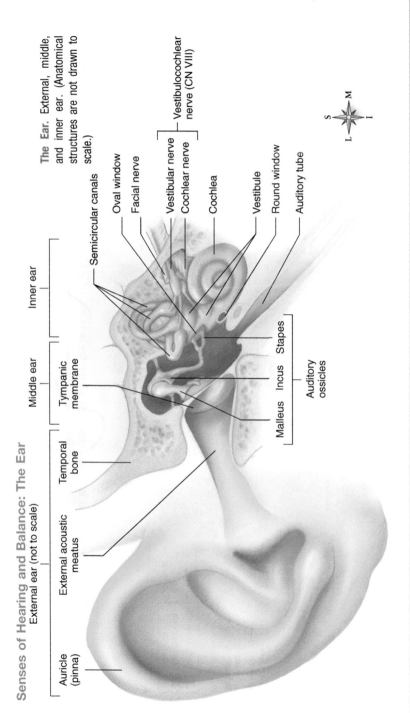

The Ear. External, middle, and inner ear. (Anatomical structures are not drawn to scale.)

Semicircular canals

Oval window

Facial nerve

Vestibular nerve

Cochlear nerve

Vestibulocochlear nerve (CN VIII)

Cochlea

Vestibule

Round window

Auditory tube

Inner ear

Middle ear

Tympanic membrane

Temporal bone

External acoustic meatus

Auricle (pinna)

Stapes

Incus

Malleus

Auditory ossicles

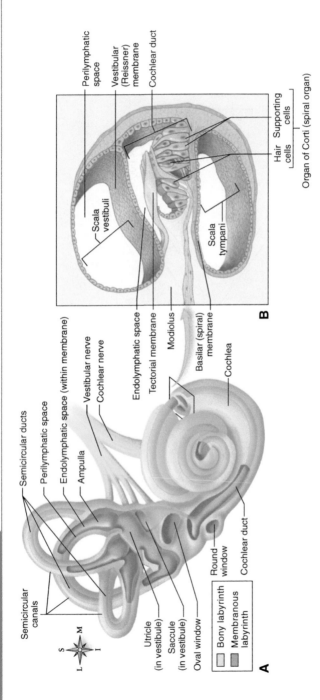

The Inner Ear. A, The bony labyrinth *(bone colored)* is the hard outer wall of the entire inner ear and includes semicircular canals, vestibule, and cochlea. Within the bony labyrinth is the membranous labyrinth *(purple)*, which is surrounded by perilymph and filled with endolymph. Each ampulla in the vestibule contains a crista ampullaris that detects changes in head position and sends sensory impulses through the vestibular nerve to the brain. **B,** The *inset* shows a section of the membranous cochlea. Hair cells in the organ of Corti (spiral organ) detect sound and send the information through the cochlear nerve. The vestibular and cochlear nerves join to form the eighth cranial nerve.

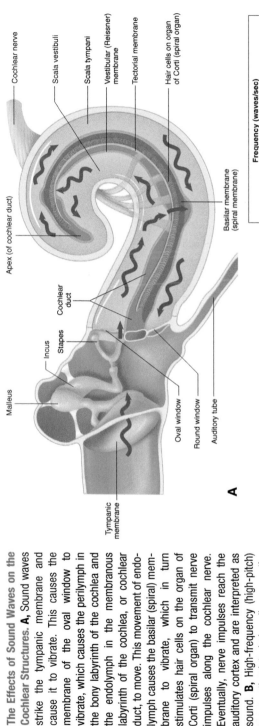

The Effects of Sound Waves on the Cochlear Structures. A, Sound waves strike the tympanic membrane and cause it to vibrate. This causes the membrane of the oval window to vibrate, which causes the perilymph in the bony labyrinth of the cochlea and the endolymph in the membranous labyrinth of the cochlea, or cochlear duct, to move. This movement of endolymph causes the basilar (spiral) membrane to vibrate, which in turn stimulates hair cells on the organ of Corti (spiral organ) to transmit nerve impulses along the cochlear nerve. Eventually, nerve impulses reach the auditory cortex and are interpreted as sound. **B,** High-frequency (high-pitch) waves stimulate hair cells nearer the stapes (oval window) and low-frequency (low-pitch) waves stimulate hair cells nearer the distal end of the cochlea. The location of peak stimulation of the hair cells allows the brain to interpret the pitch of the sound.

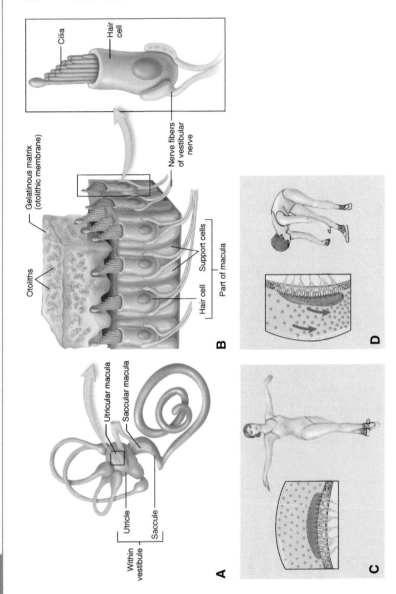

The Macula. A, Structure of vestibule showing placement of utricular and saccular maculae. **B,** Section of macula showing otoliths. **C,** Macula stationary in upright position. **D,** Macula displaced by gravity as person bends over.

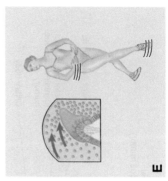

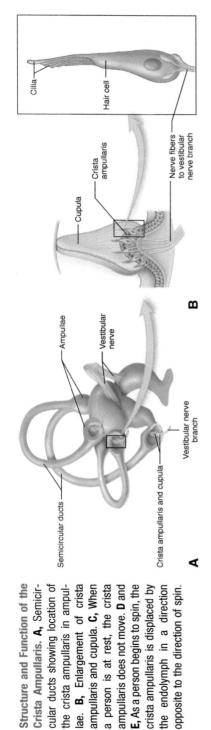

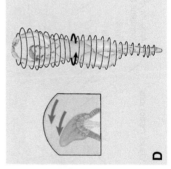

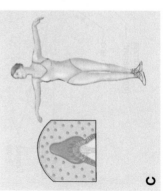

Structure and Function of the Crista Ampullaris. A, Semicircular ducts showing location of the crista ampullaris in ampullae. **B,** Enlargement of crista ampullaris and cupula. **C,** When a person is at rest, the crista ampullaris does not move. **D** and **E,** As a person begins to spin, the crista ampullaris is displaced by the endolymph in a direction opposite to the direction of spin.

Vision: The Eye

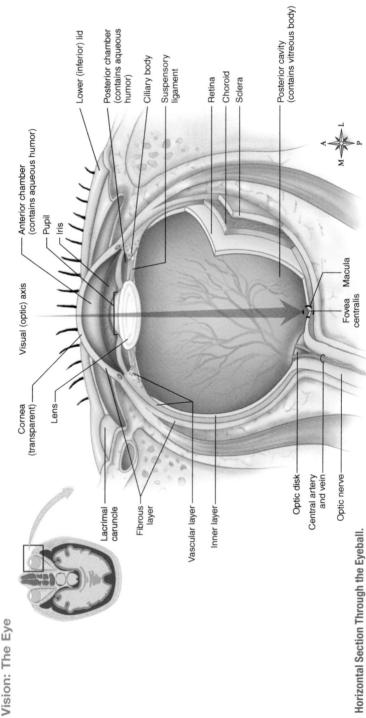

Horizontal Section Through the Eyeball.
The eye is viewed from above.

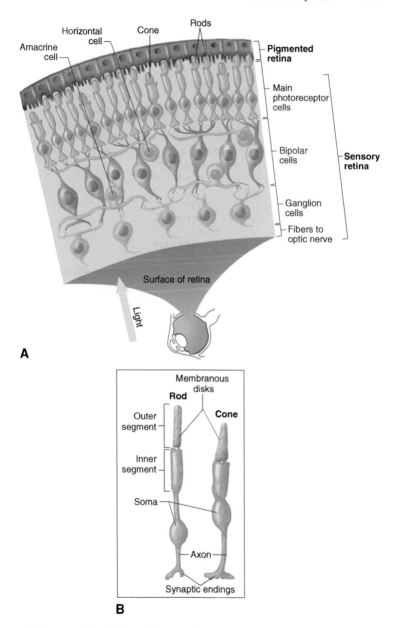

Cell Layers of the Retina. A, Pigmented and sensory layers of the retina. **B,** Rod and cone cells. Note their variation in the general structure of a neuron.

COATS OF THE EYEBALL

LOCATION	POSTERIOR PORTION	ANTERIOR PORTION	CHARACTERISTICS
Fibrous layer	Sclera	Cornea	Protective fibrous coat, cornea transparent, rest of layer white and opaque
Vascular layer	Choroid	Ciliary body, suspensory ligament, iris (pupil is hole in iris); lens suspended in suspensory ligament	Vascular, pigmented layer
Inner layer	Retinal blood vessels; optic nerve	Retna	Nervous tissue; rods and cones (receptors for second cranial nerve) located in retina

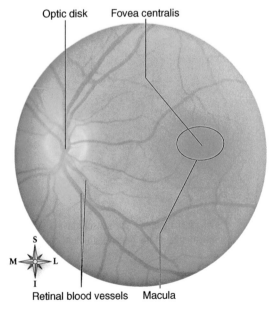

Optic disk   Fovea centralis

S
M — L
I

Retinal blood vessels   Macula

Ophthalmoscopic View of the Retina as Seen Through the Pupil.

CAVITIES OF THE EYE

CAVITY	DIVISIONS	LOCATION	CONTENTS
Anterior	Anterior chamber	Anterior to iris and posterior to cornea	Aqueous humor
	Posterior chamber	Posterior to iris and anterior to lens	Aqueous humor
Posterior	None	Posterior to lens	Vitreous body

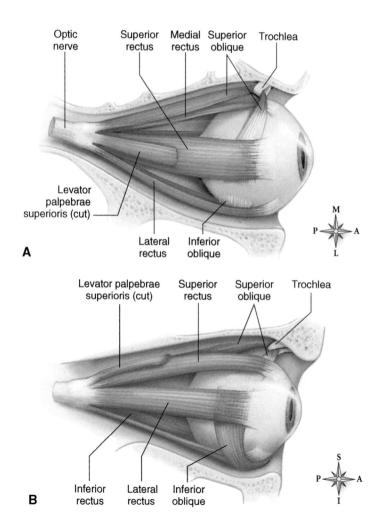

Extrinsic Muscles of the Right Eye. A, Superior view. **B,** Lateral view.

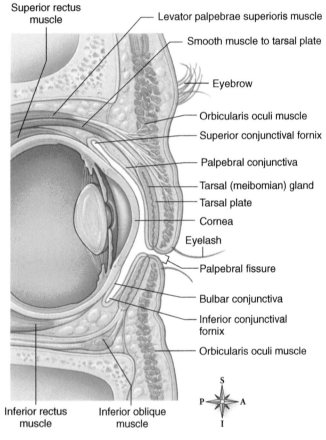

Superior rectus muscle

Levator palpebrae superioris muscle

Smooth muscle to tarsal plate

Eyebrow

Orbicularis oculi muscle

Superior conjunctival fornix

Palpebral conjunctiva

Tarsal (meibomian) gland

Tarsal plate

Cornea

Eyelash

Palpebral fissure

Bulbar conjunctiva

Inferior conjunctival fornix

Orbicularis oculi muscle

Inferior rectus muscle

Inferior oblique muscle

Accessory Structures of the Eye. Lateral view with eyelids closed.

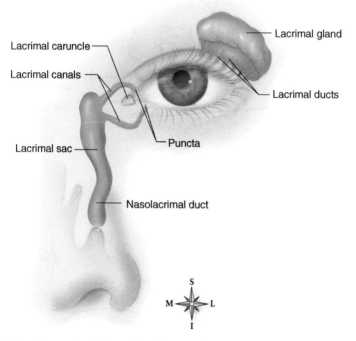

Lacrimal Apparatus. Fluid produced by lacrimal glands (tears) streams across the eye surface, enters the canals, and then passes through the lacrimal sac and nasolacrimal duct to enter the nose.

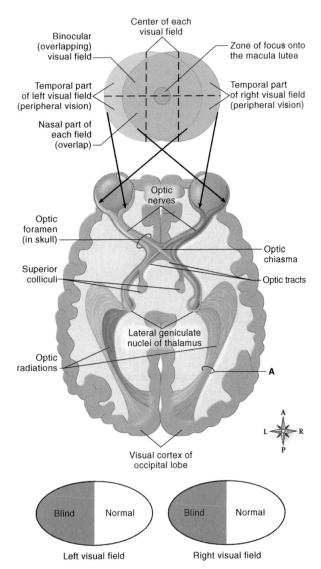

Visual Fields and Neural Pathways of the Eye. Note the structures that make up each pathway: optic nerve, optic chiasma, lateral geniculate body of thalamus, optic radiations, and visual cortex of occipital lobe. Fibers from the nasal portion of each retina cross over to the opposite side at the optic chiasma and terminate in the lateral geniculate nuclei. Location of a lesion in the visual pathway determines the resulting visual defect. Damage at point *A*, for example, would cause blindness in the right nasal and left temporal visual fields, as the ovals beneath indicate. (Trace the visual pathway from point *A* back to the visual field map to see why this is so.) What would be the effect of pressure on the optic chiasma—by a pituitary tumor, for instance? (*Answer:* It would produce blindness in both temporal visual fields. Why? Because it destroys fibers from the nasal side of both retinas.)

Endocrine System

The endocrine system and nervous system may work alone or in concert with others as a single neuroendocrine system, performing the same general functions within the body: communication, integration, and control.

Both the endocrine system and the nervous system perform their regulatory functions by means of chemical messengers sent to specific cells. In the nervous system, neurons secrete neurotransmitter molecules to signal nearby cells that have the appropriate receptor molecules. In the endocrine system, however, secreting cells send **hormone** (from the Greek *hormaein*, "to excite") molecules by way of the bloodstream to signal specific **target cells** throughout the body. Tissues and organs that contain endocrine target cells are called *target tissues and target organs*, respectively. As with postsynaptic cells, endocrine target cells must have the appropriate receptor to be influenced by the signaling chemical—a process called *signal transduction*. Many cells have receptors for neurotransmitters and hormones, so they can be influenced by both types of chemicals.

ENDOCRINE REGULATION

Organization of the Endocrine System

COMPARISON OF THE ENDOCRINE SYSTEM AND THE NERVOUS SYSTEM

FEATURE	ENDOCRINE SYSTEM	NERVOUS SYSTEM
OVERALL FUNCTION	Regulation of effectors to maintain homeostasis	Regulation of effectors to maintain homeostasis
Control by regulatory feedback loops	Yes (endocrine reflexes)	Yes (nervous reflexes)
Effector tissues	Endocrine effectors: virtually all tissues	Nervous effectors: muscle and glandular tissues only
Effector cells	Target cells (throughout the body)	Postsynaptic cells (in muscle and glandular tissue only)
CHEMICAL MESSENGER	Hormone	Neurotransmitter
Cells that secrete the chemical messenger	Glandular epithelial cells or neurosecretory cells (modified neurons)	Neurons
Distance traveled (and method of travel) by chemical messenger	Long (by way of circulating blood)	Short (across a microscopic synapse)
Location of receptor in effector cell	On the plasma membrane or within the cell	On the plasma membrane
Characteristics of regulatory effects	Slow to appear, long lasting	Appear rapidly, short lived

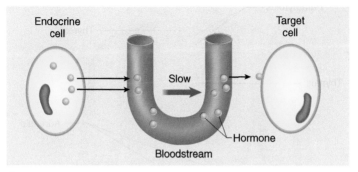

A

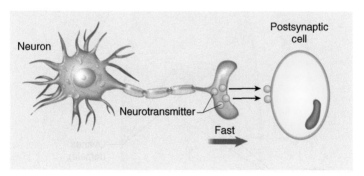

B

Mechanisms of Endocrine (A) and Nervous (B) Signals.

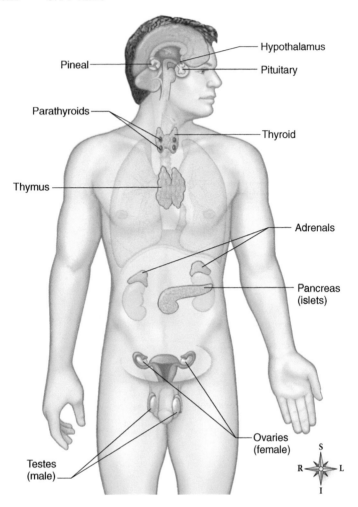

Locations of Some of the Major Endocrine Glands.

SOME OF THE MAJOR ENDOCRINE GLANDS

NAME	LOCATION
Hypothalamus	Cranial cavity (brain)
Pituitary gland	Cranial cavity
Pineal gland	Cranial cavity (brain)
Thyroid gland	Neck
Parathyroid glands	Neck
Thymus	Mediastinum
Adrenal glands	Abdominal cavity (retroperitoneal)
Pancreatic islets	Abdominal cavity (pancreas)
Ovaries	Pelvic cavity
Testes	Scrotum
Placenta	Pregnant uterus

Hormones

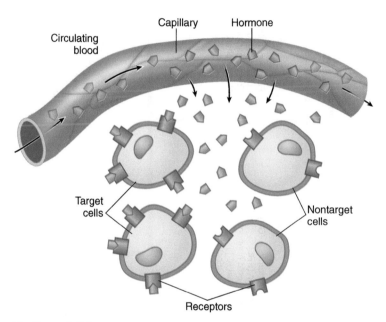

The Target Cell Concept. A hormone acts only on cells that have receptors specific to that hormone because the shape of the receptor determines which hormone can react with it. This is an example of the lock-and-key model of biochemical reactions.

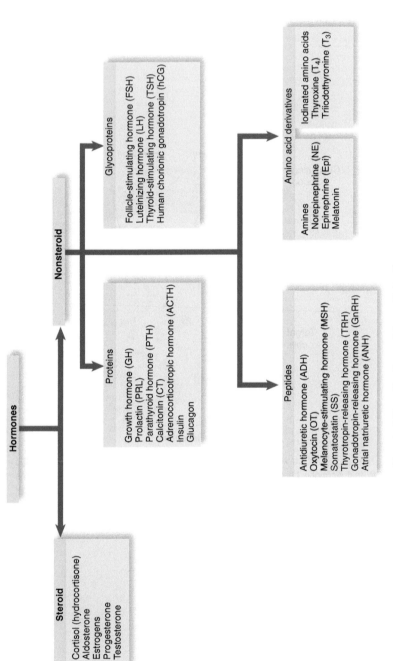

Chemical Classifications of Some Major Hormones.

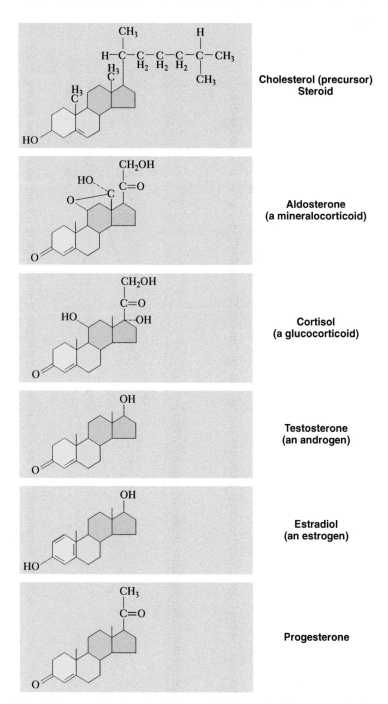

Cholesterol (precursor) Steroid

Aldosterone (a mineralocorticoid)

Cortisol (a glucocorticoid)

Testosterone (an androgen)

Estradiol (an estrogen)

Progesterone

Steroid Hormone Structure. As these examples show, steroid hormone molecules are very similar in structure to cholesterol *(top),* particularly in having a four-ring steroid nucleus at their core. Cholesterol is the precursor molecule from which the steroid hormones are all derived.

PROTEIN HORMONE (INSULIN)

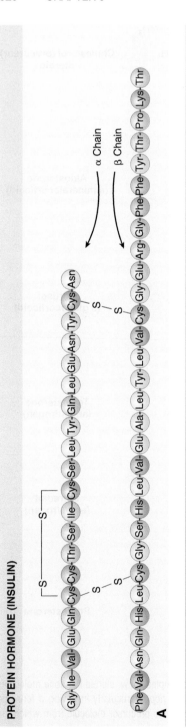

α Chain

β Chain

GLYCOPROTEIN HORMONE (HUMAN CHORIONIC GONADOTROPIN [hCG])

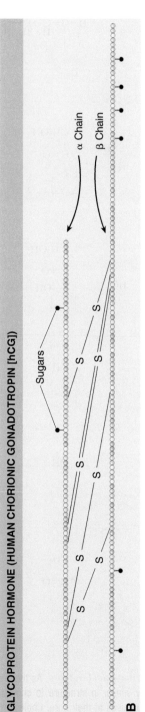

α Chain

β Chain

Sugars

Nonsteroid Hormone Structure. A, Protein hormone molecules are made of long, folded strands of amino acids. **B,** Glycoprotein hormones are long, folded strands of amino acids with attached sugar groups.

PEPTIDE HORMONE (OXYTOCIN [OT])

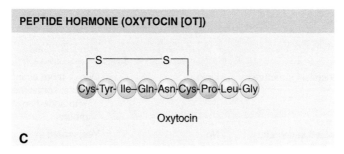

C

AMINO ACID DERIVATIVE (THYROXINE [T$_4$])

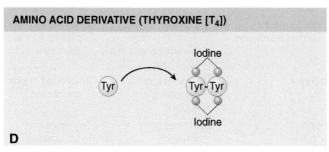

D

Nonsteroid Hormone Structure—cont'd. C, Peptide hormone molecules are smaller strands of amino acids. **D,** Amino acid derivatives are, as their name implies, derived from a single amino acid.

COMPARISON OF STEROID AND NONSTEROID HORMONES

CHARACTERISTIC	STEROID HORMONES	NONSTEROID HORMONES*
Chemical structure	Lipid	One or more amino acids, sometimes with added sugar groups
Stored in secretory cell	No	Yes; stored in secretory vesicles before release
Interaction with plasma membrane	No; simple diffusion through plasma membrane and into target cell	Yes; binds to specific plasma membrane receptors
Receptor	Mobile receptor in cytoplasm or nucleus	Embedded in plasma membrane
Action	Regulates gene activity (transcription of new proteins that eventually produce effects in the cell)	Triggers signal transduction cascade, producing internal "second messengers" that trigger rapid effects in the target cell
Response time	One hour to several days	Several seconds to a few minutes

*Some nonsteroid hormones derived from amino acids (e.g., thyroid hormones T_3 and T_4) have gene-activating actions similar to steroid hormones.

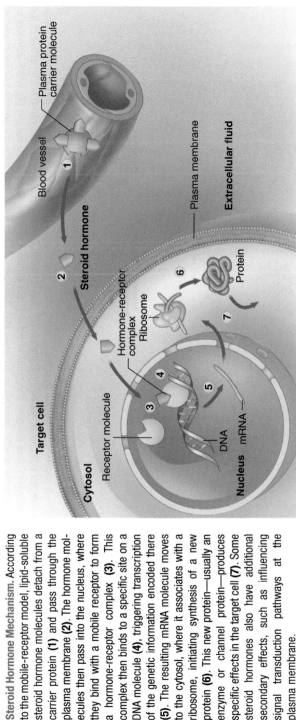

Steroid Hormone Mechanism. According to the mobile-receptor model, lipid-soluble steroid hormone molecules detach from a carrier protein **(1)** and pass through the plasma membrane **(2)**. The hormone molecules then pass into the nucleus, where they bind with a mobile receptor to form a hormone-receptor complex **(3)**. This complex then binds to a specific site on a DNA molecule **(4)**, triggering transcription of the genetic information encoded there **(5)**. The resulting mRNA molecule moves to the cytosol, where it associates with a ribosome, initiating synthesis of a new protein **(6)**. This new protein—usually an enzyme or channel protein—produces specific effects in the target cell **(7)**. Some steroid hormones also have additional secondary effects, such as influencing signal transduction pathways at the plasma membrane.

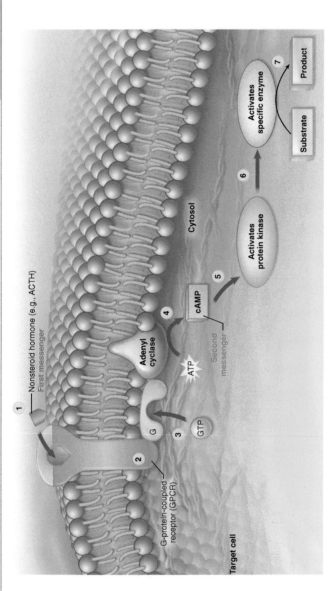

Example of a Second Messenger Mechanism. A nonsteroid hormone (first messenger) binds to a fixed G-protein–coupled receptor (GPCR) in the plasma membrane of the target cell (1). The hormone-receptor complex activates the G protein (2). The activated G protein reacts with GTP, which in turn activates the membrane-bound enzyme adenyl cyclase (3). Adenyl cyclase removes phosphates from ATP, converting it to cAMP (second messenger) (4). cAMP activates or inactivates protein kinases (5). Protein kinases activate specific intracellular enzymes (6). These activated enzymes then influence specific cellular reactions, thus producing the target cell's response to the hormone (7). *GTP,* Guanosine triphosphate; *ATP,* adenosine triphosphate; *cAMP,* cyclic adenosine monophosphate

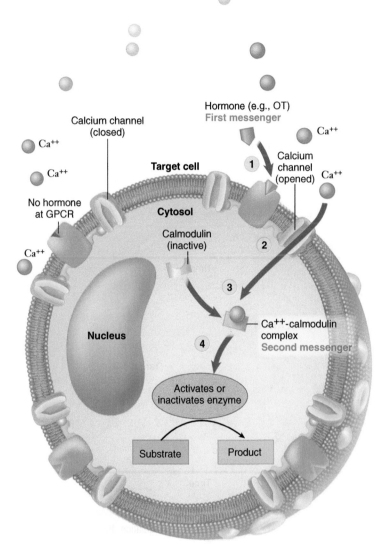

Calcium-Calmodulin as a Second Messenger. In this example of a second messenger mechanism, a nonsteroid hormone (first messenger) first binds to a fixed receptor (G-protein–coupled receptor, GPCR) in the plasma membrane **(1)**, which activates membrane-bound proteins (G protein and PIP_2) that trigger the opening of calcium channels **(2)**. Calcium ions, which are normally at a higher concentration in the extracellular fluid, diffuse into the cell and bind to a calmodulin molecule **(3)**. The Ca^{++}-calmodulin complex thus formed is a second messenger that binds to an enzyme to produce an allosteric effect that promotes or inhibits the enzyme's regulatory effect in the target cell **(4)**. *PIP_2,* Phosphatidylinositol 4,5-biphosphate.

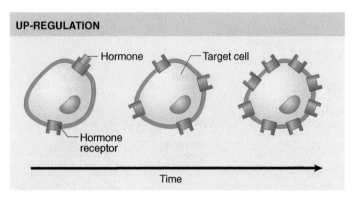

A

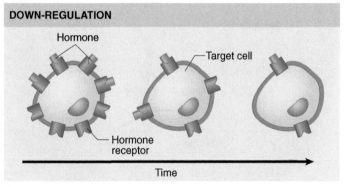

B

Regulation of Target Cell Sensitivity. A, Up-regulation. **B,** Down-regulation.

LOCAL HORMONES

The classical view of hormones is that they are secreted from a tissue into the bloodstream and have their effects in target cells at some distance from their source. This is the standard definition of an **endocrine hormone** (part A of figure). That is, hormones have "global" effects in the body. However, some hormones and related agents have primarily local effects—that is, effects *within* the source tissue. To distinguish classical endocrine hormones from local regulators such as prostaglandins and related compounds, scientists often use more precise terms for "local" hormones. Here are examples of terms used to designate local regulators:

- **Paracrine hormones**—hormones that regulate activity in nearby cells within the same tissue as their source (part B of figure)
- **Autocrine hormones**—hormones that regulate activity in the secreting cell itself (part C of figure)

To avoid confusion, scientists most often refer only to endocrine hormones simply as "hormones." For local regulators, scientists use general terms such as "tissue hormone" or "local regulator"—or more specific terms such as "paracrine" or "autocrine" factor.

Continued

LOCAL HORMONES—cont'd

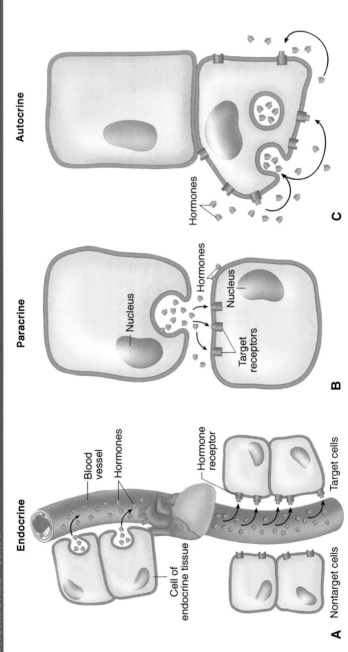

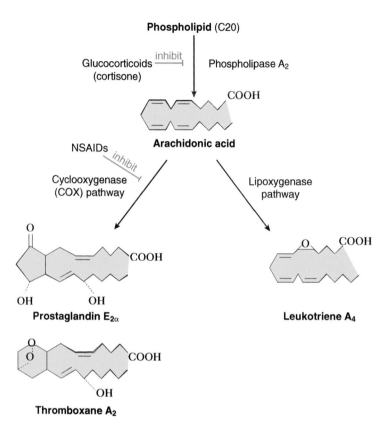

Formation of Prostaglandin and Related Molecules. Membrane phospholipids containing the 20-carbon fatty acid arachidonic acid are enzymatically broken apart (C20, 20-carbon). Therapeutic use of glucocorticoids such as cortisone can inhibit this pathway, thus reducing the amount (and effects) of any of the resulting regulator molecules. Arachidonic acid is then converted by the COX pathway to either prostaglandins or thromboxanes *(left)*. This step can be therapeutically inhibited by NSAIDs (nonsteroidal anti-inflammatory drugs). Arachidonic acid may alternatively be converted by the lipoxygenase pathway to a leukotriene *(right)*.

PROSTAGLANDINS AND RELATED HORMONES

HORMONE	SOURCE	TARGET	PRINCIPAL ACTION
Prostaglandins (PGs)	Many diverse tissues of the body	Local cells within the source tissue	Diverse local (paracrine/autocrine) effects such as regulation of inflammation, muscle contraction in blood vessels
Thromboxanes (TXs)	Platelets	Other platelets; muscles in blood vessel walls	Increase stickiness of platelets; promote blood clotting; cause constriction of blood vessels
Leukotrienes	Several types of white blood cells (leukocytes)	Local cells of various types	Regulate local inflammation triggered by allergens, including constriction of airways (as in asthma) and other inflammatory responses

ENDOCRINE GLANDS

Pituitary Gland

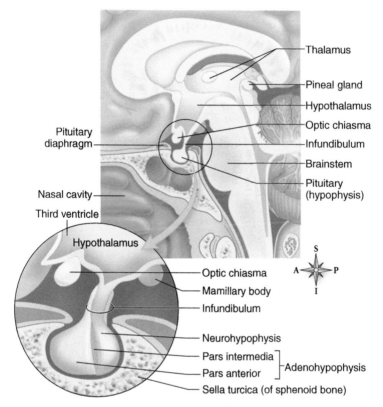

Thalamus

Pineal gland

Hypothalamus

Optic chiasma

Infundibulum

Brainstem

Pituitary (hypophysis)

Pituitary diaphragm

Nasal cavity

Third ventricle

Hypothalamus

Optic chiasma

Mamillary body

Infundibulum

Neurohypophysis

Pars intermedia ⎤
Pars anterior ⎦ Adenohypophysis

Sella turcica (of sphenoid bone)

Location and Structure of the Pituitary Gland. The pituitary gland is located within the sella turcica of the skull's sphenoid bone and is connected to the hypothalamus by a stalklike infundibulum. The infundibulum passes through a gap in the portion of the dura mater that covers the pituitary (the pituitary diaphragm). The *inset* shows that the pituitary is divided into an anterior portion, the *adenohypophysis,* and a posterior portion, the *neurohypophysis.* The adenohypophysis is further subdivided into the pars anterior and pars intermedia. The pars intermedia is almost absent in the adult pituitary.

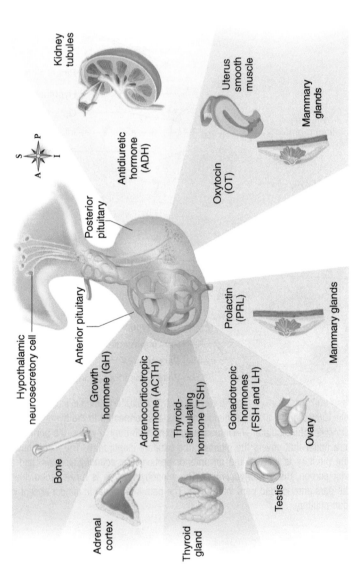

Pituitary Hormones. Some of the major hormones of the adenohypophysis and neurohypophysis and their principal target organs.

HORMONES OF THE HYPOTHALAMUS

HORMONE	SOURCE	TARGET	PRINCIPAL ACTION
Growth hormone–releasing hormone (GHRH)	Hypothalamus	Adenohypophysis (somatotrophs)	Stimulates secretion (release) of growth hormone
Growth hormone–inhibiting hormone (GHIH), or somatostatin	Hypothalamus	Adenohypophysis (somatotrophs)	Inhibits secretion of growth hormone
Corticotropin-releasing hormone (CRH)	Hypothalamus	Adenohypophysis (corticotrophs)	Stimulates release of adrenocorticotropic hormone (ACTH)
Thyrotropin-releasing hormone (TRH)	Hypothalamus	Adenohypophysis (thyrotrophs)	Stimulates release of thyroid-stimulating hormone (TSH)
Gonadotropin-releasing hormone (GnRH)	Hypothalamus	Adenohypophysis (gonadotrophs)	Stimulates release of gonadotropins (FSH and LH)
Prolactin-releasing hormone (PRH)	Hypothalamus	Adenohypophysis (corticotrophs)	Stimulates secretion of prolactin
Prolactin-inhibiting hormone (PIH)	Hypothalamus	Adenohypophysis (corticotrophs)	Inhibits secretion of prolactin

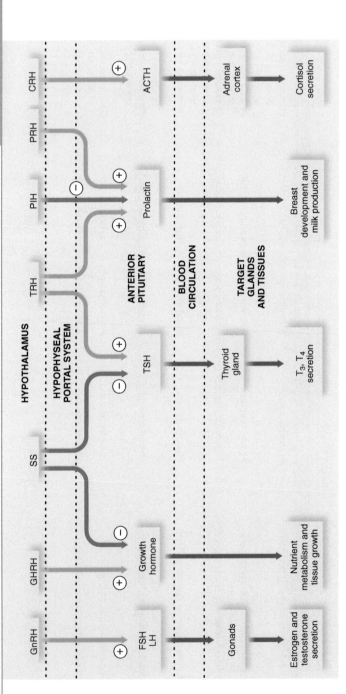

Actions of Hypothalamic Hormones. Hypothalamic hormones have releasing or inhibiting effects on the various cells of the anterior pituitary, thus regulating anterior pituitary secretion—and thus ultimately regulating the effects of anterior pituitary hormones throughout the body. *GnRH*, Gonadotropin-releasing hormone; *GHRH*, growth hormone–releasing hormone; *SS*, somatostatin; *TRH*, thyroid-releasing hormone; *PIH*, prolactin-inhibiting hormone; *PRH*, prolactin-releasing hormone; *CRH*, corticotropin-releasing hormone; *FSH*, follicle-stimulating hormone; *LH*, luteinizing hormone; *TSH*, thyroid-stimulating hormone; *ACTH*, adreno-corticotropic hormone; T_3, triiodothyronine; T_4, thyroxine.

HORMONES OF THE PITUITARY GLAND

HORMONE	SOURCE	TARGET	PRINCIPAL ACTION
Growth hormone (GH) (somatotropin [STH])	Adenohypophysis (somatotrophs)	General	Promotes growth by stimulating protein anabolism and fat mobilization
Prolactin (PRL) (lactogenic hormone)	Adenohypophysis (lactotrophs)	Mammary glands (alveolar secretory cells)	Promotes milk secretion
Thyroid-stimulating hormone (TSH)*	Adenohypophysis (thyrotrophs)	Thyroid gland	Stimulates development and secretion in the thyroid gland
Adrenocorticotropic hormone (ACTH)*	Adenohypophysis (corticotrophs)	Adrenal cortex	Promotes development and secretion in the adrenal cortex
Follicle-stimulating hormone (FSH)*	Adenohypophysis (gonadotrophs)	Gonads (primary sex organs)	*Female:* promotes development of ovarian follicle; stimulates estrogen secretion. *Male:* promotes development of testes; stimulates sperm production
Luteinizing hormone (LH)*	Adenohypophysis (gonadotrophs)	Gonads	*Female:* triggers ovulation; promotes development of corpus luteum. *Male:* stimulates production of testosterone
Antidiuretic hormone (ADH), or arginine vasopressin (AVP)	Neurohypophysis	Kidney	Promotes water retention by kidney tubules; raises blood pressure by stimulating muscles in walls of small arteries
Oxytocin (OT)	Neurohypophysis	Uterus and mammary glands	Stimulates uterine contractions; stimulates ejection of milk into ducts of mammary glands; involved in social bonding

*Tropic hormones.

Thyroid Gland

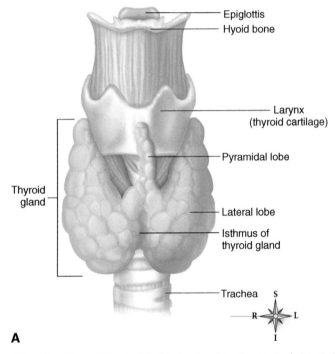

Epiglottis
Hyoid bone
Larynx (thyroid cartilage)
Pyramidal lobe
Thyroid gland
Lateral lobe
Isthmus of thyroid gland
Trachea

A

Thyroid and Parathyroid Glands. A, In this drawing of the thyroid gland, the relationship of the thyroid to the larynx (voice box) and to the trachea is easily seen.

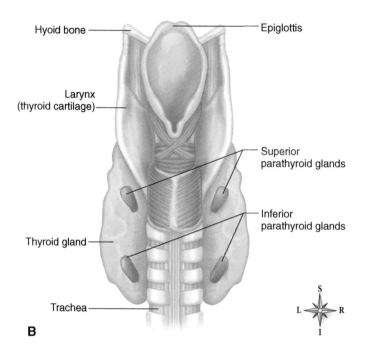

Hyoid bone

Epiglottis

Larynx
(thyroid cartilage)

Superior
parathyroid glands

Inferior
parathyroid glands

Thyroid gland

Trachea

B

S

L — R

I

Thyroid and Parathyroid Glands—cont'd. B, In this drawing of the parathyroid glands from a posterior view, note the relationship of the parathyroid glands to each other, to the thyroid gland, to the larynx (voice box), and to the trachea.

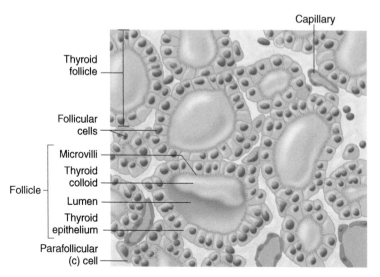

Capillary

Thyroid
follicle

Follicular
cells

Microvilli

Thyroid
colloid

Follicle

Lumen

Thyroid
epithelium

Parafollicular
(c) cell

Thyroid Gland Tissue. Note that each of the thyroid follicles is filled with colloid.

HORMONES OF THE THYROID AND PARATHYROID GLANDS

HORMONE	SOURCE	TARGET	PRINCIPAL ACTION
Triiodothyronine (T_3)	Thyroid gland (follicular cells)	General	Increases rate of metabolism
Tetraiodothyronine (T_4) or thyroxine	Thyroid gland (follicular cells)	General	Increases rate of metabolism (usually converted to T_3 first)
Calcitonin (CT)	Thyroid gland (parafollicular cells)	Bone tissue	Increases calcium storage in bone, lowering blood Ca^{++} levels
Parathyroid hormone (PTH) or parathormone	Parathyroid glands	Bone tissue and kidneys	Increases calcium removal from storage in bone and produces the active form of vitamin D in the kidneys, increasing absorption of calcium by intestines and increasing blood Ca^{++} levels

ADH, Antidiuretic hormone.

Adrenal Glands

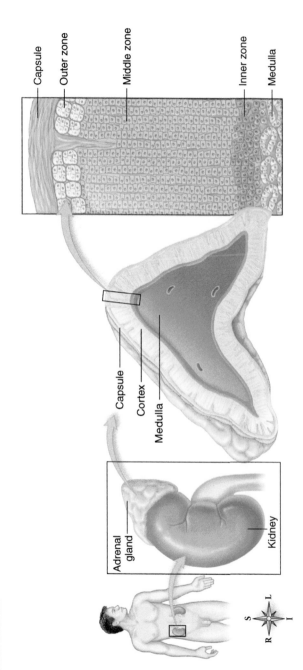

Structure of the Adrenal Gland. The zona glomerulosa of the cortex secretes aldosterone. The zona fasciculata secretes abundant amounts of glucocorticoids, chiefly cortisol. The zona reticularis secretes minute amounts of sex hormones and glucocorticoids. A portion of the medulla is visible at *lower right* at the bottom of the drawing.

HORMONES OF THE ADRENAL GLANDS

HORMONE	SOURCE	TARGET	PRINCIPAL ACTION
Aldosterone	Adrenal cortex (zona glomerulosa)	Kidney	Stimulates kidney tubules to conserve sodium, which in turn triggers the release of ADH and the resulting conservation of water by the kidney
Cortisol (hydrocortisone)	Adrenal cortex (zona fasciculata)	General	Influences metabolism of food molecules; in large amounts, it has an anti-inflammatory effect
Adrenal androgens	Adrenal cortex (zona reticularis)	Sex organs, other effectors	Exact role uncertain but may support sexual function
Adrenal estrogens	Adrenal cortex (zona reticularis)	Sex organs	Thought to be physiologically insignificant
Epinephrine (Epi) (adrenaline)	Adrenal medulla	Sympathetic effectors	Enhances and prolongs the effects of the sympathetic division of the autonomic nervous system
Norepinephrine (NE)	Adrenal medulla	Sympathetic effectors	Enhances and prolongs the effects of the sympathetic division of the autonomic nervous system

Pancreatic Islets

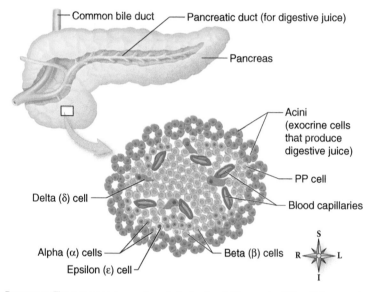

Common bile duct
Pancreatic duct (for digestive juice)
Pancreas
Acini (exocrine cells that produce digestive juice)
PP cell
Delta (δ) cell
Blood capillaries
Alpha (α) cells
Beta (β) cells
Epsilon (ε) cell
S
R — L
I

Pancreas. The pancreas is an elongated gland weighing up to 100 g (3.5 ounces). The "head" of the gland lies in the C-shaped beginning of the small intestine (duodenum), with its body extending horizontally behind the stomach and its tail touching the spleen. The endocrine portion of the pancreas is composed of both endocrine and exocrine tissues. The endocrine portion is made up of scattered, tiny islands of cells, called *pancreatic islets.* A pancreatic islet, or hormone-producing area, is evident among the pancreatic cells that produce the pancreatic digestive juice. The pancreatic islets are more abundant in the tail of the pancreas than in the body or head.

HORMONES OF THE PANCREATIC ISLETS

HORMONE	SOURCE	TARGET	PRINCIPAL ACTION
Glucagon	Pancreatic islets (alpha [α] cells, or A cells)	General	Promotes movement of glucose from storage and into the blood
Insulin	Pancreatic islets (beta [β] cells, or B cells)	General	Promotes movement of glucose out of the blood and into cells
Somatostatin (SS)	Pancreatic islets (delta [δ] cells, or D cells)	Pancreatic cells and other effectors	Can have general effects in the body, but primary role seems to be regulation of secretion of other pancreatic hormones
Pancreatic polypeptide (PP)	Pancreatic islets (pancreatic polypeptide [PP] or F cells)	Intestinal cells and other effectors	Exact function uncertain but seems to influence absorption in the digestive tract
Ghrelin (GHRL)	Stomach mucosa, pancreatic islets (epsilon [ε] cells)	Hypothalamus; other diverse tissues	Stimulates hypothalamus to boost appetite; affects energy balance in various tissues

Hormones Produced by Gonads

EXAMPLES OF ADDITIONAL HORMONES OF THE BODY

HORMONE	SOURCE	TARGET	PRINCIPAL ACTION
Cholecalciferol (vitamin D₃)	Skin, liver, kidney (in progressive steps)	Intestines, bones, most other tissues	Promotes calcium absorption from food, regulates mineral balance in bones, regulates growth and differentiation of many cell types
Dehydroepiandrosterone (DHEA)	Adrenal gland, testis, ovary, other tissues	Converted to other hormones	Eventually converted to estrogens, testosterone, or both
Melatonin	Pineal gland	Timekeeping tissues of the nervous system	Helps "set" the biological clock mechanisms of the body by signaling light changes during the day, month, and seasons; may help induce sleep
Testosterone	Testis (small amounts in adrenal and ovary)	Sperm-producing tissues of testis, muscles, other tissues	Stimulates sperm production, stimulates growth and maintenance of male sexual characteristics, promotes muscle growth
Estrogen, including estradiol (E₂) and estrone	Ovary and placenta (small amounts in adrenal and testis)	Uterus, breasts, other tissues	Stimulates development of female sexual characteristics, breast development, bone and nervous system maintenance
Progesterone	Ovary and placenta	Uterus, mammary glands, other tissues	Helps maintain proper conditions for pregnancy
Human chorionic gonadotropin (hCG)	Placenta	Ovary	Stimulates secretion of estrogen and progesterone during pregnancy
Human placental lactogens (hPLs)	Placenta	Mammary glands; pancreas and other tissues	Promote development of mammary glands during pregnancy; help regulate energy balance in fetus

Continued

EXAMPLES OF ADDITIONAL HORMONES OF THE BODY—cont'd

HORMONE	SOURCE	TARGET	PRINCIPAL ACTION
Relaxin	Placenta	Uterus and joints	Inhibits uterine contractions during pregnancy and softens pelvic joints to facilitate childbirth
Thymosins and thymopoietins	Thymus gland	Certain lymphocytes (type of white blood cell)	Stimulate development of T lymphocytes, which are involved in immunity
Gastrin	Stomach mucosa	Exocrine glands of stomach	Triggers increased gastric juice secretion
Secretin	Intestinal mucosa	Stomach and pancreas	Increases alkaline secretions of the pancreas and slows emptying of stomach; helps regulate water homeostasis
Cholecystokinin (CCK)	Intestinal mucosa	Gallbladder and pancreas	Triggers the release of bile from gallbladder and enzymes from the pancreas
Atrial natriuretic hormone (ANH) and other atrial natriuretic peptides (ANPs)	Heart muscle	Kidney	Promotes loss of sodium from body into urine, thus promoting water loss from the body and a resulting decrease in blood volume and pressure
Inhibins	Ovary and testis	Hypothalamus and adenohypophysis (anterior pituitary)	Inhibit secretion of GnRH by hypothalamus and FSH by the anterior pituitary, thus helping to regulate the female reproductive cycle
Leptin	Adipose tissue	Hypothalamus; other diverse tissues	Affects energy balance, perhaps as a signal of how much fat is stored; affects various immune, neuroendocrine, and developmental functions throughout body
Resistin	Adipose tissue and macrophages	Liver and other tissues	Reduces sensitivity to insulin (a pancreatic islet hormone), thus increasing blood glucose levels
Insulin-like growth factor 1 (IGF-1)	Liver, kidney, and other tissues	Bone, muscle, and other tissues	Secreted in response to growth hormone (GH), IGF-1 carries out many of the functions attributed to GH

Cardiovascular System

10

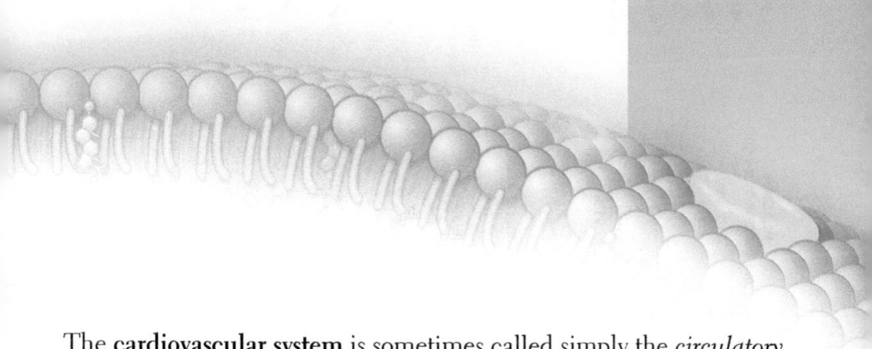

The **cardiovascular system** is sometimes called simply the *circulatory system*. It consists of the **heart**, which is a muscular pumping device, and a closed system of vessels that include:

Arteries and **arterioles**—vessels that carry blood away from the heart

Veins and **venules**—vessels that carry blood toward the heart

Capillaries—thin, microscopic vessels that carry blood through the tissues to connect

Blood is a complex connective tissue that serves multiples purposes, such as carrying oxygen and carbon dioxide (blood gases), nutrients, water, metabolic wastes, hormones, agents of immunity, heat, and more.

As the name implies, blood contained in the circulatory system is pumped by the heart around a closed circle or circuit of vessels as it passes again and again through the various organs of the body. Many factors influence the blood flow generated by the heart, some of which are described in the diagrams and tables of this chapter.

BLOOD

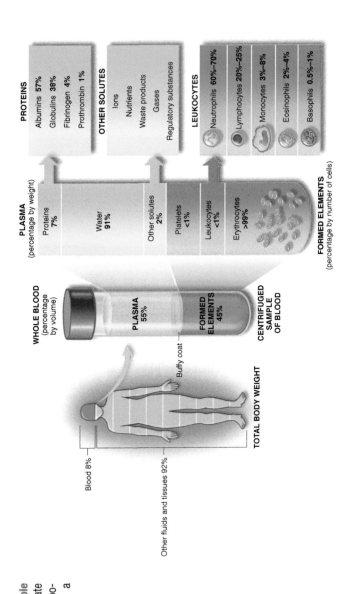

Composition of Whole Blood. Approximate values for the components of blood in a normal adult.

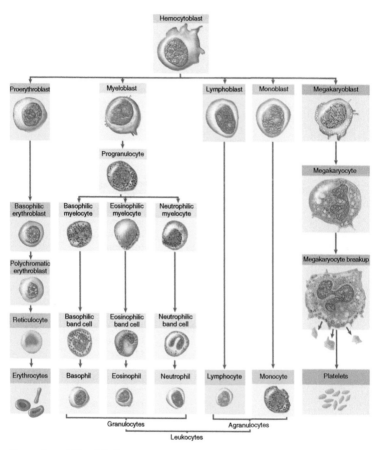

Formation of Blood Cells. The hematopoietic stem cell, called the *hemocytoblast,* serves as the original stem cell from which all formed elements of the blood are derived. Note that all five precursor cells, which ultimately produce the different components of the formed elements, are derived from the hematopoietic stem cell called a *hemocytoblast.*

CLASSES OF BLOOD CELLS

CELL TYPE	DESCRIPTION	FUNCTION	LIFE SPAN
Erythrocyte	7 µm in diameter; concave disk shape; entire cell stains pale pink; no nucleus	Transportation of respiratory gases (O_2 and CO_2)	105-120 days
Neutrophil	12-15 µm in diameter; spherical shape; multilobed nucleus; small, pink-purple–staining cytoplasmic granules	Cellular defense—phagocytosis of small pathogenic microorganisms	Hours to 3 days
Basophil	11-14 µm in diameter; spherical shape; generally two-lobed nucleus; large purple-staining cytoplasmic granules	Secretes heparin (anticoagulant) and histamine (important in inflammatory response)	Hours to 3 days
Eosinophil	10-12 µm in diameter; spherical shape; generally two-lobed nucleus; large, orange-red–staining cytoplasmic granule	Cellular defense—some phagocytosis; chemical attack of large pathogenic microorganisms (such as protozoa) and parasitic worms; helps regulate allergic reactions and other inflammatory responses	10-12 days
Lymphocyte	6-9 µm in diameter; spherical shape; round (single-lobed) nucleus; small lymphocytes have scant cytoplasm	Humoral defense—secretes antibodies; involved in immune system response and regulation	Days to years

CLASSES OF BLOOD CELLS—cont'd

CELL TYPE	DESCRIPTION	FUNCTION	LIFE SPAN
Monocyte	12-17 µm in diameter; spherical shape; nucleus generally kidney-bean or horseshoe shaped with convoluted surface; ample cytoplasm often "steel blue" in color	Capable of migrating out of the blood to enter tissue spaces as a macrophage— an aggressive phagocytic cell capable of ingesting bacteria, cellular debris, and cancerous cells	Months
Platelet	2-5 µm in diameter; irregularly shaped fragments; cytoplasm contains very small, pink-staining granules	Releases clot-activating substances and helps in formation of actual blood clot by forming platelet "plugs"	7-10 days

DIFFERENTIAL COUNT OF WHITE BLOOD CELLS

CLASS	DIFFERENTIAL COUNT*	
	NORMAL RANGE (%)	TYPICAL VALUE (%)†
Neutrophils	65-75	65
Lymphocytes (large and small)	20-25	25
Monocytes	3-8	6
Eosinophils	2-5	3
Basophils	½-1	1
TOTAL	100	100

*In any differential count, the sum of the percentages of the different kinds of white blood cells (WBCs) must, of course, total 100%.
†The following mnemonic phrase may help you remember percent values in decreasing order by class of WBC: "**N**ever **L**et **M**onkeys **E**at **B**ananas."

Recipient's blood		Reactions with donor's blood			
RBC antigens	Plasma antibodies	Donor type O	Donor type A	Donor type B	Donor type AB
None (Type O)	Anti-A Anti-B				
A (Type A)	Anti-B				
B (Type B)	Anti-A				
AB (Type AB)	(None)				

Results of Cross-Matching Different Combinations (Types) of Donor and Recipient Blood. The *left columns* show the antigen and antibody characteristics that define the recipient's blood type, and the top row shows the donor's blood type. Cross-matching identifies either a compatible combination of donor-recipient blood (no agglutination) or an incompatible combination (agglutinated blood). Photo inset shows drops of blood showing appearance of agglutinated and nonagglutinated red blood cells.

COAGULATION FACTORS:
STANDARD NOMENCLATURE AND SYNONYMS

FACTOR	COMMON SYNONYMS
Factor I	Fibrinogen
Factor II	Prothrombin
Factor III	Thromboplastin
	Thrombokinase
Factor IV (now obsolete)	Calcium
Factor V	Proaccelerin
	Labile factor
Factor VI (now obsolete)	Activated factor V
Factor VII	Serum prothrombin conversion accelerator (SPCA)
Factor VIII	Antihemophilic globulin (AHG)
	Antihemophilic factor (AHF)
Factor IX	Plasma thromboplastin component (PTC)
	Christmas factor
Factor X	Stuart factor
Factor XI	Plasma thromboplastin antecedent (PTA)
Factor XII	Hageman factor
Factor XIII	Fibrin-stabilizing factor

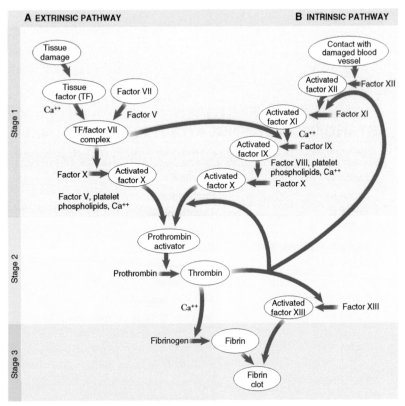

Clot Formation. A, Extrinsic clotting pathway. *Stage 1:* Damaged tissue releases tissue factor, which with factor VII and calcium ions activates factor X. Activated factor X, factor V, phospholipids, and calcium ions form prothrombin activator (prothrombinase). *Stage 2:* Prothrombin is converted to thrombin by prothrombin activator. *Stage 3:* Fibrinogen is converted to fibrin by thrombin. Fibrin forms a clot. **B,** Intrinsic clotting pathway. *Stage 1:* Damaged vessels cause activation of factor XII. Activated factor XII activates factor XI, which activates factor IX. Factor IX, along with factor VIII and platelet phospholipids, activates factor X. Activated factor X, factor V, phospholipids, and calcium ions form prothrombin activator. Stages 2 and 3 take the same course as the extrinsic clotting pathway.

BLOOD, PLASMA, AND SERUM VALUES

TEST	NORMAL VALUES*	SIGNIFICANCE OF A CHANGE
Acid phosphatase	*Women:* 0.01-0.56 sigma U/ml *Men:* 0.13-0.63 sigma U/ml	↑ in prostate cancer ↑ in kidney disease ↑ after trauma and in fever
Alkaline phosphatase	*Adult:* 13-39 IU/L *Child:* up to 104 IU/L	↑ in bone disorders ↑ in liver disease ↑ during pregnancy ↑ in hypothyroidism
Bicarbonate	22-26 mEq/L	↑ in metabolic alkalosis ↑ in respiratory alkalosis ↑ in metabolic acidosis ↑ in respiratory alkalosis
Blood urea nitrogen (BUN)	5-25 mg/100 ml	↑ with increased protein intake ↑ in kidney failure
Blood volume	*Women:* 65 ml/kg body weight *Men:* 69 ml/kg body weight	↓ during hemorrhage
Calcium	8.4-10.5 mg/100 ml	↑ in hypervitaminosis D ↑ in hyperparathyroidism ↑ in bone cancer and other bone diseases ↓ in severe diarrhea ↓ in hypoparathyroidism ↓ in avitaminosis D (rickets and osteomalacia)
Carbon dioxide content	24-32 mEq/L	↑ in severe vomiting ↑ in respiratory disorders ↑ in obstruction of intestines ↓ in acidosis ↓ in severe diarrhea ↓ in kidney disease
Chloride	96-107 mEq/L	↑ in hyperventilation ↑ in kidney disease ↑ in Cushing syndrome ↓ in diabetic acidosis ↓ in severe diarrhea ↓ in severe burns ↓ in Addison disease
Clotting time	5-10 min	↓ in hemophilia ↓ (occasionally) in other clotting disorders
Copper	100-200 µg/100 ml	↑ in some liver disorders

Continued

BLOOD, PLASMA, AND SERUM VALUES—cont'd

TEST	NORMAL VALUES*	SIGNIFICANCE OF A CHANGE
Creatine phosphokinase (CPK)	*Women:* 5-35 mU/ml *Men:* 5-55 mU/ml	↑ in Duchenne muscular dystrophy ↑ during myocardial infarction ↑ in muscle trauma
Creatine	0.6-1.5 mg/100 ml	↑ in some kidney disorders
Glucose	70-110 mg/100 ml (fasting)	↑ in diabetes mellitus ↑ in kidney disease ↑ in liver disease ↑ during pregnancy ↑ in hyperthyroidism ↓ in hypothyroidism ↓ in Addison disease ↓ in hyperinsulinism
Hematocrit (packed cell volume)	*Women:* 38%-47% *Men:* 40%-54%	↑ in polycythemia ↑ in severe dehydration ↓ in anemia ↓ in leukemia ↓ in hyperthyroidism ↓ in cirrhosis of liver
Hemoglobin	*Women:* 12-16 g/100 ml *Men:* 13-18 g/100 ml *Newborn:* 14-20 g/100 ml	↑ in polycythemia ↑ in chronic obstructive pulmonary disease ↑ in congestive heart failure ↓ in anemia ↓ in hyperthyroidism ↓ in cirrhosis of liver
Iron	50-150 µg/100 ml (can be higher in men)	↑ in liver disease ↑ in anemia (some forms) ↓ in iron-deficiency anemia
Lactic dehydrogenase (LDH)	60-120 U/ml	↑ during myocardial infarction ↑ in anemia (several forms) ↑ in liver disease ↑ in acute leukemia and other cancers
Lipids—total Cholesterol— total High-density lipoprotein (HDL) Low-density lipoprotein (LDL) Triglycerides Phospholipids Fatty acids	450-1000 mg/100 ml 120-220 mg/100 ml >40 mg/100 ml <180 mg/100 ml 40-150 mg/100 ml 145-200 mg/100 ml 190-420 mg/100 ml	↑ (total) in diabetes mellitus ↑ (total) in kidney disease ↑ (total) in hypothyroidism ↓ (total) in hyperthyroidism ↑ in inherited hypercholesterolemia ↑ (cholesterol) in chronic hepatitis ↓ (cholesterol) in acute hepatitis ↑ (HDL) with regular exercise

BLOOD, PLASMA, AND SERUM VALUES—cont'd

TEST	NORMAL VALUES*	SIGNIFICANCE OF A CHANGE
Mean corpuscular volume	82-98 μL	↑ or ↓ in various forms of anemia
Osmolality	285-295 mOsm/L	↑ or ↓ in fluid and electrolyte imbalances
Pco₂	35-43 mm Hg	↑ in severe vomiting ↑ in respiratory disorders ↑ in obstruction of intestines ↓ in acidosis ↓ in severe diarrhea ↓ in kidney disease
pH	7.35-7.45	↑ during hyperventilation ↑ in Cushing syndrome ↓ during hypoventilation ↓ in acidosis ↓ in Addison disease
Phosphorus	2.5-4.5 mg/100 ml	↑ in hypervitaminosis D ↑ in kidney disease ↑ in hypoparathyroidism ↑ in acromegaly ↓ in hyperparathyroidism ↓ in hypovitaminosis D (rickets and osteomalacia)
Plasma volume	*Women:* 40 ml/kg body weight *Men:* 39 ml/kg body weight	↑ or ↓ in fluid and electrolyte imbalances ↓ during hemorrhage
Platelet count	150,000-400,000/mm³	↑ in heart disease ↑ in cancer ↑ in cirrhosis of liver ↑ after trauma ↓ in anemia (some forms) ↓ during chemotherapy ↓ in some allergies
Po₂	75-100 mm Hg (breathing standard air)	↑ in polycythemia ↓ in anemia ↓ in chronic obstructive pulmonary disease
Potassium	3.8-5.1 mEq/L	↑ in hypoaldosteronism ↑ in acute kidney failure ↓ in vomiting or diarrhea ↓ in starvation

Protein—total
  Albumin
  Globulin
	6-8.4 g/100 ml
	3.5-5 g/100 ml
	2.3-3.5 g/100 ml
		↑ (total) in severe dehydration
		↓ (total) during hemorrhage
		↓ (total) in starvation

Continued

BLOOD, PLASMA, AND SERUM VALUES—cont'd

TEST	NORMAL VALUES*	SIGNIFICANCE OF A CHANGE
Red blood cell count	*Women:* 4.2-5.4 million/mm³ *Men:* 4.5-6.2 million/mm³	↑ in polycythemia ↑ in dehydration ↓ in anemia (several forms) ↓ in Addison's disease ↓ in systemic lupus erythematosus
Reticulocyte count	25,000-75,000/mm³ (0.5%-1.5% of red blood cell count)	↑ in hemolytic anemia ↑ in leukemia and metastatic carcinoma ↓ in pernicious anemia ↓ in iron-deficiency anemia ↓ during radiation therapy
Sodium	136-145 mEq/L	↑ in dehydration ↑ in trauma or disease of the central nervous system ↑ or ↓ in kidney disorders ↓ in excessive sweating, vomiting, or diarrhea ↓ in burns (sodium shift into cells)
Specific gravity	1.058	↑ or ↓ in fluid imbalances
Transaminase	10-40 U/ml	↑ during myocardial infarction ↑ in liver disease
Uric acid	*Women:* 2.5-7.5 mg/100 ml *Men:* 3-9 mg/100 ml	↑ in gout ↑ in toxemia of pregnancy ↑ during trauma
Viscosity	1.4-1.8 times the viscosity of water	↑ in polycythemia ↑ in dehydration
White blood cell count (total) Neutrophils Eosinophils Basophils Lymphocytes Monocytes	4500-11,000/mm³ 60%-70% of total 2%-4% of total 0.5%-1% of total 20%-25% of total 3%-8% of total	↑ (total) in acute infections ↑ (total) in trauma ↑ (total) some cancers ↑ (total) in anemia (some forms) ↑ (total) during chemotherapy ↑ (neutrophil) in acute infection ↑ (eosinophil) in allergies ↓ (basophil) in severe allergies ↑ (lymphocyte) during antibody reactions ↑ (monocyte) in chronic infections

*Values vary with the analysis method used; 100 ml = 1 dl.

CONVERSION FACTORS (SI UNITS)

COMPONENT	NORMAL RANGE IN UNITS AS CUSTOMARILY REPORTED	CONVERSION FACTOR	NORMAL RANGE IN SI UNITS, MOLECULAR UNITS, INTERNATIONAL UNITS, OR DECIMAL FRACTIONS
BIOCHEMICAL COMPONENTS OF BLOOD			
Acetoacetic acid (S)	0.2-1.0 mg/dl	98	19.6-98.0 µmol/L
Acetone (S)	0.3-2.0 mg/dl	172	51.6-344.0 µmol/L
Albumin (S)	3.2-4.5 g/dl	10	32-45 g/L
Ammonia (P)	20-120 µg/dl	0.588	11.7-70.5 µmol/L
Amylase (S)	60-160 Somogyi units/dl	1.85	111-296 U/L
Base, total (S)	145-160 mEq/L	1	145-160 mmol/L
Bicarbonate (P)	21-28 mEq/L	1	21-28 mmol/L
Bile acids (S)	0.3-3.0 mg/dl	10	3-30 mg/L
		2.547	0.8-7.6 µmol/L
Bilirubin, direct (S)	≤0.3 mg/dl	17.1	≤5.1 µmol/L
Bilirubin, indirect (S)	0.1-1.0 mg/dl	17.1	1.7-17.1 µmol/L
Blood gases (B)			
Pco_2 arterial	35-40 mm Hg	0.133	4.66-5.32 kPa
Po_2 arterial	95-100 mm Hg	0.133	12.64-13.30 kPa
Calcium (S)	8.5-10.5 mg/dl	0.25	2.1-2.6 mmol/L
Chloride (S)	95-103 mEq/L	1	95-103 mmol/L
Creatine (S)	0.1-0.4 mg/dl	76.3	7.6-30.5 µmol/L
Creatinine (S)	0.6-1.2 mg/dl	88.4	53-106 µmol/L
Creatinine clearance (P)	107-139 ml/min	0.0167	1.78-2.32 ml/s
Fatty acids (total) (S)	8-20 mg/dl	0.01	0.08-2.00 mg/L

Continued

CONVERSION FACTORS (SI UNITS)—cont'd

COMPONENT	NORMAL RANGE IN UNITS AS CUSTOMARILY REPORTED	CONVERSION FACTOR	NORMAL RANGE IN SI UNITS, MOLECULAR UNITS, INTERNATIONAL UNITS, OR DECIMAL FRACTIONS
Fibrinogen (P)	200-400 mg/dl	0.01	2.00-4.00 g/L
Gamma globulin (S)	0.5-1.6 g/dl	10	5-16 g/L
Globulins (total) (S)	2.3-3.5 g/dl	10	23-35 g/L
Glucose (fasting) (S)	70-110 mg/dl	0.055	3.85-6.05 mmol/L
Insulin (radioimmunoassay) (P)	4.24 µIU/ml	0.0417	0.17-1.00 µg/L
	0.20-0.84 µg/L	172.2	35-145 mol/L
Iodine, BEI (S)	3.5-6.5 µg/dl	0.079	0.28-0.51 µmol/L
Iodine, PBI (S)	4.0-8.0 µg/dl	0.079	0.32-0.63 µmol/L
Iron, total (S)	60-150 µg/dl	0.179	11-27 µmol/L
Iron-binding capacity (S)	300-360 µg/dl	0.179	54-64 µmol/L
17-Ketosteroids (P)	25-125 µg/dl	0.01	0.25-1.25 mg/L
Lactic dehydrogenase (S)	80-120 units at 30°C	0.48	38-62 U/L at 30°C
	Lactate → pyruvate	1	100-190 U/L at 37°C
Lipase (S)	0-1.5 U/ml	278	0-417 U/L
	Cherry-Crandall		
Lipids (total) (S)	400-800 mg/dl	0.01	4.00-8.00 g/L
Cholesterol	150-250 mg/dl	0.026	3.9-6.5 mmol/L
Triglycerides	75-165 mg/dl	0.0114	0.85-1.89 mmol/L
Phospholipids	150-380 mg/dl	0.01	1.50-380 g/L
Free fatty acids	9.0-15.0 mM/L	1	9.0-15.0 mmol/L
Nonprotein nitrogen (S)	20-35 mg/dl	0.714	14.3-25.0 mmol/L
Phosphatase (P)			

Acid (units/dl)	Cherry-Crandall	2.77	0-5.5 U/L
Alkaline (units/dl)	King-Armstrong	1.77	0-5.5 U/L
	Bodansky	5.37	0-5.5 U/L
	King-Armstrong	1.77	30-120 U/L
	Bodansky	5.37	30-120 U/L
	Bessey-Lowry-Brock	16.67	30-120 U/L
Phosphorus, inorganic (S)	3.0-4.5 mg/dl	0.323	0.97-1.45 mmol/L
Potassium (P)	3.8-5.0 mEq/L	1	3.8-5.0 mmol/L
Proteins, total (S)	6.0-7.8 g/dl	10	60-78 g/L
Albumin	3.2-4.5 g/dl	10	32-45 g/L
Globulin	2.3-3.5 g/dl	10	23-35 g/L
Sodium (P)	136-142 mEq/L	1	136-142 mmol/L
Testosterone:			1
Male (S)	300-1200 ng/dl	0.035	0.5-42.0 nmol/L
Female	30-95 ng/dl	0.035	1.0-3.3 nmol/L
Thyroid tests (S)			
Thyroxine (T_4)	4-11 µg/dl	12.87	51-142 nmol/L
T_4 expressed as iodine	3.2-7.2 µg/dl	79.0	253-569 nmol/L
T_3 resin uptake	25%-38% relative uptake	0.01	0.25%-0.38% relative uptake
Thyroid-stimulating hormone (S)	10 µU/ml	1	<10^{-3} IU/L
Urea nitrogen (S)	8-23 mg/dl	0.357	2.9-8.2 mmol/L
Uric acid (S)	2-6 mg/dl	59.5	0.120-0.360 mmol/L
Vitamin B_{12} (S)	160-195 pg/ml	0.74	118-703 pmol/L

Continued

CONVERSION FACTORS (SI UNITS)—cont'd

COMPONENT	NORMAL RANGE IN UNITS AS CUSTOMARILY REPORTED	CONVERSION FACTOR	NORMAL RANGE IN SI UNITS, MOLECULAR UNITS, INTERNATIONAL UNITS, OR DECIMAL FRACTIONS
HEMATOLOGY VALUES*			
Red cell volume (male)	25-35 ml/kg body weight	0.001	0.025-0.035 L/kg body weight
Hematocrit	40%-50%	0.01	0.40-0.50
Hemoglobin	13.5-18.0 g/dl	10	135-180 g/L
Hemoglobin	13.5-18.0 g/dl	0.155	2.09-2.79 mmol/L
Red blood cell count	$4.5\text{-}6 \times 10^6/\mu L$	1	$4.6\text{-}6 \times 10^{12}/L$
White blood cell count	$4.5\text{-}10 \times 10^3/\mu L$	1	$4.5\text{-}10 \times 10^9/L$
Mean corpuscular volume	80-96 μm^3	1	80-96 fL

*The International Committee for Standardization in Hematology recommends that the numbers remain the same but that the units change, so that hemoglobin is expressed as grams per deciliter (g/dl) even though other measurements are expressed as units per liter (U/L).
A *femtoliter (fL)* is one quadrillionth (or one thousand trillionth) of a liter.

ANATOMY OF THE CARDIOVASCULAR SYSTEM

The Heart

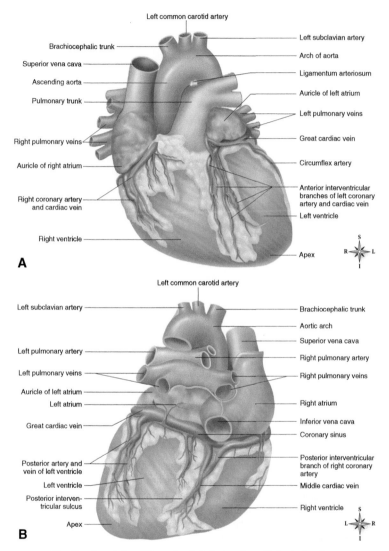

The Heart and Great Vessels. A, Anterior view. **B,** Posterior view.

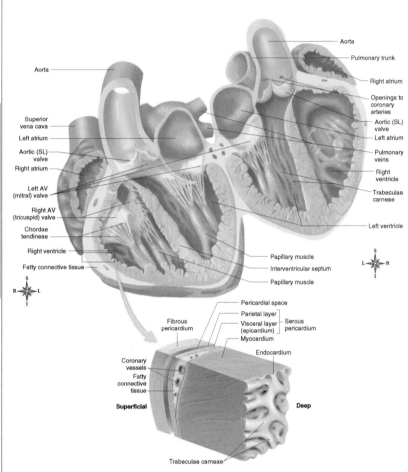

Interior of the Heart. The heart as it would appear if it were cut along a frontal plane and opened like a book. The front portion of the heart lies to the reader's right; the back portion of the heart lies to the reader's left. The four chambers of the heart—two **atria** and two **ventricles**—are easily seen. The *inset* shows a small slice of the ventricular wall, revealing the layers of the **heart wall** and layers of the **pericardium.**

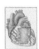

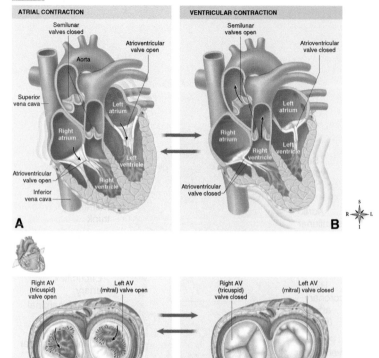

Chambers and Valves of the Heart. A, During atrial contraction, cardiac muscle in the atrial wall contracts, forcing blood through the atrioventricular (AV) valves and into the ventricles. Bottom illustration shows superior view of all four valves, with semilunar (SL) valves closed and AV valves open. **B,** During ventricular contraction that follows, the AV valves close, and the blood is forced out of the ventricles through the SL valves and into the arteries. Bottom illustration shows superior view of SL valves open and AV valves closed.

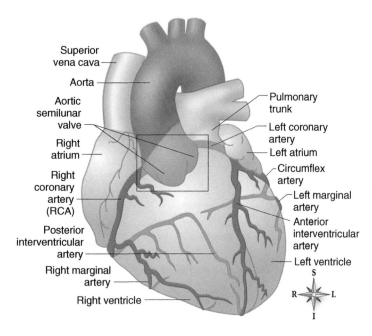

Coronary Arteries. Diagram showing the major coronary arteries (anterior view). Clinicians often refer to the interventricular arteries as *descending arteries.* Thus, a cardiologist would refer to the *left anterior descending (LAD) artery,* and an anatomist would refer to the same vessel as the *anterior interventricular artery.*

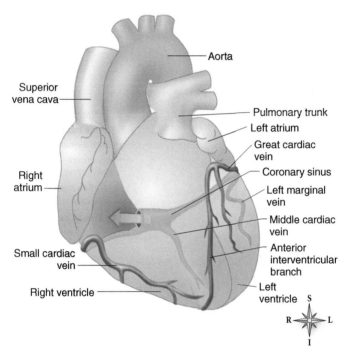

Coronary Veins. Diagram showing the major veins of the coronary circulation (anterior view). Vessels near the anterior surface are more darkly colored than vessels of the posterior surface seen through the heart.

Blood Vessels

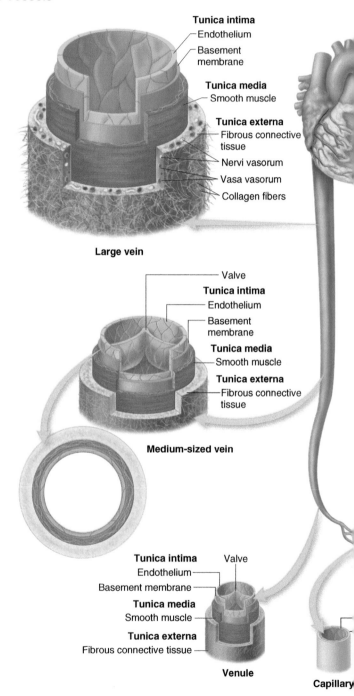

Large vein

Tunica intima
- Endothelium
- Basement membrane

Tunica media
- Smooth muscle

Tunica externa
- Fibrous connective tissue
- Nervi vasorum
- Vasa vasorum
- Collagen fibers

Medium-sized vein

Valve

Tunica intima
- Endothelium
- Basement membrane

Tunica media
- Smooth muscle

Tunica externa
- Fibrous connective tissue

Venule

Tunica intima
- Endothelium
- Basement membrane

Tunica media
- Smooth muscle

Tunica externa
- Fibrous connective tissue

Valve

Capillary

Structure of Blood Vessels. The tunica externa of the veins are shown in *blue,* and the arteries are *red.*

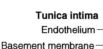

Tunica intima
Endothelium
Basement membrane

Tunica media
Elastic tissue
and smooth muscle

Tunica externa
Fibrous connective
tissue
Nervi vasorum
Vasa vasorum
Collagen fibers

Elastic artery

Tunica intima
Endothelium
Basement membrane

Tunica media
Internal elastic
membrane
Smooth muscle

Tunica externa
External elastic
membrane
Fibrous connective
tissue

Muscular artery

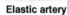

Tunica intima
Endothelium
Basement membrane

Tunica media
Smooth muscle

Tunica externa
Fibrous connective tissue

Endothelium
Basement
membrane

Arteriole

STRUCTURE OF BLOOD VESSELS

	TYPICAL DIAMETER	TYPICAL WALL THICKNESS	TUNICA INTIMA	TUNICA MEDIA	TUNICA EXTERNA
Typical histology			Endothelium	Smooth muscle; elastic fibers	Collagen fibers
Arteries	Aorta: 25 mm Small artery: 4 mm Arteriole: 30 μm	Aorta: 2 mm Small artery: 1 mm Arteriole: 8 μm	Smooth lining	Allows constriction and dilation of vessels; thicker than in veins; muscle innervated by autonomic fibers	Provides flexible support that resists collapse or injury; thicker than in veins; thinner than tunica media
Veins	Vena cava: 30 mm Vein: 5 mm Venule: 20 μm	Vena cava: 1.5 mm Vein: 0.5 mm Venule: 1 μm	Smooth lining with valves to ensure one-way flow	Allows constriction and dilation of vessels; thinner than in arteries; muscle innervated by autonomic fibers	Provides flexible support that resists collapse or injury; thinner than in arteries; thicker than tunica media
Capillaries	5 μm	0.5 μm	Makes up entire wall of capillary; thinness permits ease of transport across vessel wall	(Absent)	(Absent)

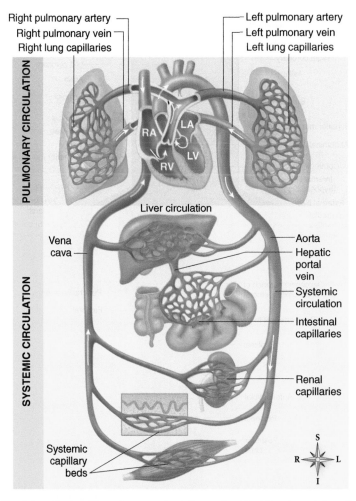

Circulatory Routes. The pulmonary circulation routes blood flow to and from the gas-exchange tissues of the lungs. The systemic circulation, on the other hand, routes blood flow to and from the oxygen-consuming tissues of the body.

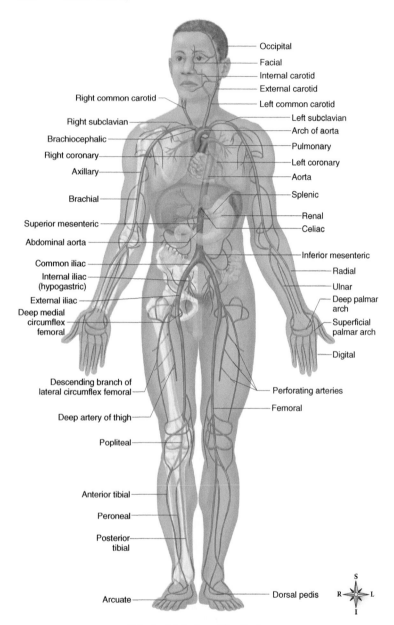

Occipital
Facial
Internal carotid
External carotid
Right common carotid
Left common carotid
Right subclavian
Left subclavian
Brachiocephalic
Arch of aorta
Right coronary
Pulmonary
Axillary
Left coronary
Aorta
Brachial
Splenic
Superior mesenteric
Renal
Abdominal aorta
Celiac
Common iliac
Inferior mesenteric
Internal iliac (hypogastric)
Radial
External iliac
Ulnar
Deep medial circumflex femoral
Deep palmar arch
Superficial palmar arch
Digital
Descending branch of lateral circumflex femoral
Perforating arteries
Deep artery of thigh
Femoral
Popliteal
Anterior tibial
Peroneal
Posterior tibial
Arcuate
Dorsal pedis

S
R L
I

Principal Arteries of the Body.

MAJOR SYSTEMIC ARTERIES

ARTERY*	REGION SUPPLIED
ASCENDING AORTA	
Coronary arteries	Myocardium
ARCH OF AORTA	
Brachiocephalic (innominate)	Head, upper extremity
Right common carotid	Head, neck
Right internal carotid†	Brain, eye, forehead, nose
Right external carotid†	Thyroid, tongue, tonsils, ear, etc.
Right subclavian	Head, upper extremity
Right vertebral†	Spinal cord, brain
Right axillary (continuation of subclavian)	Shoulder, chest, axillary region
Right brachial (continuation of axillary)	Arm, hand
Right radial	Forearm, hand (lateral)
Right ulnar	Forearm, hand (medial)
Superficial and deep palmar arches (formed by anastomosis of branches of radial and ulnar)	Hand, fingers
Digital	Fingers
Left common carotid	Head, neck
Left internal carotid†	Brain, eye, forehead, nose
Left external carotid†	Thyroid, tongue, tonsils, ear, etc.
Left subclavian	Head, upper extremity
Left vertebral†	Spinal cord, brain
Left axillary (continuation of subclavian)	Shoulder, chest, axillary region
Left brachial (continuation of axillary)	Arm, hand
Left radial	Forearm, hand (lateral)
Left ulnar	Forearm, hand (medial)
Superficial and deep palmar arches (formed by anastomosis of branches of radial and ulnar)	Hand, fingers
Digital	Fingers
DESCENDING THORACIC AORTA	
Visceral Branches	Thoracic viscera
Bronchial	Lungs, bronchi
Esophageal	Esophagus
Parietal Branches	Thoracic walls
Intercostal	Lateral thoracic walls (rib cage)
Superior phrenic	Superior surface of diaphragm

*Branches of each artery are indented below its name.
†See text and/or figures for branches of the artery.

Continued

MAJOR SYSTEMIC ARTERIES—cont'd

ARTERY*	REGION SUPPLIED
DESCENDING ABDOMINAL AORTA	
Visceral Branches	Abdominal viscera
Celiac artery (trunk)	Abdominal viscera
Left gastric	Stomach, esophagus
Common hepatic	Liver
Splenic	Spleen, pancreas, stomach
Superior mesenteric	Pancreas, small intestine, colon
Inferior mesenteric	Descending colon, rectum
Suprarenal	Adrenal (suprarenal) gland
Renal	Kidney
Ovarian	Ovary, uterine tube, ureter
Testicular	Testis, ureter
Parietal Branches	Walls of abdomen
Inferior phrenic	Inferior surface of diaphragm, adrenal gland
Lumbar	Lumbar vertebrae, muscles of back
Median sacral	Lower vertebrae
Common iliac (formed by terminal branches of aorta)	Pelvis, lower extremity
External iliac	Thigh, leg, foot
Femoral **(continuation of external iliac)**	Thigh, leg, foot
Popliteal **(continuation of femoral)**	Leg, foot
Anterior tibial	Leg, foot
Posterior tibial	Leg, foot
Plantar arch **(formed by anastomosis of branches of anterior and posterior tibial arteries)**	Foot, toes
Digital	Toes
Internal iliac	Pelvis
Visceral Branches	Pelvic viscera
Middle rectal	Rectum
Vaginal	Vagina, uterus
Uterine	Uterus, vagina, uterine tube, ovary
Parietal Branches	Pelvic wall, external regions
Lateral sacral	Sacrum
Superior gluteal	Gluteal muscles
Obturator	Pubic region, hip joint, groin
Internal pudendal	Rectum, external genitals, floor of pelvis
Inferior gluteal	Lower gluteal region, coccyx, upper thigh

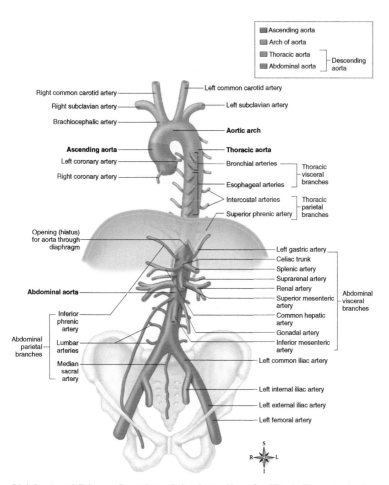

Ascending aorta
Arch of aorta
Thoracic aorta ⎤
Abdominal aorta ⎦ Descending aorta

Right common carotid artery
Right subclavian artery
Brachiocephalic artery

Left common carotid artery
Left subclavian artery
Aortic arch

Ascending aorta
Left coronary artery
Right coronary artery

Thoracic aorta
Bronchial arteries ⎤ Thoracic
Esophageal arteries ⎦ visceral branches

Intercostal arteries ⎤ Thoracic
Superior phrenic artery ⎦ parietal branches

Opening (hiatus) for aorta through diaphragm

Abdominal aorta

Abdominal parietal branches
  Inferior phrenic artery
  Lumbar arteries
  Median sacral artery

Left gastric artery
Celiac trunk
Splenic artery
Suprarenal artery
Renal artery
Superior mesenteric artery
Common hepatic artery
Gonadal artery
Inferior mesenteric artery
Left common iliac artery

Abdominal visceral branches

Left internal iliac artery
Left external iliac artery
Left femoral artery

S
R ✴ L
I

Divisions and Primary Branches of the Aorta (Anterior View). The aorta is the main systemic artery, serving as a trunk from which other arteries branch. Blood is conducted from the heart first through the ascending aorta, then through the arch of the aorta, and then through the thoracic and abdominal segments of the descending aorta. Note the designation of visceral and parietal branches in the thoracic and abdominal aortic divisions.

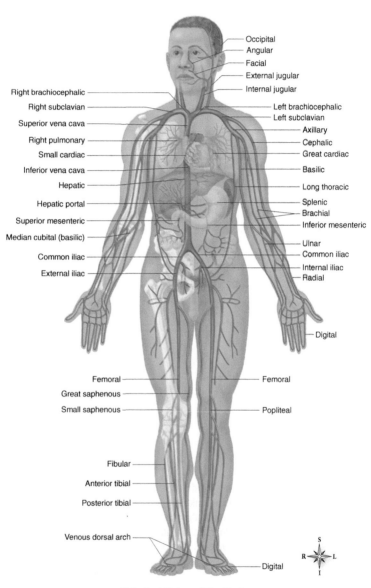

Occipital
Angular
Facial
External jugular
Internal jugular
Right brachiocephalic
Right subclavian
Superior vena cava
Right pulmonary
Small cardiac
Inferior vena cava
Hepatic
Hepatic portal
Superior mesenteric
Median cubital (basilic)
Common iliac
External iliac
Left brachiocephalic
Left subclavian
Axillary
Cephalic
Great cardiac
Basilic
Long thoracic
Splenic
Brachial
Inferior mesenteric
Ulnar
Common iliac
Internal iliac
Radial
Digital
Femoral
Great saphenous
Small saphenous
Femoral
Popliteal
Fibular
Anterior tibial
Posterior tibial
Venous dorsal arch
Digital

Principal Veins of the Body.

MAJOR SYSTEMIC VEINS

VEIN*	REGION DRAINED
SUPERIOR VENA CAVA	Head, neck, thorax, upper extremity
Brachiocephalic (innominate)	Head, neck, upper extremity
Internal jugular (continuation of sigmoid sinus)	Brain
Lingual	Tongue, mouth
Superior thyroid	Thyroid, deep face
Facial	Superficial face
Sigmoid sinus (continuation of transverse sinus; direct tributary of internal jugular)	Brain, meninges, skull
Superior and inferior petrosal sinuses	Anterior brain, skull
Cavernous sinus	Anterior brain, skull
Ophthalmic veins	Eye, orbit
Transverse sinus (direct tributary of sigmoid sinus)	Brain, meninges, skull
Occipital sinus	Inferior, central region of cranial cavity
Straight sinus	Central region of brain, meninges
Inferior sagittal sinus	Central region of brain, meninges
Superior sagittal (longitudinal) sinus	Superior region of cranial cavity
External jugular	Superficial, posterior head, neck
Subclavian (continuation of axillary; direct tributary of brachiocephalic)	Axilla, lower extremity
Cephalic	Lateral arm and forearm, hand
Axillary (continuation of basilic; direct tributary of subclavian)	Axilla, lower extremity
Brachial	Deep arm
Radial	Deep lateral forearm
Ulnar	Deep medial forearm
Basilic (direct tributary of axillary)	Medial arm and forearm, hand
Median cubital (formed by anastomosis of cephalic and basilic)	Forearm, hand

*Tributaries of each vein are identified below its name; deep veins are printed in dark blue, and superficial veins are printed in light blue.

Continued

MAJOR SYSTEMIC VEINS—cont'd

VEIN*	REGION DRAINED
Deep and superficial palmar venous arches (formed by anastomosis of cephalic and basilic)	Hand
Digital	Fingers
Azygos (anastomoses with right ascending lumbar)	Right posterior wall of thorax and abdomen, esophagus, bronchi, pericardium, mediastinum
Hemiazygos (anastomoses with left renal)	Left inferior posterior wall of thorax and abdomen, esophagus, mediastinum
Accessory hemiazygos	Left superior posterior wall of thorax
INFERIOR VENA CAVA	Lower trunk and extremity
Phrenic	Diaphragm
Hepatic portal system	Upper abdominal viscera
Hepatic veins (continuations of liver venules and sinusoids and ultimately the hepatic portal vein)	Liver
Hepatic portal vein	Gastrointestinal organs, pancreas, spleen, gallbladder
Cystic	Gallbladder
Gastric	Stomach
Splenic	Spleen
Inferior mesenteric	Descending colon, rectum
Pancreatic	Pancreas
Superior mesenteric	Small intestine, most of colon
Gastroepiploic	Stomach
Renal	Kidneys
Suprarenal	Adrenal (suprarenal) gland
Left ovarian	Left ovary
Left testicular	Left testis
Left ascending lumbar (anastomoses with hemiazygos)	Left lumbar region
Right ovarian (gonadal)	Right ovary
Right testicular (gonadal)	Right testis
Right ascending lumbar (anastomoses with azygos)	Right lumbar region

MAJOR SYSTEMIC VEINS—cont'd

VEIN*	REGION DRAINED
Common iliac (continuation of external iliac; common iliacs unite to form inferior vena cava)	Lower extremity
External iliac (continuation of femoral direct tributary of common iliac)	Thigh, leg, foot
Femoral (continuation of popliteal direct tributary of external iliac)	Thigh, leg, foot
Popliteal	Leg, foot
Small (external, short) saphenous	Superficial posterior leg, lateral foot
Dorsal veins of foot (also drain into great saphenous)	Anterior (dorsal) foot, toes
Medial and lateral plantar	Sole of foot
Anterior tibial	Anterior leg, foot
Fibular (peroneal)	Lateral and anterior leg, foot
Posterior tibial	Deep posterior leg
Great (internal, long) saphenous	Superficial medial and anterior thigh, leg, foot
Dorsal veins of foot	Anterior (dorsal) foot, toes
Dorsal venous arch	Anterior (dorsal) foot, toes
Digital	Toes
Internal iliac (unites with external iliac to form common iliac)	Pelvic region

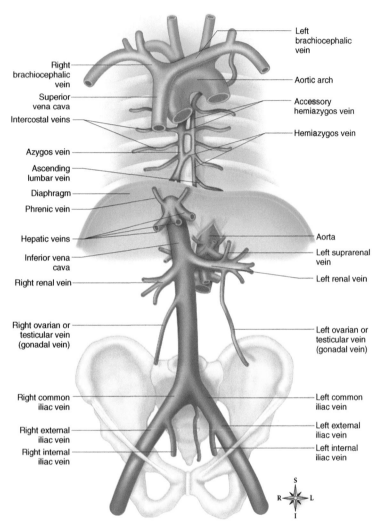

Left brachiocephalic vein

Right brachiocephalic vein

Aortic arch

Superior vena cava

Accessory hemiazygos vein

Intercostal veins

Hemiazygos vein

Azygos vein

Ascending lumbar vein

Diaphragm

Phrenic vein

Hepatic veins

Aorta

Inferior vena cava

Left suprarenal vein

Right renal vein

Left renal vein

Right ovarian or testicular vein (gonadal vein)

Left ovarian or testicular vein (gonadal vein)

Right common iliac vein

Left common iliac vein

Right external iliac vein

Left external iliac vein

Right internal iliac vein

Left internal iliac vein

Inferior Vena Cava and Its Abdominopelvic Tributaries. Anterior view of the ventral body cavity with many of the viscera removed. Note the close anatomical relationship between the inferior vena cava and the descending aorta. Smaller veins of the thorax drain blood into the inferior vena cava or into the azygos vein—both are shown here. The hemiazygos vein and accessory hemiazygos vein on the *left* drain into the azygos vein on the *right*.

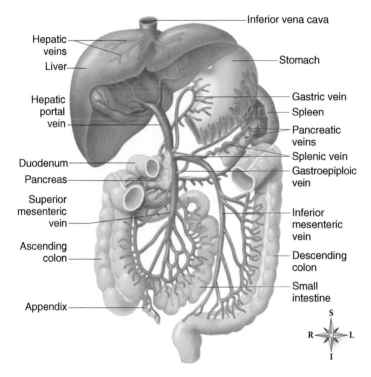

Hepatic veins

Liver

Hepatic portal vein

Duodenum

Pancreas

Superior mesenteric vein

Ascending colon

Appendix

Inferior vena cava

Stomach

Gastric vein

Spleen

Pancreatic veins

Splenic vein

Gastroepiploic vein

Inferior mesenteric vein

Descending colon

Small intestine

Hepatic Portal Circulation. In this unusual circulatory route, a vein is located between two capillary beds. The hepatic portal vein collects blood from capillaries in visceral structures located in the abdomen and empties it into the liver. Hepatic veins return blood to the inferior vena cava.

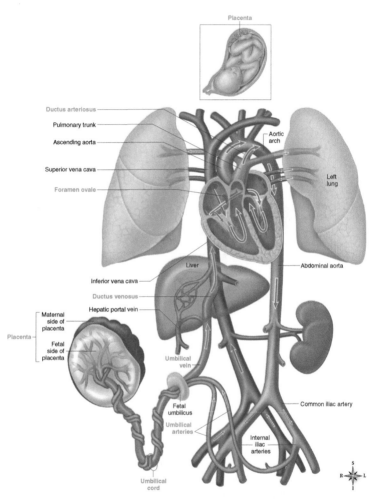

Placenta

Ductus arteriosus
Pulmonary trunk
Ascending aorta
Superior vena cava
Foramen ovale

Aortic arch

Left lung

Abdominal aorta

Liver
Inferior vena cava
Ductus venosus
Hepatic portal vein

Maternal side of placenta
Fetal side of placenta

Placenta

Umbilical vein

Fetal umbilicus
Umbilical arteries

Common iliac artery

Internal iliac arteries

Umbilical cord

Plan of Fetal Circulation. Before birth, the human circulatory system has several special features that adapt the body to life in the womb. These features (labeled in red type) include two umbilical arteries, one umbilical vein, ductus venosus, foramen ovale, ductus arteriosus, and umbilical cord. The placenta, another essential feature of the fetal circulatory plan, is shown in greater detail on p. 562.

PHYSIOLOGY OF THE CARDIOVASCULAR SYSTEM

The Heart as a Pump

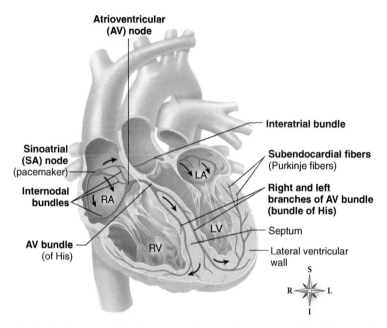

Conduction System of the Heart. Specialized cardiac muscle cells (boldface type) in the wall of the heart rapidly initiate or conduct an electrical impulse throughout the myocardium. This sketch of the conduction system shows the origin and path of conduction. The signal is initiated by the SA node (pacemaker) and spreads to the rest of the right atrial myocardium directly, to the left atrial myocardium by way of a bundle of interatrial conducting fibers, and to the AV node by way of three internodal bundles. The AV node then initiates a signal that is conducted through the ventricular myocardium by way of the AV bundle (of His) and subendocardial branches (Purkinje fibers).

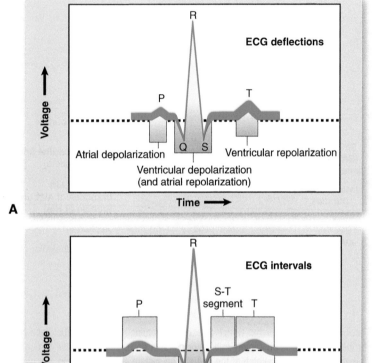

Electrocardiogram. A, Idealized ECG deflections represent depolarization and repolarization of cardiac muscle tissue. **B,** Principal ECG intervals between P, QRS, and T waves. Note that the P-R interval is measured from the start of the P wave to the start of the Q wave.

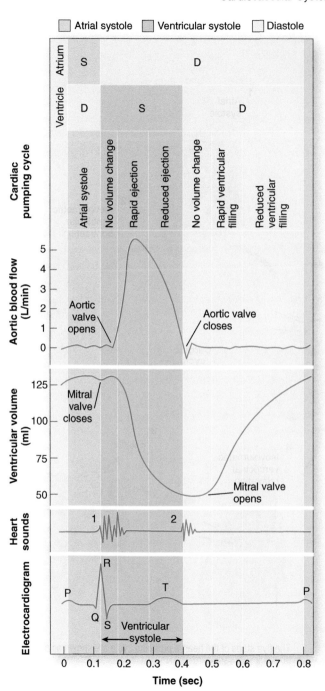

Composite Chart of Heart Functions. This chart is a composite of several diagrams of heart function during rest (72 beats/min). Along the top, *S* represents systole and *D* represents diastole of each heart chamber. Below that, details of the cardiac pumping cycle, aortic blood flow, ventricular volume, valve actions, heart sounds, and ECG are all adjusted to the same time scale. Although it appears daunting at first glance, this "stack of graphs," will be a valuable reference tool as you proceed through the rest of this chapter and try to "put it all together."

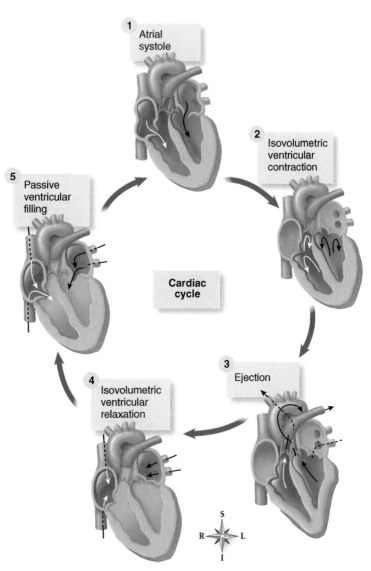

The Cardiac Cycle. The five steps of the heart's pumping cycle are shown as a series of changes in the heart wall and valves.

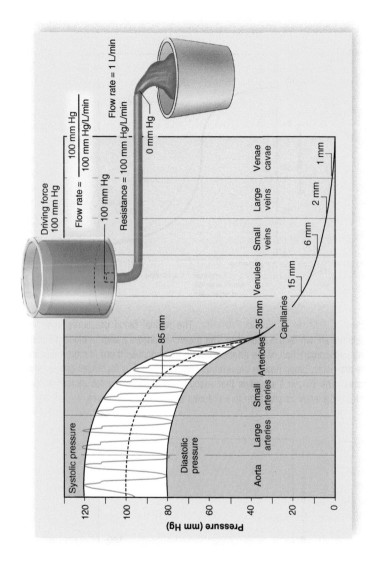

The Primary Principle of Circulation. Fluid always travels from an area of high pressure to an area of low pressure. In the *inset*, fluid flows from an area of high pressure in the tank (100 mm Hg) toward the area of low pressure above the bucket (0 mm Hg). In the graph, blood tends to move from an area of high pressure at the beginning of the aorta (100 mm Hg) toward the area of lowest pressure at the end of the venae cavae (0 mm Hg). Blood flow between any two points in the circulatory system can always be predicted by the pressure gradient.

Arterial Blood Pressure

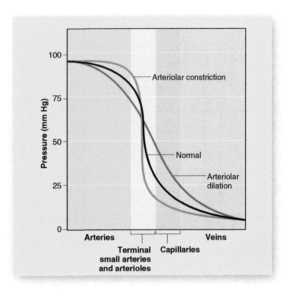

Vasomotor Effects on Blood Pressure. The normal blood pressures in various vessels are shown by the *black line*. The *green line* shows a shift in blood pressures during vasoconstriction of the arterioles. Note that because there is more resistance in the arterioles, blood flow in the arteries backs up and thus increases arterial blood pressure. The *purple line* shows that vasodilation of the arterioles increases blood flow from the arteries and therefore reduces arterial blood pressure.

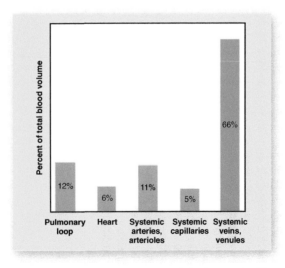

Relative Blood Volumes. The relative volumes of blood at rest in different parts of the adult cardiovascular system expressed as percentages of total blood volume. Note that at rest most of the body's blood supply is in the systemic veins and venules.

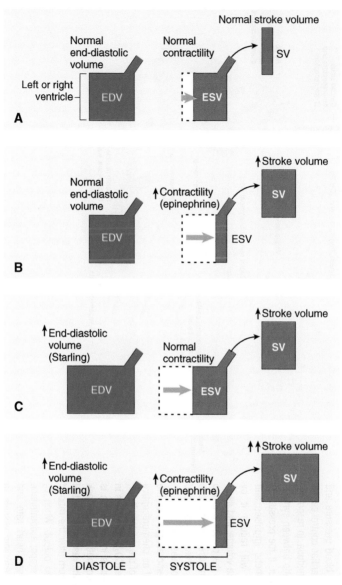

Stroke Volume. Changes in stroke volume caused by increasing the end-diastolic volume (EDV) and/or contractility. **A,** Normal stroke volume (no external influences). **B,** When EDV remains constant and contractility increases (from epinephrine), then the stroke volume increases. **C,** When contractility remains constant and EDV increases, then the stroke volume increases (Starling's law of the heart). **D,** When both EDV and contractility increase, a combined effect increases the stroke volume even more. *EDV,* End-diastolic volume; *ESV,* end-systolic volume; *SV,* stroke volume.

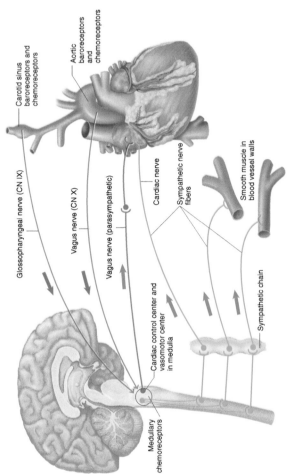

Glossopharyngeal nerve (CN IX)

Carotid sinus baroreceptors and chemoreceptors

Aortic baroreceptors and chemoreceptors

Vagus nerve (CN X)

Vagus nerve (parasympathetic)

Cardiac nerve

Sympathetic nerve fibers

Smooth muscle in blood vessel walls

Cardiac control center and vasomotor center in medulla

Sympathetic chain

Medullary chemoreceptors

Vasomotor Pressoreflexes. Carotid sinus and aortic baroreceptors detect changes in blood pressure and feed the information back to the cardiac control center and the vasomotor center in the medulla. In response, these control centers alter the ratio between sympathetic and parasympathetic output. If the pressure is too high, increased parasympathetic impulses and reduced sympathetic impulses will reduce it by slowing heart rate, reducing stroke volume, and dilating blood "reservoir" vessels. If the pressure is too low, an increase in sympathetic impulses will increase it by increasing heart rate and stroke volume and constricting arterioles and reservoir vessels.

Vasomotor Chemoreflexes. Chemoreceptors in the carotid and aortic bodies, as well as chemoreceptive neurons in the vasomotor center of the medulla itself, detect increases in carbon dioxide (CO_2), decreases in blood oxygen (O_2), and/or decreases in pH (which is really an increase in H^+). This information feeds back to the cardiac control center and the vasomotor control center of the medulla, which in turn alter the ratio of parasympathetic and sympathetic output. When O_2 drops, CO_2 increases, and/or pH drops, a dominance of sympathetic impulses increases heart rate and stroke volume and constricts reservoir vessels in response.

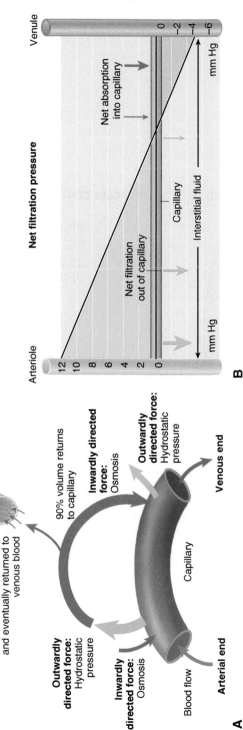

Starling's Law of the Capillaries. A, At the arterial end of a capillary the outward driving force of blood pressure (hydrostatic pressure of blood) is larger than the inwardly directed force of osmosis—thus fluid moves out of the vessel. At the venous end of a capillary the inward driving force of osmosis is greater than the outward directed force of hydrostatic pressure—thus fluid enters the vessel. About 90% of the fluid leaving the capillary at the arterial end is recovered by the blood before it leaves the venous end. The remaining 10% is recovered by the venous blood eventually, by way of the lymphatic vessels. **B,** Graph showing the shift in net filtration force along the length of a capillary, according to Starling's law of the capillaries. At the arterial end, net movement of fluid is *out of* the capillary; at the venous end, net movement of fluid shifts *into* the capillary.

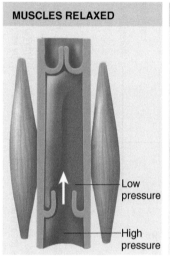
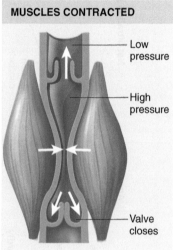

MUSCLES RELAXED

Low pressure

High pressure

A

MUSCLES CONTRACTED

Low pressure

High pressure

Valve closes

B

Venous Valves. In veins, one-way valves aid circulation by preventing backflow of venous blood when pressure in a local area is low. **A,** Local high blood pressure pushes the flaps of the valve to the side of the vessel, allowing easy flow. **B,** When pressure below the valve drops, blood begins to flow backward but fills the "pockets" formed by the valve flaps, pushing the flaps together and thus blocking further backward flow.

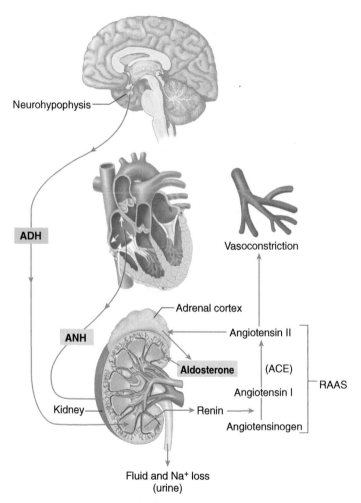

Three Mechanisms That Influence Total Plasma Volume. The antidiuretic hormone (ADH) mechanism and renin-angiotensin-aldosterone system (RAAS) tend to increase water retention and thus increase total plasma volume. The atrial natriuretic hormone (ANH) mechanism antagonizes these mechanisms by promoting water loss and thus promoting a decrease in total plasma volume. *ACE,* Angiotensinogen-converting enzyme.

Minute Volume of Blood

Factors That Influence the Flow of Blood. The flow of blood, expressed as volume of blood flowing per minute (or *minute volume*), is determined by various factors. This chart shows only some of the major factors that influence blood flow. Note that some factors appear more than once in the chart, indicating that they can influence blood flow in several ways. *ADH,* Antidiuretic hormone; *ANH,* atrial natriuretic hormone.

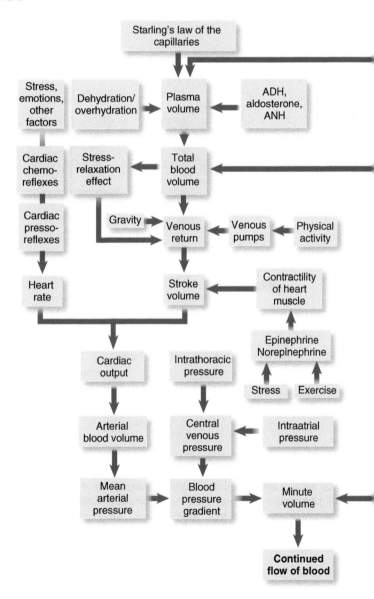

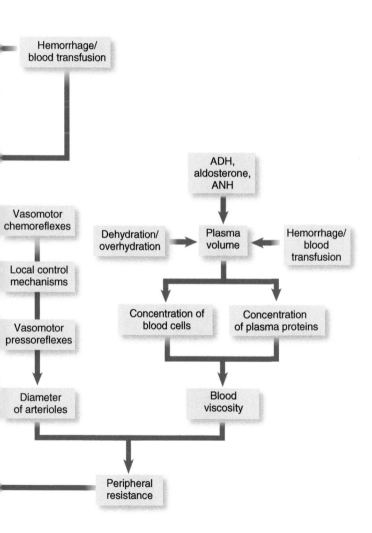

Pulse

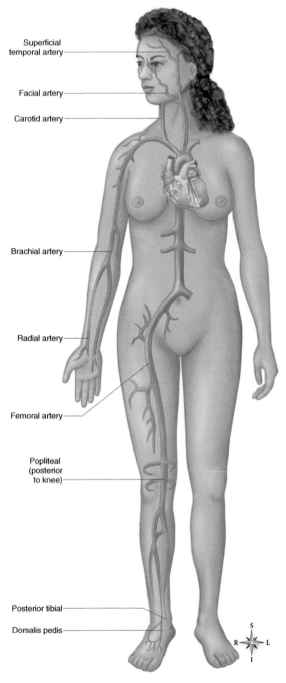

Pulse Points. Each pulse point is named after the artery with which it is associated. (Some arteries in the figure have been enlarged to clarify the location of pulse points.)

Lymphatic and Immune Systems

11

The **lymphatic system** serves various functions in the body. The two most important functions of this system are maintenance of fluid balance in the internal environment and **immunity**. A third, somewhat less important, function of the lymphatic system is the absorption of lipids from digested food in the small intestine and its transport to the large systemic veins.

The lymphatic system maintains the body's fluid balance by collecting tissue fluid that fails to return to the blood and would otherwise cause tissue swelling. The lymphatic system is often considered to be a component of the circulatory system because it consists of a moving fluid (**lymph**) derived from the blood and tissue fluid and a group of vessels (**lymphatics**) that return the lymph to the blood. In general, the lymphatic vessels that drain the peripheral areas of the body parallel the venous return.

The immune system functions as an internal "security force" using components of blood, **lymphoid tissue** of the lymphatic organs, and other agents to protect the body. Immunity can help the body counteract harmful effects of microbes (such as bacteria), cancer cells, burns, chemical toxins, and other damaging insults to the body.

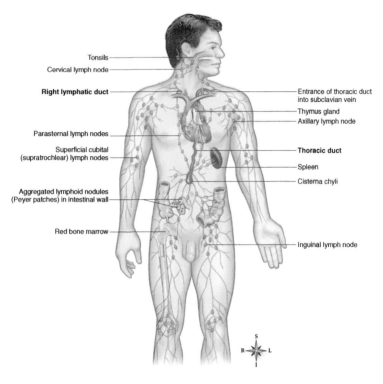

Tonsils

Cervical lymph node

Right lymphatic duct

Parasternal lymph nodes

Superficial cubital
(supratrochlear) lymph nodes

Aggregated lymphoid nodules
(Peyer patches) in intestinal wall

Red bone marrow

Entrance of thoracic duct
into subclavian vein

Thymus gland

Axillary lymph node

Thoracic duct

Spleen

Cisterna chyli

Inguinal lymph node

Principal Organs of the Lymphatic System.

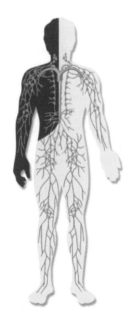

Lymphatic Drainage. The right lymphatic duct drains lymph from the upper right quadrant *(dark blue)* of the body into the right subclavian vein. The thoracic duct drains lymph from the rest of the body *(yellow)* into the left subclavian vein. The lymphatic fluid is thus returned to the systemic blood just before entering the heart.

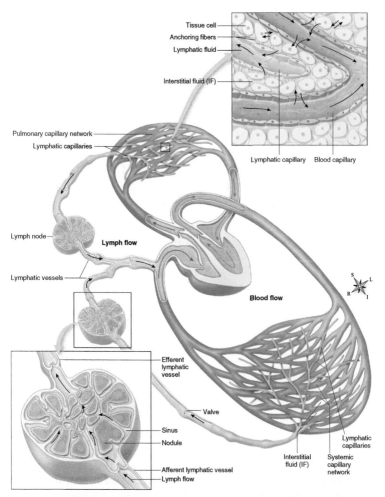

Circulation Plan of Lymphatic Fluid. This diagram outlines the general scheme for lymphatic circulation. Fluids from the systemic and pulmonary capillaries leave the bloodstream and enter the interstitial space, thus becoming part of the interstitial fluid (IF). The IF also exchanges materials with the surrounding tissues. Often, because less fluid is returned to the blood capillary than had left it, IF pressure increases—causing IF to flow into the lymphatic capillary. The fluid is then called *lymph* (lymphatic fluid) and is carried through one or more lymph nodes and finally to large lymphatic ducts. The lymph enters a subclavian vein, where it is returned to the systemic blood plasma. Thus fluid circulates through blood vessels, tissues, and lymphatic vessels in a sort of "open circulation."

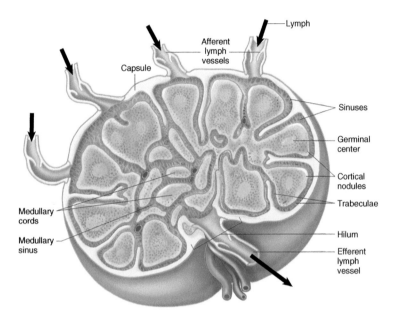

Capsule

Lymph

Afferent
lymph
vessels

Sinuses

Germinal
center

Cortical
nodules

Trabeculae

Medullary
cords

Medullary
sinus

Hilum

Efferent
lymph
vessel

Internal Structure of a Lymph Node. Several afferent valved lymphatics bring lymph to the node. In this example, a single efferent lymphatic leaves the node at a concave area called the *hilum.* Note that the artery and vein also enter and leave at the hilum. *Arrows* show direction of lymph flow.

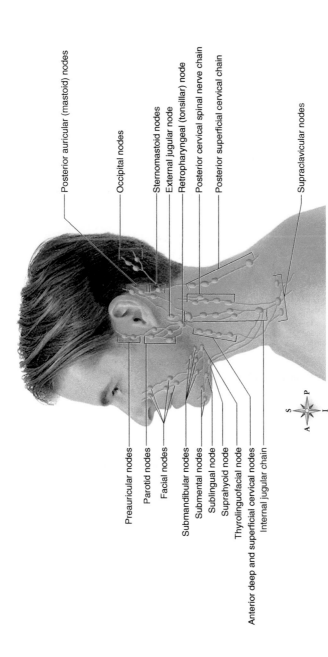

Posterior auricular (mastoid) nodes

Occipital nodes

Sternomastoid nodes

External jugular node

Retropharyngeal (tonsillar) node

Posterior cervical spinal nerve chain

Posterior superficial cervical chain

Supraclavicular nodes

Preauricular nodes

Parotid nodes

Facial nodes

Submandibular nodes

Submental nodes

Sublingual node

Suprahyoid node

Thyrolinguofacial node

Anterior deep and superficial cervical nodes

Internal jugular chain

Lymphatic Drainage of the Head and Neck. The head and neck contain many lymph nodes (and associated lymphatic vessels) that are often of clinical significance in certain infections and cancers.

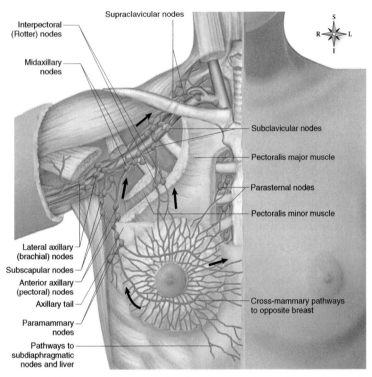

Lymphatic Drainage of the Breast. Note the extensive network of lymphatic vessels and nodes that receive lymph from the breast.

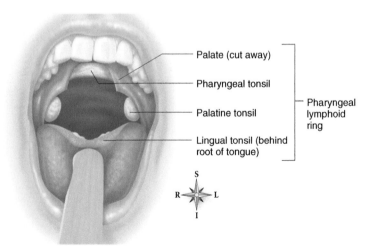

Location of the Tonsils. Small segments of the roof and floor of the mouth have been removed to show the protective ring of tonsils (pharyngeal lymphoid ring) around the internal openings of the nose and throat. Tubal tonsils are not visible in this view.

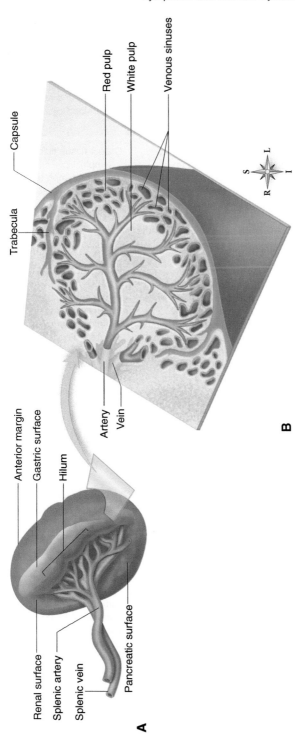

Capsule

Trabecula

Red pulp

White pulp

Venous sinuses

Artery

Vein

Anterior margin

Gastric surface

Hilum

Renal surface

Splenic artery

Splenic vein

Pancreatic surface

A

B

S

L

I

R

Structure of the Spleen. A, Medial aspect of the spleen. Notice the concave surface that fits against the stomach within the abdominopelvic cavity. **B,** Section showing the internal organization of the spleen.

MAJOR LYMPHATIC ORGANS

ORGAN	STRUCTURE	FUNCTION
Lymphatic vessels	Thin-walled vessels with numerous valves that ensure one-way flow of lymphatic fluid (lymph); larger vessels have three layers (similar to veins)	Collect fluids draining from tissues of the body (lymph) and return it to the blood circulation
Lymphatic capillaries	Microscopic, blind-end vessels, made up of single endothelial layer having many gaps	Collect tissue fluid (forming lymph) Transport lymph to larger lymphatic vessels
Lymphatic ducts	Large lymphatic vessels formed by many tributaries throughout the body; connect to the subclavian veins	Collect lymph from network of lymphatic vessels and drain it into the blood circulation
Lymphoid organs	Have a significant component of lymphoid tissue (developing white blood cells)	Hematopoiesis (white blood cells) Immunity Filter body fluids
Lymph nodes	Fibrous capsule surrounding a maze of sinuses, each with lymphoid tissue nodule suspended by reticular fibers	Filtration of lymph before it enters bloodstream Mechanical filtration: removing particles Biological filtration: cells destroy and remove particles
Aggregated lymph nodules (tonsils, Peyer patches)	Groupings of nodules (lumps of lymphoid tissue) embedded in mucous membranes	Immunity at common points of entry for pathogenic microbes
Thymus	Two pyramid-shaped lobes subdivided into smaller lobules containing lymphoid tissue	Hematopoiesis—site of T-lymphocyte (T-cell) development Hormone production—thymosin regulates T-cell development
Spleen	Ovoid fibrous capsule with internal maze of sinuses containing dense lymphoid tissue (white pulp) surrounded by blood sinusoids having cords of lymphoid tissue (red pulp)	Hematopoiesis (white blood cells) Immunity Filtration of blood Tissue repair Destruction of old red blood cells and platelets Blood reservoir

IMMUNE SYSTEM

INNATE AND ADAPTIVE IMMUNITY

		INNATE IMMUNITY	ADAPTIVE IMMUNITY
SYNONYMS	Frequently used alternate terminology	Nonspecific immunity, native immunity, genetic immunity	Specific immunity, acquired immunity
CHARACTERISTICS			
Specificity	Unique antigens produce unique responses of the immune system	Not specific— recognizes variety of different groups of foreign cells or particles	Specific— recognizes specific antigens on specific cells or particles
Speed of reaction	Reaction time of the immune responses	Rapid: immediate up to several hours	Slower: several hours to several days
Memory	Enhanced responses to repeated exposures to the same antigen	None	Yes
Does not react to self	Prevents injury to the individual's own cells*	Yes	Yes
COMPONENTS			
Barriers	Prevent entry of harmful particles	Skin, mucosa, antimicrobial chemicals	Lymphocytes in epithelia; antibodies released at epithelial surfaces
Blood proteins	Circulate throughout body, providing wide area of protection	Complement, interferon (IFN), others	Antibodies
Cells	Types of leukocytes involved in immunity	Phagocytes (macrophages, neutrophils), natural killer (NK) cells	Lymphocytes (B cells and T cells)

*Assumes healthy function. Anti-self immunity (autoimmunity) is a characteristic of many disorders.

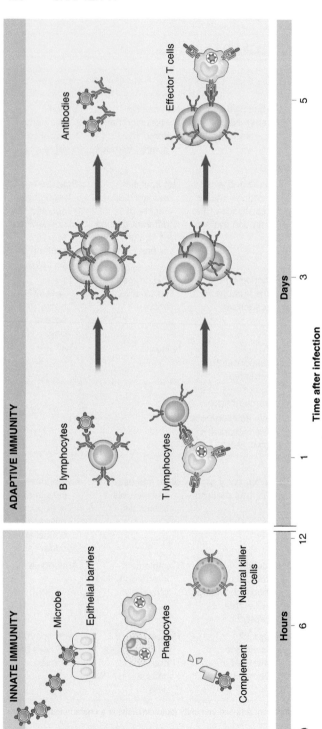

Innate and Adaptive Immunity. Innate (nonspecific) immune mechanisms are "built in" and ready for action—thus providing the initial defense against infections and other assaults on the body. Adaptive (specific) immune mechanisms develop later, as lymphocytes are activated to work against specific foreign or abnormal cells and particles. The timeframes are generalizations.

MECHANISMS OF INNATE DEFENSE

MECHANISM	DESCRIPTION
Species Resistance	Genetic characteristics of the human species protect the body from certain pathogens
Mechanical and Chemical Barriers	Physical impediments to the entry of foreign cells or substances
Skin and mucosa	Forms a continuous wall that separates the internal environment from the external environment, preventing the entry of pathogens
Secretions	Secretions such as sebum, mucus, acids, and enzymes chemically inhibit the activity of pathogens
Inflammation	The inflammatory response isolates the pathogens and stimulates the speedy arrival of large numbers of immune cells
Fever	Fever may enhance immune reactions and inhibit pathogens
Phagocytosis	Ingestion and destruction of pathogens by phagocytic cells
Neutrophils	Granular leukocytes that are usually the first phagocytic cells to arrive at the scene of an inflammatory response
Macrophages	Monocytes that have enlarged to become giant phagocytic cells capable of consuming many pathogens; often called by other, more specific names when found in specific tissues of the body
Natural Killer (NK) Cells	Group of lymphocytes that kill many different types of cancer cells and virus-infected cells
Interferon	Protein produced by cells after they become infected by a virus; inhibits the spread or further development of a viral infection
Complement	Group of plasma proteins (inactive enzymes) that produce a cascade of chemical reactions that ultimately causes lysis (rupture) of a foreign cell; the complement cascade can be triggered by adaptive or innate immune mechanisms
Toll-like Receptors (TLRs)	Membrane receptors that recognize nonspecific patterns in microbial molecules (not human molecules) and trigger a variety of innate immune responses (many of those listed in this table)

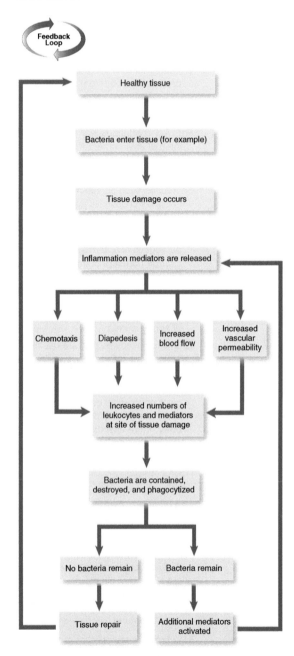

Example of the Inflammatory Response. Tissue damage caused by bacteria triggers a series of events that produces the inflammatory response and promotes phagocytosis at the site of injury. These responses tend to inhibit or destroy the bacteria, eventually bringing the tissue back to its healthy state. Similar reactions will occur in the presence of other abnormal or injurious particles or conditions.

EXAMPLES OF PHAGOCYTE LOCATIONS

PHAGOCYTES	LOCATION
Circulating phagocytes	Bloodstream
Osteoclasts; bone marrow (fixed) phagocytes	Bone and bone marrow
Microglia	Central nervous system
Histiocytes	Connective tissues
Epidermal dendritic cells	Epidermis
Kupffer cells	Liver
Alveolar macrophages (dust cells); dendritic cells	Lung
Fixed and free lymphoid macrophages; dendritic cells	Lymph nodes
Pleural macrophages; peritoneal macrophages	Serous fluids
Splenic macrophages	Spleen

TYPES OF ADAPTIVE IMMUNITY

TYPE	DESCRIPTION OR EXAMPLE
NATURAL IMMUNITY	Exposure to the causative agent is not deliberate
Active (exposure)	A child develops measles and acquires an immunity to a subsequent infection
Passive (exposure)	A fetus receives protection from the mother through the placenta, or an infant receives protection through the mother's milk
ARTIFICIAL IMMUNITY	Exposure to the causative agent is deliberate
Active (exposure)	Injection of the causative agent, such as a vaccination against polio, confers immunity
Passive (exposure)	Injection of protective material (antibodies) that was developed by another individual's immune system

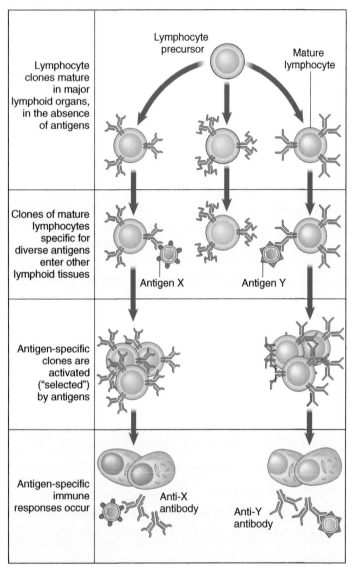

The Clonal Selection Theory. This theory of immunity states that each specific antigen (here shown as *X* and *Y*) activates—selects—a previously produced clone of lymphocytes. The clone is "selected" because it is specifically targeted at the selecting antigen. The clone, when thus activated, produces effector cells that attack the antigen. B cells are shown here, but the same principle also applies to T cells.

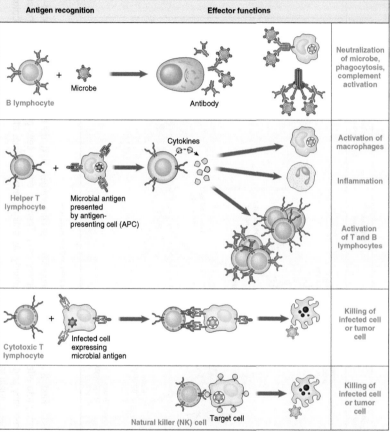

Lymphocyte Functions. This diagram summarizes, in a simplified way, the main functions of the major classes of lymphocytes. B and T lymphocytes participate in adaptive immunity and NK cells participate in innate immunity.

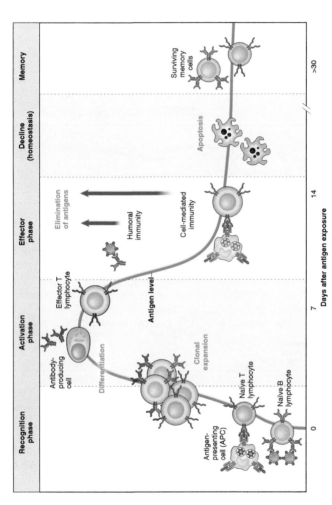

Stages of the Adaptive Immune Response. First, B cells and T cells recognize a specific antigen. Next, the B and T cells are activated—expanding their population (clonal expansion) while differentiating into effector cells and memory cells. Then the effector cells get to work attacking the source or sources of the antigen—humoral (antibody-mediated) immunity and cell-mediated immunity. As antigen levels decline, effector cells die off (apoptosis). Memory cells then remain—ready to quickly engage the antigen again later.

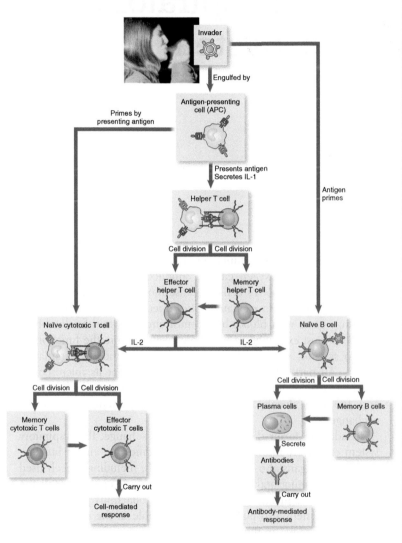

Summary of Adaptive Immunity. Flowchart summarizing an example of adaptive immune response when exposed to a microbial pathogen.

12

Respiratory System

The **respiratory system** functions as an air distributor and a gas exchanger so that oxygen can be supplied to and carbon dioxide removed from the body's cells. Because most of our trillions of cells lie too far from air to exchange gases directly with it, air must first exchange gases with blood, blood must circulate, and finally, blood and cells must exchange gases. These events require the functioning of two systems, namely, the respiratory system and the circulatory system. All parts of the respiratory system—except its microscopic-sized sacs called alveoli—function as air distributors. Only the alveoli and the tiny alveolar ducts that open into them serve as gas exchangers.

In addition to air distribution and gas exchange, the respiratory system effectively filters, warms, and humidifies the air we breathe. Respiratory organs also help produce sounds, including speech used in communicating oral language. Special sensory epithelium in the respiratory tract makes the sense of smell (olfaction) possible. The respiratory system also plays an important role in the regulation, or homeostasis, of pH in the body.

ANATOMY OF THE RESPIRATORY SYSTEM

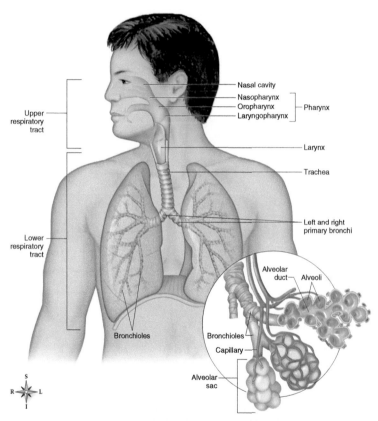

Structural Plan of the Respiratory System. The *inset* shows the alveolar sacs, where the interchange of oxygen and carbon dioxide takes place through the walls of the grapelike alveoli.

Upper Respiratory Tract.

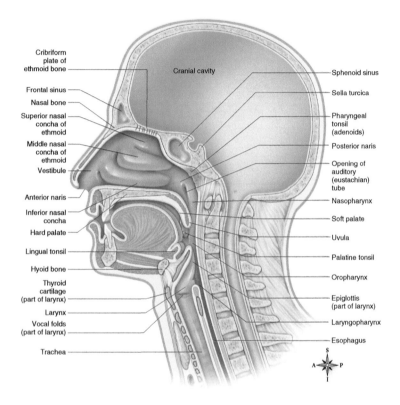

Cribriform plate of ethmoid bone

Frontal sinus

Nasal bone

Superior nasal concha of ethmoid

Middle nasal concha of ethmoid

Vestibule

Anterior naris

Inferior nasal concha

Hard palate

Lingual tonsil

Hyoid bone

Thyroid cartilage (part of larynx)

Larynx

Vocal folds (part of larynx)

Trachea

Cranial cavity

Sphenoid sinus

Sella turcica

Pharyngeal tonsil (adenoids)

Posterior naris

Opening of auditory (eustachian) tube

Nasopharynx

Soft palate

Uvula

Palatine tonsil

Oropharynx

Epiglottis (part of larynx)

Laryngopharynx

Esophagus

Upper Respiratory Tract. In this midsagittal section through the upper respiratory tract, the nasal septum has been removed to reveal the turbinates (nasal conchae) of the lateral wall of the nasal cavity. The three divisions of the pharynx (nasopharynx, oropharynx, and laryngopharynx) are also visible.

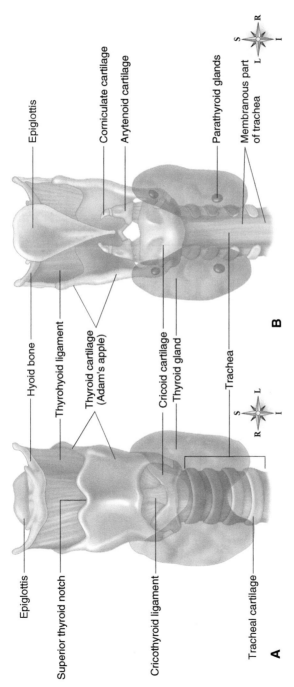

Laryngeal Cartilages. Some softer tissues of the larynx and surrounding structures have been removed to make it possible to see the cartilages of the larynx. Note the position of the nearby thyroid gland. **A,** Anterior view. **B,** Posterior view.

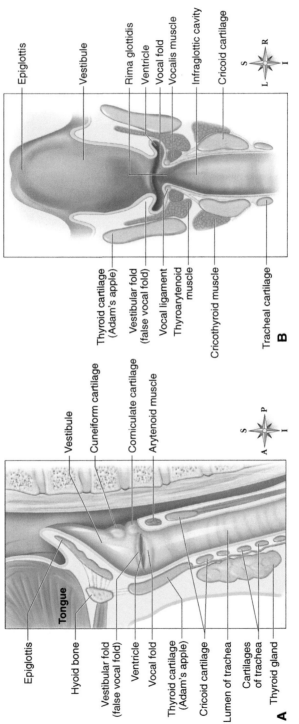

Larynx. These illustrations depict the mucosal lining of the larynx, with its folds and underlying muscles and ligaments visible. **A,** Sagittal section. **B,** Frontal section, viewed from behind.

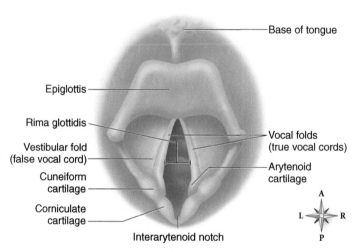

Vocal Folds. Vocal folds viewed from above.

Lower Respiratory Tract.

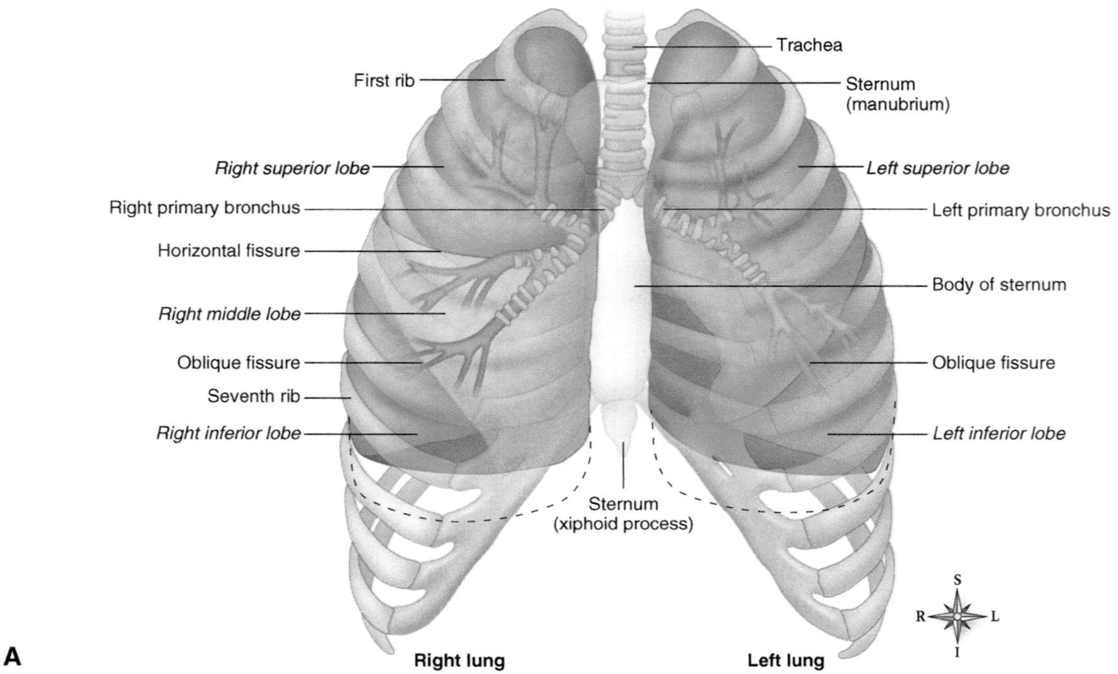
Trachea
First rib
Sternum
(manubrium)
Right superior lobe
Left superior lobe
Right primary bronchus
Left primary bronchus
Horizontal fissure
Body of sternum
Right middle lobe
Oblique fissure
Oblique fissure
Seventh rib
Right inferior lobe
Left inferior lobe
Sternum
(xiphoid process)
S
R
L
I
A
Right lung
Left lung

Lobes and Segments of the Lungs. A. Anterior view of the lungs, bronchi, and trachea.

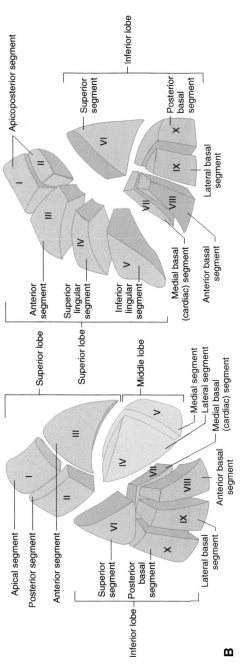

Lobes and Segments of the Lungs—cont'd. B, Expanded diagram showing the bronchopulmonary segments.

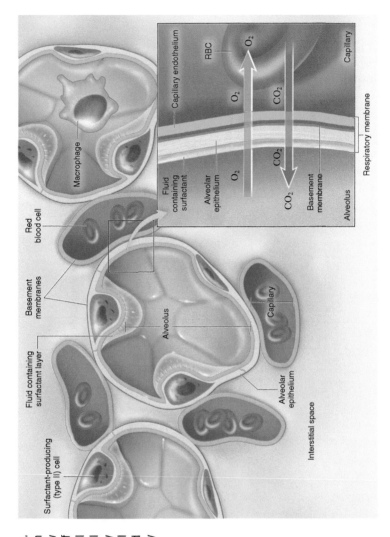

Gas Exchange Structures of the Lung. Each alveolus is continually ventilated with fresh air. The *inset* shows a magnified view of the respiratory membrane composed of the alveolar wall (fluid coating, epithelial cells, and basement membrane), interstitial fluid, and the wall of a pulmonary capillary (basement membrane and endothelial cells). The gases—CO_2 (carbon dioxide) and O_2 (oxygen)—diffuse across the respiratory membrane.

Structures of the Respiratory Tract

SUMMARY OF RESPIRATORY TRACT STRUCTURES*

STRUCTURE	DESCRIPTION	FUNCTION
UPPER RESPIRATORY TRACT	Portion of the respiratory tract outside the thoracic cavity	Processing of incoming air Conducts air to/from lungs Vocalization and phonation Olfaction
Nasal cavity	Lumen of nose, separated into left and right portions by nasal septum supported by cartilage, vomer, and perpendicular plate of ethmoid; supported laterally by nasal conchae	Conducts air between atmosphere (external environment) and pharynx Warms, humidifies, cleans inspired air
Anterior nares (external nares)	Nostrils External openings of nasal cavity	Boundary between external environment and nasal cavity
Vestibule	Extends from the anterior nares to the inferior meatus Supported by cartilage of septum and ala Lined with skin epidermis (keratinized stratified squamous epithelium) with vibrissae (hairs)	Conducts air between external environment and respiratory portion of nasal cavity Vibrissae prevent entry of large contaminants
Respiratory portion	Extends from vestibule to posterior nares Supported by bones of septum and nasal conchae, which curve to form meatuses Lined with highly vascular respiratory mucosa (pseudostratified ciliated columnar epithelium) Olfactory epithelium in superior lining contains numerous sensory receptors	Conducts air between vestibule and pharynx Meatuses create turbulence to assist processing of inspired air Mucosa warms, humidifies, and cleans inspired air Olfaction

Continued

SUMMARY OF RESPIRATORY TRACT STRUCTURES*—cont'd

STRUCTURE	DESCRIPTION	FUNCTION
Paranasal sinuses	Four pairs of air-filled spaces within frontal, maxillary, ethmoid, and sphenoid bones of skull Lined with pseudostratified ciliated columnar epithelium Drain into the nasal cavity	Reduce weight of skull Help warm and humidify air
Posterior nares (internal nares)	Openings from the nasal cavity into the pharynx	Boundary between nasal cavity and pharynx
Pharynx	Throat Extends from posterior nares to the esophagus Supported by occipital bone and skeletal muscle Lined with mucous membrane (nonkeratinized stratified squamous epithelium)	Conducts air between nasal cavity and larynx
Nasopharynx	Segment of pharynx posterior to nasal cavity Pharyngeal tonsils in posterior wall	Conducts air between posterior nares and oropharynx
Oropharynx	Segment of pharynx posterior to oral cavity Pair of palatine tonsils in lateral walls Lingual tonsils in anterior wall, at base of tongue	Conducts air between nasopharynx and/or oral cavity and laryngopharynx
Laryngopharynx	Segment of pharynx posterior to opening of larynx and superior to opening of esophagus	Conducts air between oropharynx and larynx
Tonsils	Ring of individual aggregations of lymphoid nodules	Immune protection of respiratory and digestive mucosa

Continued

Larynx	Voice box Extends from laryngopharynx to trachea Supported by nine cartilages connected by muscle and ligaments Lined with mucosa (pseudostratified ciliated columnar epithelium, except epiglottis and vocal folds)	Conducts air between the pharynx and trachea Prevents food from entering lower airways Vocalization Ciliary escalator removes contaminants
Epiglottis	Flexible "lid" of larynx Covered/lined with nonkeratinized stratified squamous epithelium, transitioning through simple columnar to pseudostratified ciliated columnar epithelium at border with vestibule	Flexes during swallowing to cover larynx and prevent food from entering lower airways
Vestibule	Extends from base of epiglottis to vestibular folds	Conducts air between pharynx and vestibular folds
Vestibular folds (false vocal folds)	Superior pair of lateral mucosal folds	Slow contaminants dripping toward lower airways
Ventricle (laryngeal ventricle)	Space between the vestibular folds and vocal folds	Conducts air between mucosal folds of larynx
Vocal folds (true vocal folds or vocal cords)	Inferior pair of lateral mucosal folds Each fold supported by skeletal muscle and strong *vocal ligament* at medial edge Covered with nonkeratinized stratified squamous epithelium Glottis: vocal folds and space between them (rima glottidis)	Prevent contaminants from entering lower airways Produce vibrations when pulled together during expiration (vocalization)
Infraglottic cavity	Segments below glottis, between vocal folds and trachea	Conducts air between vocal folds and trachea

SUMMARY OF RESPIRATORY TRACT STRUCTURES*—cont'd

STRUCTURE	DESCRIPTION	FUNCTION
LOWER RESPIRATORY TRACT		
Trachea	Portion of respiratory tract within the thoracic cavity Also called *bronchial tree*	Conducts air to/from gas-exchange tissues of lungs
	Windpipe Extends from larynx to primary bronchi Supported by C-shaped cartilage rings Lined with respiratory mucosa (pseudostratified ciliated columnar epithelium)	Conducts air between the larynx and bronchi Ciliary escalator removes contaminants
Bronchi	Treelike branching of airways (23 levels of branching), producing a huge number of individual airways Supported by cartilage rings (incomplete outside lungs; complete inside lungs) Lined with respiratory mucosa (pseudostratified ciliated columnar epithelium)	Conduct air between trachea and lungs Ciliary escalator removes contaminants
Primary bronchi	Left and right branch from trachea, one to each lung	Conduct air to/from the lungs
Secondary bronchi (lobar bronchi)	Branches of the primary bronchi; three from the right, two from the left	Conduct air to/from the lobes of lungs
Tertiary bronchi (segmental bronchi)	Branches of the secondary bronchi	Conduct air to/from the various bronchopulmonary segments of lungs
Bronchioles	Smallest branches (20 levels of branching)	Conduct air to/from alveoli
Alveoli	Microscopic air spaces at terminals of bronchial tree Lined with simple squamous epithelium that joins with pulmonary capillary endothelium to form the respiratory membrane	Exchange of gases (CO_2, O_2) between air and pulmonary blood Surfactant lining alveoli prevents collapse of air spaces

*Listed in order of airflow during inspiration.

PHYSIOLOGY OF THE RESPIRATORY SYSTEM

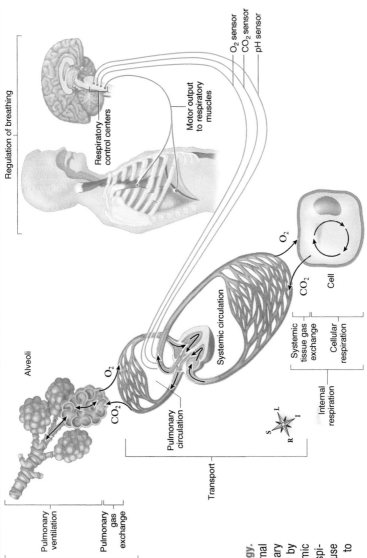

Overview of Respiratory Physiology.
Respiratory function includes external respiration (ventilation and pulmonary gas exchange), transport of gases by blood, and internal respiration (systemic tissue gas exchange and cellular respiration). Regulatory mechanisms use feedback from blood gas sensors to regulate ventilation.

Pulmonary Ventilation.

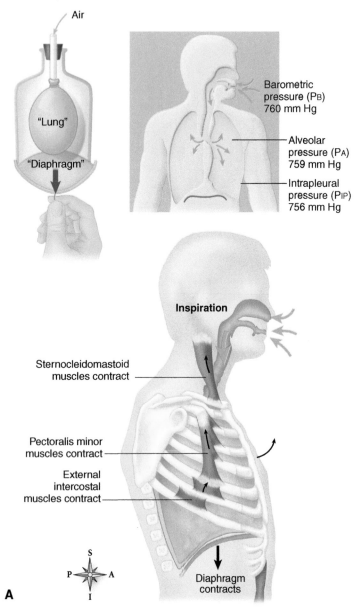

Mechanics of Ventilation. **A,** During **inspiration,** the diaphragm contracts downward, increasing the volume of the thoracic cavity. The increased volume results in decreased alveolar pressure (P_A), which causes air to rush into the lungs. During heavy breathing, additional inspiratory muscles assist the diaphragm to enlarge the thorax even more and thereby produce a greater drop in alveolar pressure to increase air flow into the lungs.

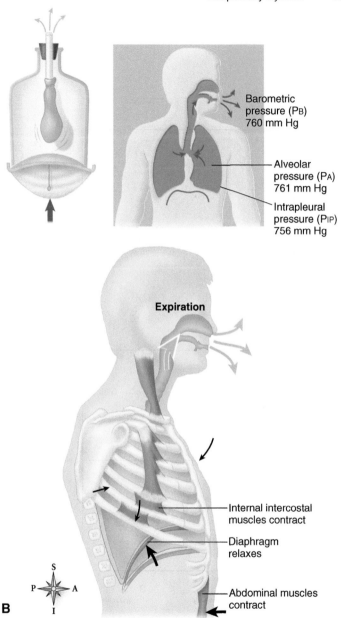

Barometric
pressure (P$_B$)
760 mm Hg

Alveolar
pressure (P$_A$)
761 mm Hg

Intrapleural
pressure (P$_{IP}$)
756 mm Hg

Expiration

Internal intercostal
muscles contract

Diaphragm
relaxes

Abdominal muscles
contract

B

S
P ✦ A
I

Mechanics of Ventilation—cont'd. B, During **expiration,** the diaphragm recoils upward, reducing the volume (thereby increasing the alveolar pressure) in the thoracic cavity, which forces air out of the lungs. During heavy breathing, additional expiratory muscles may compress the thorax and thereby produce a greater increase in alveolar pressure to increase air flow out of the lungs. Insets show the classic model in which a jar represents the rib cage, a rubber sheet represents the diaphragm, and a balloon represents the lungs.

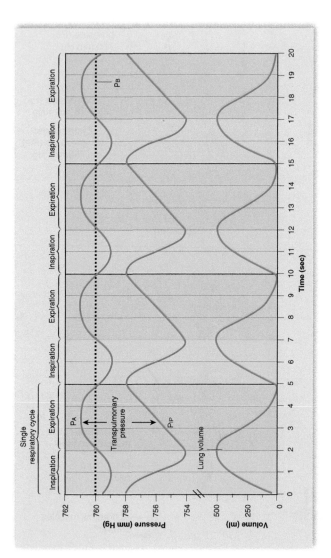

Rhythm of Ventilation. Respiratory cycles repeat continuously in normal, quiet breathing. Notice the rhythmic rise and fall of the intrapleural pressure (P_{IP}) and alveolar pressure (P_A). You can easily see that P_{IP} is always lower than P_A (negative transpulmonary pressure), which helps keep the alveoli inflated. The *lowest line* shows the change in air volumes during the respiratory cycle.

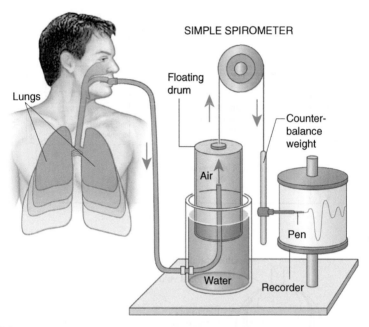

SIMPLE SPIROMETER

Lungs

Floating drum

Counter-balance weight

Air

Pen

Water   Recorder

Spirometer. Spirometers are devices that measure the volume of gas that the lungs inhale and exhale, usually as a function of time. A diagram of a classic spirometer design showing how the volume of air exhaled and inhaled is recorded as a rising and falling line.

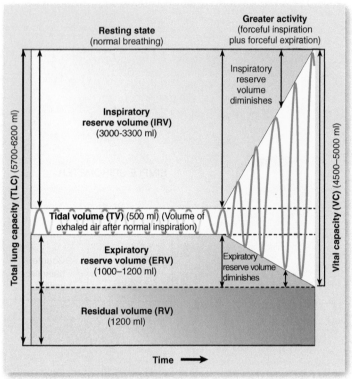

A

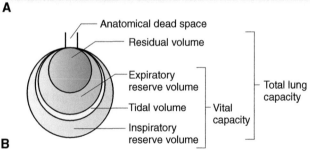

B

Pulmonary Ventilation Volumes and Capacities. A, Spirogram. **B,** Pulmonary volumes (at rest) represented as relative proportions of an inflated balloon. During normal, quiet respirations, the atmosphere and lungs exchange about 500 ml of air (TV). With forcible inspiration, about 3300 ml more air can be inhaled (IRV). After a normal inspiration and normal expiration, approximately 1000 ml more air can be forcibly expired (ERV). Vital capacity is the amount of air that can be forcibly expired after a maximal inspiration and therefore indicates the largest amount of air that can enter and leave the lungs during respiration. Residual volume is the air that remains trapped in the alveoli.

PULMONARY VOLUMES AND CAPACITIES

VOLUME	DESCRIPTION	TYPICAL VALUE	CAPACITY	FORMULA	TYPICAL VALUE
Tidal volume (TV)	Volume moved into or out of the respiratory tract during a normal respiratory cycle	500 ml (0.5 L)	Vital capacity (VC)	TV + IRV + ERV	4500–5000 ml (4.5–5.0 L)
Inspiratory reserve volume (IRV)	Maximum volume that can be moved into the respiratory tract after a normal inspiration	3000–3300 ml (3.0–3.3 L)	Inspiratory capacity (IC)	TV + IRV	3500–3800 ml (3.5–3.8 L)
Expiratory reserve volume (ERV)	Maximum volume that can be moved out of the respiratory tract after a normal expiration	1000–1200 ml (1.0–1.2 L)	Functional residual capacity (FRC)	ERV + RV	2200–2400 ml (2.2–2.4 L)
Residual volume (RV)	Volume remaining in the respiratory tract after maximum expiration	1200 ml (1.2 L)	Total lung capacity (TLC)	TV + IRV + ERV + RV	5700–6200 ml (5.7–6.2 L)

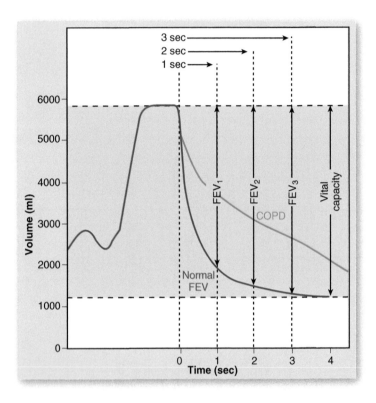

Forced Expiratory Volume (FEV). A normal individual forcefully exhales about 83% of the vital capacity (VC) during the first second, 94% at the end of 2 seconds, and 97% by the end of 3 seconds. The *red line* shows the results from a person with COPD (chronic obstructive pulmonary disease) who cannot forcefully exhale a large percentage of the vital capacity as quickly as a person without pulmonary obstruction.

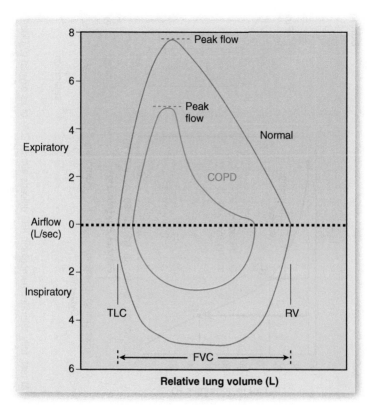

Flow-Volume Loops. The top of the loop represents expiratory flow (vertically) and volume (horizontally). The bottom of the loop represents inspiratory flow and volume. Notice that a person with COPD (chronic obstructive pulmonary disease) will produce a smaller loop with a "scooped-out" shape at the end of the expiratory curve. *FVC,* Forced vital capacity; *TLC,* Total lung capacity; *RV,* residual volume.

How Blood Transports Gases.

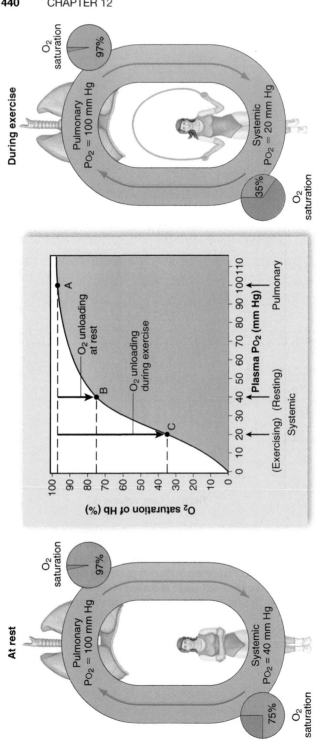

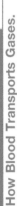

Oxygen Unloading at Rest and During Exercise. At rest, fully saturated hemoglobin (Hb) unloads almost 25% of its oxygen (O_2) load when it reaches the low-PO_2 (40 mm Hg) environment in systemic tissues *(left inset)*. During exercise, the tissue PO_2 is even lower (20 mm Hg)—thus causing fully saturated Hb to unload about 70% of its O_2 load *(right inset)*. As you can see in the graph, a slight drop in tissue PO_2—from point *B* to point *C*—causes a large increase in O_2 unloading. PO_2, Oxygen pressure; *mm Hg*, millimeters of mercury.

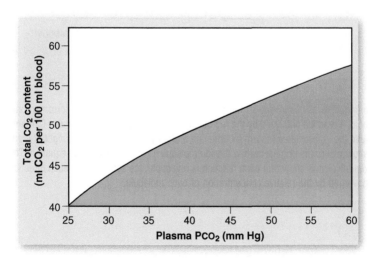

Carbon Dioxide–Hemoglobin Reaction. Carbon dioxide can bind to an amine group (NH_2) in an amino acid within a hemoglobin (Hb) molecule to form carbaminohemoglobin ($HbNCOOH^-$) and a hydrogen ion. The *highlighted areas* show where the original carbon dioxide molecule is in each part of the equation.

Carbon Dioxide Dissociation Curve. The relationship between carbon dioxide pressure (P_{CO_2}) and total CO_2 content (ml CO_2 per 100 ml blood) is graphed as a nearly straight line. Notice that the CO_2-carrying capacity of blood increases as the plasma P_{CO_2} increases.

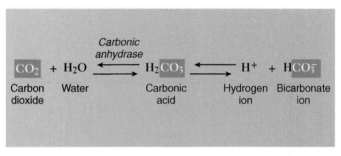

Formation of Bicarbonate. Carbon dioxide can react with water to form carbonic acid, a reaction catalyzed by the red blood cell enzyme carbonic anhydrase. Carbonic acid then dissociates to form bicarbonate and a hydrogen ion. The *highlighted areas* show where the original carbon dioxide molecule is in each part of the equation. The *double arrows* show that each reaction is reversible, the actual rate in each direction governed by the relative concentration of each molecule.

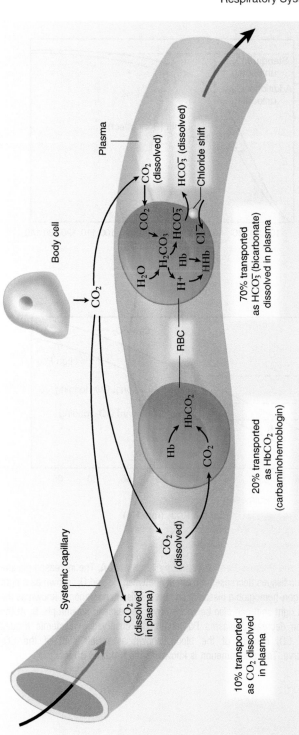

Carbon Dioxide Transport in the Blood. As the illustration shows, CO_2 dissolves in the plasma. Some of the dissolved CO_2 enters red blood cells (RBCs) and combines with hemoglobin (Hb) to form carbaminohemoglobin ($HbCO_2$). Some of the CO_2 entering RBCs combines with H_2O to form carbonic acid (H_2CO_3), a process facilitated by the enzyme carbonic anhydrase (CA) present inside each cell. Carbonic acid then dissociates to form H^+ and bicarbonate (HCO_3^-). The H^+ combines with Hb, whereas the HCO_3^- diffuses down its concentration gradient into the plasma. As HCO_3^- leaves each RBC, Cl^- enters and prevents an imbalance in charge——a phenomenon called the *chloride shift*.

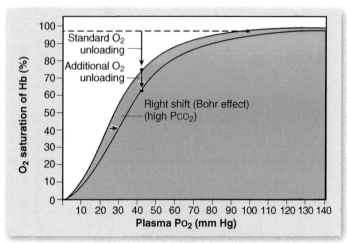

A

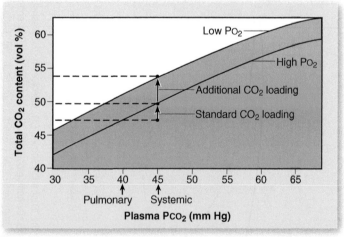

B

Effects of Po_2 and Pco_2 on Gas Transport by the Blood. **A,** The increased plasma Pco_2 in systemic tissues decreases the affinity between Hb and O_2, shown as a right shift of the oxygen-hemoglobin dissociation curve. This phenomenon is known as the **Bohr effect.** A right shift can also be caused by a decrease in plasma pH. **B,** At the same time, the decreased plasma Po_2 commonly observed in systemic tissues increases the CO_2 content of the blood, shown as a left shift of the CO_2 dissociation curve. This phenomenon is known as the **Haldane effect.**

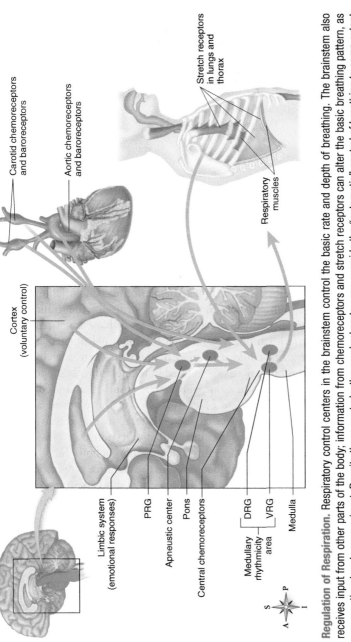

Carotid chemoreceptors and baroreceptors

Aortic chemoreceptors and baroreceptors

Stretch receptors in lungs and thorax

Respiratory muscles

Cortex (voluntary control)

Limbic system (emotional responses)

PRG

Apneustic center

Pons

Central chemoreceptors

Medullary rhythmicity area — DRG / VRG

Medulla

Regulation of Respiration. Respiratory control centers in the brainstem control the basic rate and depth of breathing. The brainstem also receives input from other parts of the body; information from chemoreceptors and stretch receptors can alter the basic breathing pattern, as can emotional and sensory input. Despite these controls, the cerebral cortex can override the "automatic" control of breathing to some extent to accomplish activities such as singing or blowing up a balloon. *Green arrows* show the flow of regulatory information as it flows into the respiratory control centers. The *purple arrow* shows the flow of regulatory information from the control centers to the respiratory muscles that provide the power needed for breathing.

13

Digestive System

The organs of the **digestive system** together perform a vital function—that of preparing nutrients for absorption and for use by the millions of body cells. Most food when eaten is in a form that cannot reach the cells (because it cannot pass through the intestinal mucosa into the bloodstream), nor could it be used by the cells even if it could reach them. It must therefore be modified in both chemical composition and physical state so that nutrients can be absorbed and used by the body cells. The complete process of altering the physical and chemical composition of ingested food material so that it can be absorbed and used by the body cells is called **digestion.**

The complex process of digestion is the function of both the digestive tract and accessory organs that make up the digestive system. The process of digestion depends on both endocrine and exocrine secretions and the controlled movement of ingested food materials through the tract so that absorption can occur.

ANATOMY OF THE DIGESTIVE SYSTEM

Organization of the Digestive System

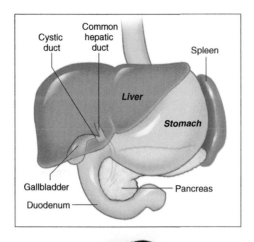

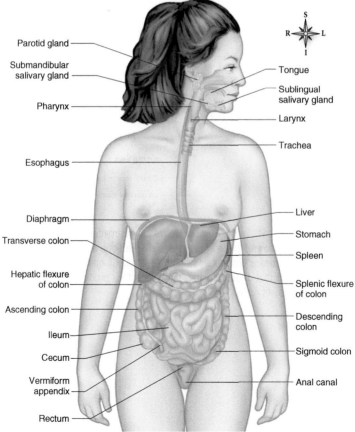

Location of the Digestive Organs.

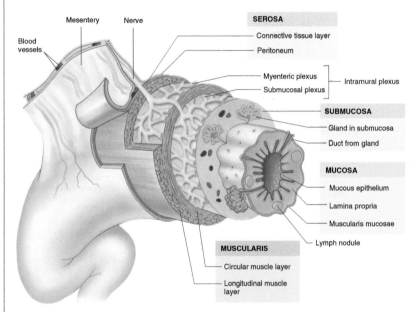

Wall of the Gastrointestinal Tract. The wall of the gastrointestinal (GI) tract is made up of four layers, shown here in a generalized diagram of a segment of the GI tract. Notice that the serosa is continuous with a fold of serous membrane called a *mesentery*. Notice also that digestive glands may empty their products into the lumen of the GI tract by way of ducts.

MODIFICATIONS OF LAYERS OF THE DIGESTIVE TRACT WALL

ORGAN	MUCOSA	MUSCULARIS	SEROSA
Esophagus	Stratified squamous epithelium resists abrasion	Two layers—inner one of circular fibers and outer one of longitudinal fibers; striated muscle in the upper part and smooth muscle in the lower part of the esophagus and in the rest of the tract	Outer layer, fibrous (adventitia); serous around part of the esophagus in the thoracic cavity
Stomach	Arranged in flexible longitudinal folds called *rugae*; allow for distention; contains gastric pits with microscopic gastric glands	Has three layers instead of the usual two—circular, longitudinal, and oblique fibers; two sphincters—lower esophageal sphincter at the entrance of the stomach and pyloric sphincter at its exit, formed by circular fibers	Outer layer, visceral peritoneum; hangs in a double fold from the lower edge of the stomach over the intestines and forms an apronlike structure; greater omentum; lesser omentum connects the stomach to the liver
Small intestine	Contains permanent circular folds, *plicae circulares* Microscopic fingerlike projections, villi with brush border Crypts (of Lieberkühn) Microscopic duodenal (Brunner) mucous glands Aggregated lymphoid nodules (Peyer patches) Numerous single lymphoid nodules called *solitary nodules*	Two layers—inner one of circular fibers and outer one of longitudinal fibers	Outer layer, visceral peritoneum, continuous with the mesentery
Large intestine	Solitary lymph nodes Intestinal mucous glands Anal columns form in the anal region	Outer longitudinal layer condensed to form three tapelike strips (taeniae coli); small sacs (haustra) give the rest of the wall of the large intestine a puckered appearance; internal anal sphincter formed by circular smooth fibers; external anal sphincter formed by striated fibers	Outer layer, visceral peritoneum, continuous with mesocolon

Mouth

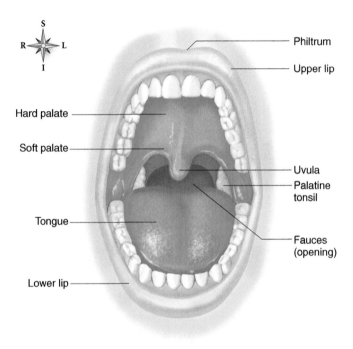

The Oral Cavity.

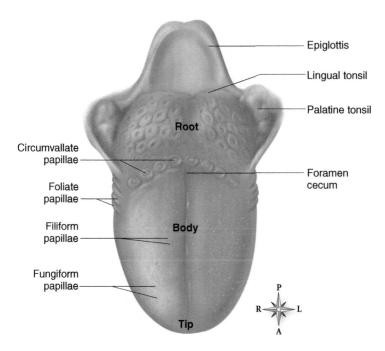

Dorsal Surface of the Tongue. Sketch showing the three divisions of the tongue.

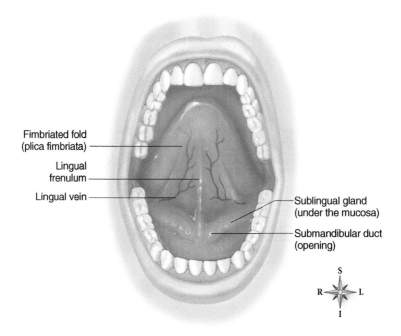

Floor of the Mouth. Floor of mouth and ventral surface of tongue.

Salivary Glands

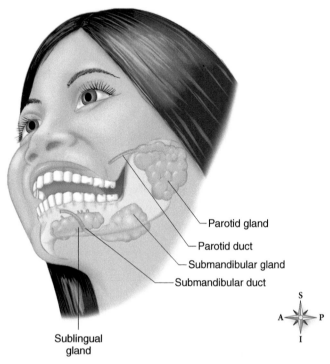

Parotid gland

Parotid duct

Submandibular gland

Submandibular duct

Sublingual gland

Salivary Glands. Locations of the salivary glands.

Teeth

DENTITION

NAME OF TOOTH	NUMBER PER JAW (UPPER OR LOWER)	
	DECIDUOUS SET	PERMANENT SET
Central incisors	2	2
Lateral incisors	2	2
Canines (cuspids)	2	2
Premolars (bicuspids)	0	4
First molars (tricuspids)	2	2
Second molars	2	2
Third molars (wisdom teeth)	0	2
TOTAL (per jaw)	10	16
TOTAL (per set)	20	32

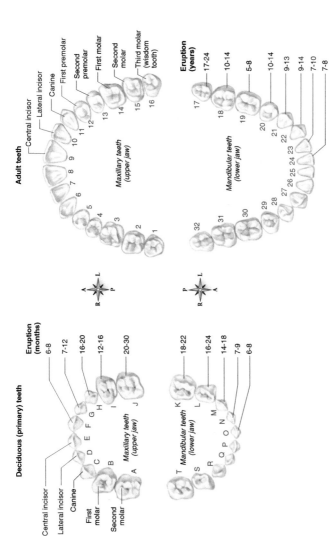

Adult teeth

Central incisor
Lateral incisor
Canine
First premolar
Second premolar
First molar
Second molar
Third molar (wisdom tooth)

6 7 8 9 10 11 12 13 14 15 16
5
4
3
2
1

Maxillary teeth (upper jaw)

L
A   P
R

Eruption (years)

17 17-24
18 10-14
19 5-8
20 10-14
21 9-13
22 9-14
23 7-10
24 7-8
25
26
27
28
29
30
31
32

Mandibular teeth (lower jaw)

P   L
R   A

Deciduous (primary) teeth

Eruption (months)

Central incisor   6-8
Lateral incisor   7-12
Canine   16-20
First molar   12-16
Second molar   20-30

C D E F G H
B   I
A   J

Maxillary teeth (upper jaw)

18-22   K
16-24   L
14-18   M
7-9   N
6-8   O

T S R Q P

Mandibular teeth (lower jaw)

Dentition. In the deciduous set, where letters are used in place of numbers, there are no premolars and only two pairs of molars in each jaw. Generally, the lower teeth erupt before the corresponding upper teeth.

Stomach

Stomach. A portion of the anterior wall has been cut away to reveal the muscle layers of the stomach wall. Notice that the mucosa lining the stomach forms folds called *rugae*.

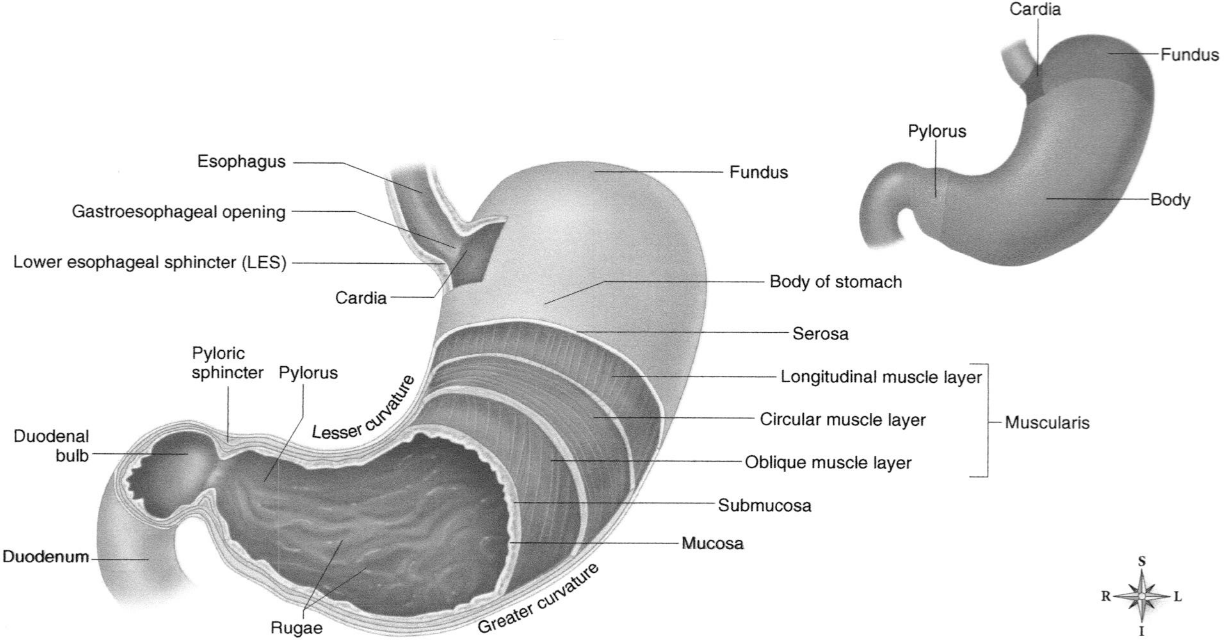

Fundus

Body

Cardia

Pylorus

Body of stomach

Serosa

Longitudinal muscle layer

Circular muscle layer

Oblique muscle layer

Muscularis

Submucosa

Mucosa

Greater curvature

Rugae

Lesser curvature

Fundus

Esophagus

Gastroesophageal opening

Lower esophageal sphincter (LES)

Cardia

Pyloric sphincter

Pylorus

Duodenal bulb

Duodenum

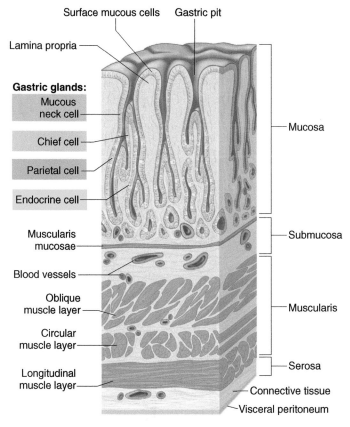

Surface mucous cells   Gastric pit

Lamina propria

Gastric glands:
Mucous neck cell

Chief cell

Parietal cell

Endocrine cell

Muscularis mucosae

Blood vessels

Oblique muscle layer

Circular muscle layer

Longitudinal muscle layer

Mucosa

Submucosa

Muscularis

Serosa

Connective tissue

Visceral peritoneum

Gastric Pits and Gastric Glands. Gastric pits are depressions in the epithelial lining of the stomach. At the bottom of each pit are one or more tubular *gastric glands.* Chief cells produce the enzymes of gastric juice, and parietal cells produce stomach acid. Endocrine cells secrete the appetite-boosting hormone ghrelin.

Small and Large Intestines

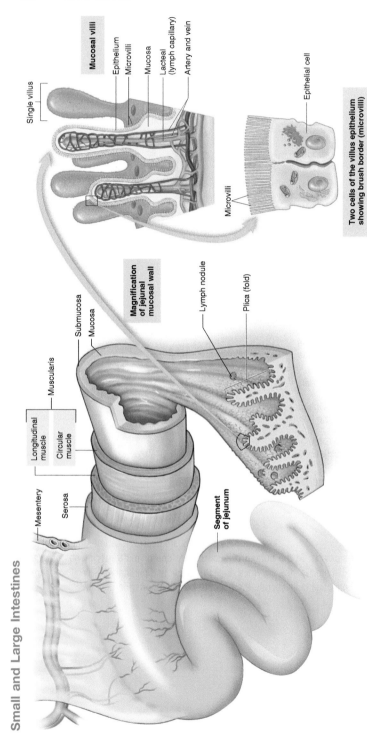

Mucosal villi

Epithelium
Microvilli
Mucosa
Lacteal
(lymph capillary)
Artery and vein

Single villus

Epithelial cell

Microvilli

Two cells of the villus epithelium showing brush border (microvilli)

Magnification of jejunal mucosal wall

Lymph nodule

Plica (fold)

Submucosa
Mucosa

Muscularis

Longitudinal muscle
Circular muscle

Mesentery

Serosa

Segment of jejunum

Wall of the Small Intestine. Note folds of mucosa are covered with villi and each villus is covered with epithelium, which increases the surface area for absorption of food.

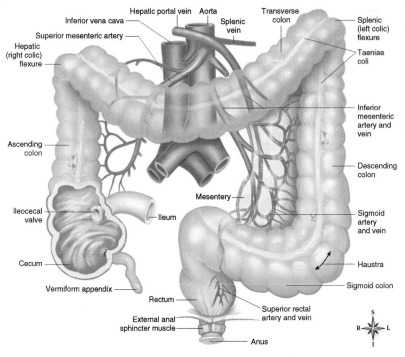

Divisions of the Large Intestine. Illustration showing divisions of the large intestine and adjacent vascular structures.

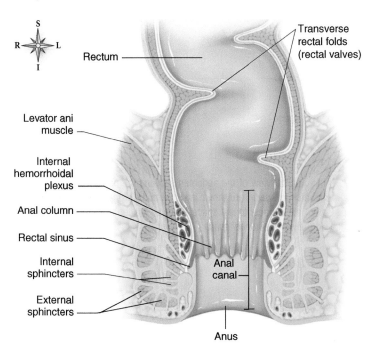

The Rectum and the Anus.

Peritoneum

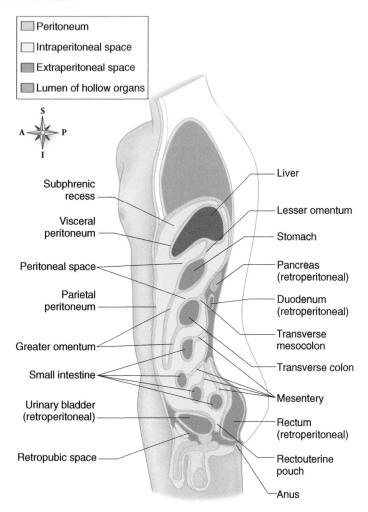

- Peritoneum
- Intraperitoneal space
- Extraperitoneal space
- Lumen of hollow organs

Subphrenic recess
Visceral peritoneum
Peritoneal space
Parietal peritoneum
Greater omentum
Small intestine
Urinary bladder (retroperitoneal)
Retropubic space

Liver
Lesser omentum
Stomach
Pancreas (retroperitoneal)
Duodenum (retroperitoneal)
Transverse mesocolon
Transverse colon
Mesentery
Rectum (retroperitoneal)
Rectouterine pouch
Anus

Peritoneum. Sagittal view of the abdomen showing the peritoneum and its reflections. *Intraperitoneal spaces* are shown in yellow and *extraperitoneal spaces* in green. The portion of the extraperitoneal space along the posterior wall of the abdomen is often called the *retroperitoneal space*.

Liver and Gallbladder

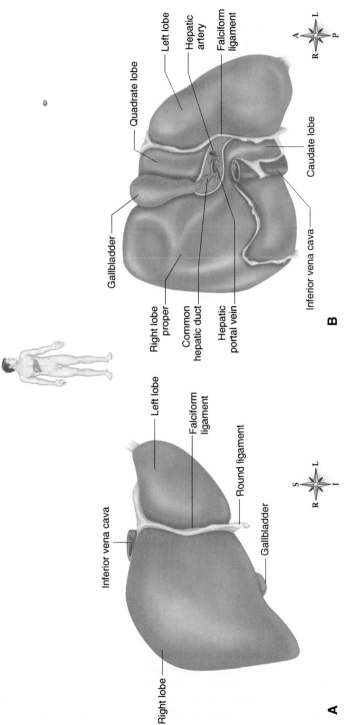

Gross Structure of the Liver. Diagrams of a normal liver. **A,** Anterior view. **B,** Inferior view.

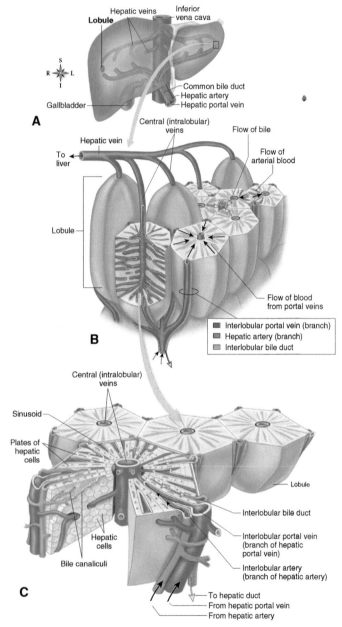

Microscopic Structure of the Liver. A, This diagram shows the location of liver lobules relative to the overall circulatory scheme of the liver. **B** and **C,** Enlarged views of several lobules show how blood from the hepatic portal veins and hepatic arteries flows through sinusoids and thus past plates of hepatic cells toward a central vein in each lobule *(black arrows)*. Hepatic cells form bile, which flows through bile canaliculi toward hepatic ducts that eventually drain the bile from the liver *(yellow arrows)*.

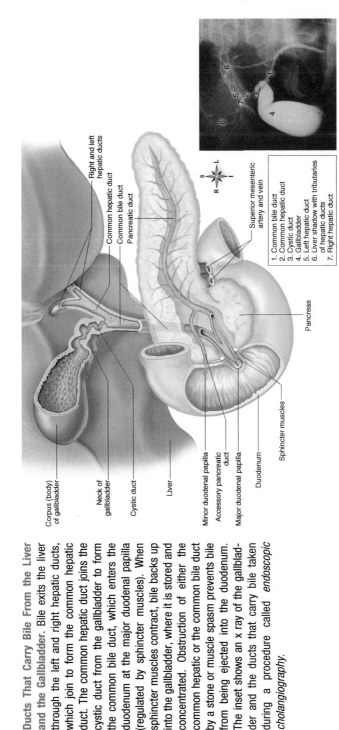

Ducts That Carry Bile From the Liver and the Gallbladder. Bile exits the liver through the left and right hepatic ducts, which join to form the common hepatic duct. The common hepatic duct joins the cystic duct from the gallbladder to form the common bile duct, which enters the duodenum at the major duodenal papilla (regulated by sphincter muscles). When sphincter muscles contract, bile backs up into the gallbladder, where it is stored and concentrated. Obstruction of either the common hepatic or the common bile duct by a stone or muscle spasm prevents bile from being ejected into the duodenum. The inset shows an x ray of the gallbladder and the ducts that carry bile taken during a procedure called *endoscopic cholangiography.*

Right and left hepatic ducts
Common hepatic duct
Common bile duct
Pancreatic duct

S
R — L
I

Superior mesenteric artery and vein

1. Common bile duct
2. Common hepatic duct
3. Cystic duct
4. Gallbladder
5. Left hepatic duct
6. Liver shadow with tributaries of hepatic ducts
7. Right hepatic duct

Pancreas

Corpus (body) of gallbladder

Neck of gallbladder

Cystic duct

Liver

Minor duodenal papilla
Accessory pancreatic duct
Major duodenal papilla
Duodenum
Sphincter muscles

PHYSIOLOGY OF THE DIGESTIVE SYSTEM

Overview of Digestive Function

PRIMARY MECHANISMS OF THE DIGESTIVE SYSTEM

MECHANISM	DESCRIPTION
Ingestion	Process of taking food into the mouth, starting it on its journey through the digestive tract
Digestion	A group of processes that break complex nutrients into simpler ones, thus facilitating their absorption; mechanical digestion physically breaks large chunks into small bits; chemical digestion breaks molecules apart
Motility	Movement by the muscular components of the digestive tube, including processes of mechanical digestion; examples include peristalsis and segmentation
Secretion	Release of digestive juices (containing enzymes, acids, bases, mucus, bile, or other products that facilitate digestion); some digestive organs also secrete endocrine hormones that regulate digestion or metabolism of nutrients
Absorption	Movement of digested nutrients through the gastrointestinal (GI) mucosa and into the internal environment
Elimination	Excretion of the residues of the digestive process (feces) from the rectum, through the anus; defecation
Regulation	Coordination of digestive activity (motility, secretion, etc.)

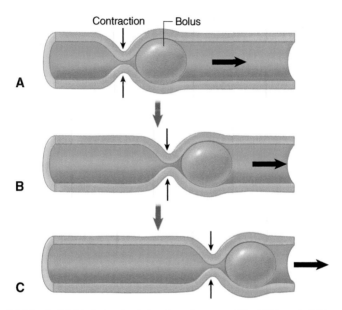

Peristalsis. Peristalsis is a progressive type of movement in which material is propelled from point to point along the gastrointestinal (GI) tract. **A,** A ring of contraction occurs where the GI wall is stretched, and the bolus is pushed forward. **B,** The moving bolus triggers a ring of contraction in the next region that pushes the bolus even farther along. **C,** The ring of contraction moves like a wave along the GI tract to push the bolus forward.

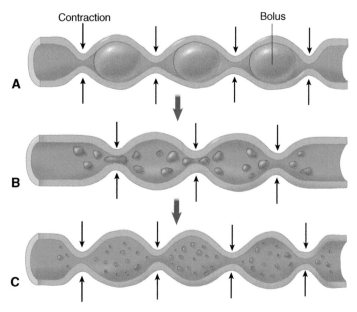

Segmentation. Segmentation is a back-and-forth action that breaks apart chunks of food and mixes in digestive juices. **A,** Ringlike regions of contraction occur at intervals along the gastrointestinal (GI) tract. **B,** Previously contracted regions relax and adjacent regions now contract, effectively "chopping" the contents of each segment into smaller chunks. **C,** The location of the contracted regions continues to alternate back and forth, chopping and mixing the contents of the GI lumen.

PROCESSES OF MECHANICAL DIGESTION

ORGAN	MECHANICAL PROCESS	NATURE OF PROCESS
Mouth (teeth and tongue)	Mastication	Chewing movements—reduce size of food particles and mix them with saliva
	Deglutition	Swallowing—movement of food from mouth to stomach
Pharynx	Deglutition	See description above
Esophagus	Deglutition	See description above
	Peristalsis	Rippling movements that squeeze food downward in digestive tract; a constricted ring forms first in one section, then the next, and so on, causing waves of contraction to spread along entire canal
Stomach	Churning	Forward and backward movement (propulsion/retropulsion) of gastric contents, mixing food with gastric juices to form chyme
	Peristalsis	Wave starting in body of stomach that occurs about three times per minute and sweeps toward closed pyloric sphincter; at intervals, strong peristaltic waves press chyme past sphincter into duodenum
Small intestine	Segmentation (mixing contractions)	Forward and backward movement within segment of intestine; purpose is to mix food and digestive juices thoroughly and to bring all digested food into contact with intestinal mucosa to facilitate absorption; purpose of peristalsis, on the other hand, is to propel intestinal contents along digestive tract
	Peristalsis	
Large intestine		
Colon	Segmentation	Churning movements within haustral sacs
	Peristalsis	See description above
Descending colon	Mass peristalsis	Entire contents moved into sigmoid colon and rectum; occurs three or four times a day, usually after a meal
Rectum	Defecation	Emptying of rectum, so-called bowel movement

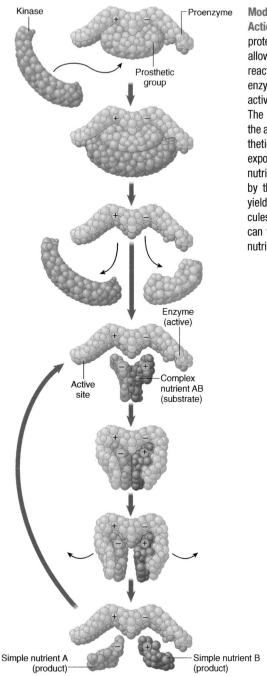

Kinase

Proenzyme

Prosthetic group

Enzyme (active)

Active site

Complex nutrient AB (substrate)

Simple nutrient A (product)

Simple nutrient B (product)

Model of Digestive Enzyme Action. Enzymes are functional proteins whose molecular shape allows them to catalyze chemical reactions. First, an inactive pro-enzyme must be altered by an activating enzyme called a *kinase*. The kinase often accomplishes the activation by removing a prosthetic group from the proenzyme, exposing an active site. A complex nutrient molecule *AB* is acted on by the active digestive enzyme, yielding simpler nutrient molecules *A* and *B*. The active enzyme can then digest another complex nutrient molecule.

CHEMICAL DIGESTION

DIGESTIVE JUICES AND ENZYMES	SUBSTANCE DIGESTED (OR HYDROLYZED)	RESULTING PRODUCT*
SALIVA		
Amylase (ptyalin)	Starch (polysaccharide)	Maltose (disaccharide)
GASTRIC JUICE		
Protease (pepsin)[†] plus hydrochloric acid	Proteins	Partially digested proteins
PANCREATIC JUICE		
Proteases (e.g., trypsin)[‡]	Proteins (intact or partially digested)	Peptides and **amino acids**
Lipases	Fats emulsified by bile	**Fatty acids, monoglycerides**, and **glycerol**
Amylase	Starch	Maltose
Nucleases	Nucleic acids (DNA, RNA)	Nucleotides
INTESTINAL ENZYMES[§]		
Peptidases	Peptides	**Amino acids**
Sucrase	Sucrose (cane sugar)	**Glucose** and **fructose**[¶] (monosaccharides)
Lactase	Lactose (milk sugar)	**Glucose** and **galactose** (monosaccharides)
Maltase	Maltose (malt sugar)	**Glucose**
Nucleotidases and phosphatases	Nucleotides	Nucleosides

*Substances in **boldface type** are end products of digestion (that is, completely digested nutrients ready for absorption).
[†]Secreted in inactive form (pepsinogen); activated by low pH (hydrochloric acid).
[‡]Secreted in inactive form (trypsinogen); activated by enterokinase, an enzyme in the intestinal brush border.
[§]Brush-border enzymes.
[¶]Glucose is also called *dextrose;* fructose is also called *levulose.*

Secretion

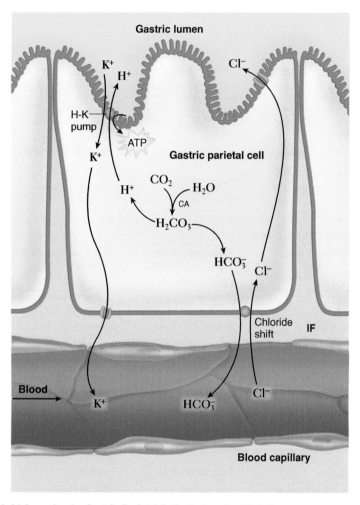

Acid Secretion by Gastric Parietal Cells. In this simplified diagram, you can see that hydrochloric acid (HCl) secretion by gastric parietal cells uses H^+ produced by the dissociation of carbonic acid (H_2CO_3). Recall that carbonic acid is produced by the reaction of water and carbon dioxide—a process enhanced by the enzyme carbonic anhydrase (CA). The chloride (Cl^-) of gastric HCl comes from a chloride shift into the cell in exchange for bicarbonate ions (HCO_3^-) produced by the same dissociation of carbonic acid that yielded the H^+. As Cl^- is shifted into the cell, the intracellular Cl^- concentration rises and produces a concentration gradient with the lumen of the gastric gland—forcing Cl^- to diffuse out of the parietal cell. The net effect is that active pumping of H^+ out of the cell by the H-K pump drives the concurrent shift of Cl^- into the cell from the blood and diffusion of Cl^- out of the cell and into the duct of the gastric gland. *IF*, Interstitial fluid.

DIGESTIVE SECRETIONS

DIGESTIVE JUICE	SOURCE	SUBSTANCE	FUNCTIONAL ROLE
Saliva	Salivary glands	Mucus	*Lubricates bolus of food; facilitates mixing of food*
		Amylase (ptyalin)	**Enzyme; begins digestion of starches**
		Sodium bicarbonate	**Increases pH** (for optimum amylase function)
		Water	*Dilutes food and other substances; facilitates mixing*
Gastric juice	Gastric glands	Pepsin	**Enzyme; digests proteins**
		Hydrochloric acid	Denatures proteins; decreases pH (for optimum pepsin function)
		Intrinsic factor	**Protects and allows later absorption of vitamin B$_{12}$**
		Mucus	*Lubricates chyme; protects stomach lining*
		Water	*Dilutes food and other substances; facilitates mixing*
Pancreatic juice	Pancreas (exocrine portion)	Proteases (trypsin, chymotrypsin, collagenase, elastase, etc.)	**Enzymes; digest proteins and polypeptides**
		Lipases (lipase, phospholipase, etc.)	**Enzymes; digest lipids**
		Colipase	**Coenzyme; helps lipase digest fats**
		Nucleases	**Enzymes; digest nucleic acids (RNA and DNA)**
		Amylase	**Enzyme; digests starches**
		Water	*Dilutes food and other substances; facilitates mixing*
		Mucus	*Lubricates*
		Sodium bicarbonate	**Increases pH** (for optimum enzyme function)

Continued

DIGESTIVE SECRETIONS—cont'd

DIGESTIVE JUICE	SOURCE	SUBSTANCE	FUNCTIONAL ROLE
Bile	Liver (stored and concentrated in gallbladder)	Lecithin and bile salts	*Emulsify lipids*
		Sodium bicarbonate	**Increases pH** (for optimum enzyme function)
		Cholesterol	Excess cholesterol from body cells, to be excreted with feces
		Products of detoxification	From detoxification of harmful substances by hepatic cells, to be excreted with feces
		Bile pigments (mainly bilirubin)	Products of breakdown of heme groups during hemolysis, to be excreted with feces
		Mucus	*Lubrication*
		Water	Dilutes food and other substances; facilitates mixing
Intestinal juice	Mucosa of small and large intestine	Mucus	*Lubrication*
		Sodium bicarbonate	**Increases pH** (for optimum enzyme function)
		Water	Small amount to carry mucus and sodium bicarbonate

****Boldface type** indicates a chemical digestive process; *italic type* indicates a mechanical process.

1 **Cephalic Phase** Sensations of thoughts about food are relayed to the brainstem, where parasympathetic signals to the gastric mucosa are initiated. This directly stimulates gastric juice secretion and also stimulates the release of gastrin, which prolongs and enhances the effect.

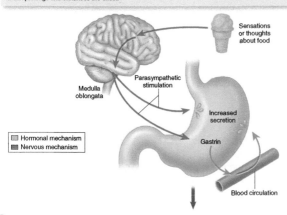

Sensations or thoughts about food

Medulla oblongata

Parasympathetic stimulation

Increased secretion

Gastrin

☐ Hormonal mechanism
☐ Nervous mechanism

Blood circulation

2 **Gastric Phase** The presence of food, specifically the distention it causes, triggers local and parasympathetic nervous reflexes that increase secretion of gastric juice and gastrin (which further amplifies gastric juice secretion).

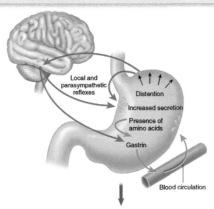

Local and parasympathetic reflexes

Distention

Increased secretion

Presence of amino acids

Gastrin

Blood circulation

3 **Intestinal Phase** As food moves into the duodenum, the presence of fats, carbohydrates, and acid stimulates hormonal and nervous reflexes that inhibit stomach activity.

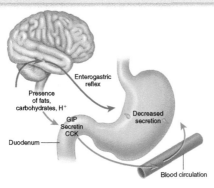

Enterogastric reflex

Presence of fats, carbohydrates, H⁺

Decreased secretion

GIP
Secretin
CCK

Duodenum

Blood circulation

Phases of Gastric Secretion.

ACTIONS OF SOME DIGESTIVE
HORMONES SUMMARIZED

HORMONE	SOURCE	ACTION
Gastrin	Secreted by gastric mucosa in presence of partially digested proteins, when stimulated by the vagus nerve, or when the stomach is stretched	Stimulates secretion of gastric juice rich in pepsin and hydrochloric acid
Gastric inhibitory peptide (GIP)	Secreted by intestinal mucosa in presence of glucose, fats, and perhaps other nutrients	Inhibits gastric secretion and motility; enhances insulin secretion by pancreas
Secretin	Secreted by intestinal mucosa in presence of acid, partially digested proteins, and fats	Inhibits gastric secretion; stimulates secretion of pancreatic juice low in enzymes and high in alkalinity (bicarbonate); enhances effects of CCK
Cholecystokinin (CCK)	Secreted by intestinal mucosa in presence of fats, partially digested proteins, and acids	Stimulates ejection of bile from gallbladder and secretion of pancreatic juice high in enzymes; relaxes sphincters that regulate flow from the common bile duct; opposes the action of gastrin, raising the pH of gastric juice

Absorption

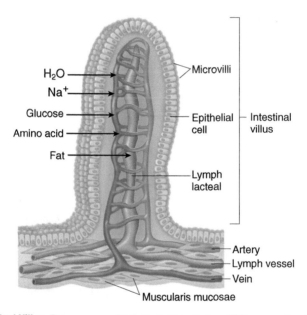

Intestinal Villus. The presence of intestinal villi and microvilli increases the absorptive surface area of the intestinal mucosa. Most absorbed substances enter the blood in intestinal capillaries, with the exception of fat, which enters lymph by way of the intestinal lacteals.

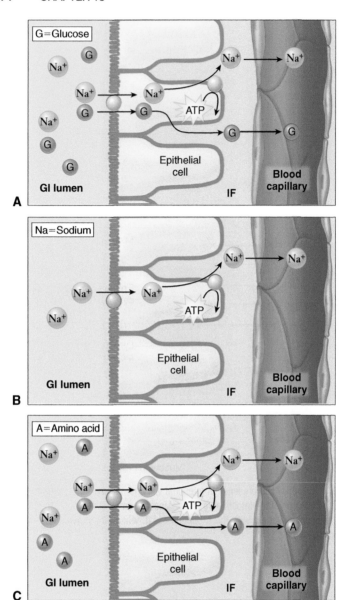

Absorption of Glucose, Sodium, and Amino Acids. Absorption of glucose **(A),** sodium **(B),** and amino acids **(C)** is a form of *secondary active transport* because each involves two carriers, one of which is active. The active carrier on the basal side of the epithelial cell maintains a sodium gradient, which facilitates passive transport of sodium, and perhaps another molecule, out of the gastrointestinal (GI) lumen via a passive carrier on the luminal side of the cell. *IF,* Interstitial fluid.

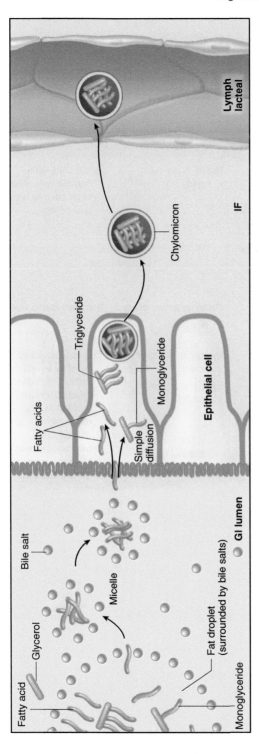

Absorption of Fats. Fats such as triglycerides are chemically digested within emulsified fat droplets, yielding fatty acids, monoglycerides, and glycerol (*left*). Fatty acids and other lipid-soluble compounds (such as cholesterol) leave the fat droplets in small spheres coated with bile salts (micelles). When a micelle reaches the plasma membrane of an absorptive cell, individual fat-soluble molecules diffuse directly into the cytoplasm. The endoplasmic reticulum of the cell resynthesizes fatty acids and monoglycerides into triglycerides. A Golgi body within the cell packages the fats into water-soluble micelles called *chylomicrons*, which then exit the absorptive cell by exocytosis and enter a lymphatic lacteal. *IF*, Interstitial fluid.

FOOD ABSORPTION

FORM ABSORBED	STRUCTURES INTO WHICH ABSORBED	CIRCULATION
Protein—as amino acids Perhaps minute quantities of some short-chain polypeptides and whole proteins are absorbed; for example, some antibodies	Blood in intestinal capillaries	Portal vein, liver, hepatic vein, inferior vena cava to heart, and so on
Carbohydrates—as simple sugars	Same as amino acids	Same as amino acids
Fats		
Glycerol and monoglycerides	Lymph in intestinal lacteals	During absorption, that is, while in epithelial cells of intestinal mucosa, glycerol and fatty acids recombine to form microscopic packages of fats (chylomicrons); lymphatics carry them by way of thoracic duct to left subclavian vein, superior vena cava, heart, and so on; some fats are transported by blood in form of phospholipids or cholesterol esters
Fatty acids combine with bile salts to form water-soluble substance	Lymph in intestinal lacteals	
Some finely emulsified, undigested fats absorbed	Small fraction enters intestinal blood capillaries	

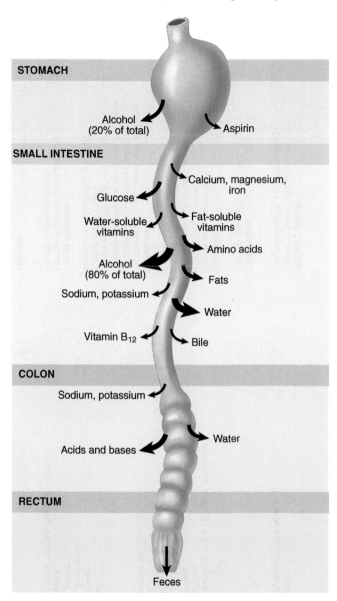

Absorption Sites in the Digestive Tract. The size of the arrow at each site indicates the relative amount of absorption of a particular substance at that site. Notice that most absorption occurs in the intestines, particularly the small intestine.

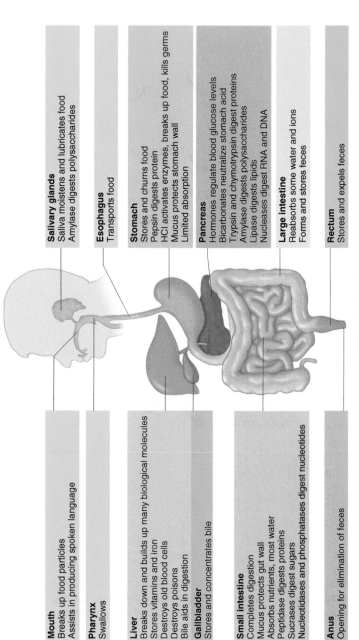

Salivary glands
Saliva moistens and lubricates food
Amylase digests polysaccharides

Esophagus
Transports food

Stomach
Stores and churns food
Pepsin digests protein
HCl activates enzymes, breaks up food, kills germs
Mucus protects stomach wall
Limited absorption

Pancreas
Hormones regulate blood glucose levels
Bicarbonates neutralize stomach acid
Trypsin and chymotrypsin digest proteins
Amylase digests polysaccharides
Lipase digests lipids
Nucleases digest RNA and DNA

Large intestine
Reabsorbs some water and ions
Forms and stores feces

Rectum
Stores and expels feces

Mouth
Breaks up food particles
Assists in producing spoken language

Pharynx
Swallows

Liver
Breaks down and builds up many biological molecules
Stores vitamins and iron
Destroys old blood cells
Destroys poisons
Bile aids in digestion

Gallbladder
Stores and concentrates bile

Small intestine
Completes digestion
Mucus protects gut wall
Absorbs nutrients, most water
Peptidase digests proteins
Sucrases digest sugars
Nucleotidases and phosphatases digest nucleotides

Anus
Opening for elimination of feces

Summary of Digestive Function.

Nutrition and Metabolism

14

Nutrition refers to the food people eat and the nutrients it contains. **Metabolism** refers to the complex, interactive set of chemical processes that make life possible. Metabolism is the use the body makes of foods after they have been digested, absorbed, and circulated to the body's cells. The nutrients from food are used by the body as an energy source and as "building blocks" for making complex chemical compounds.

Every cell in the body must maintain the operation of its *metabolic pathways* to ensure its survival. Anabolic pathways (**anabolism**) are required to build the various structural and functional components of the cells. Catabolic pathways (**catabolism**) are required to convert energy to a usable form. Catabolic pathways are also needed to degrade large molecules into small subunits that can be used in anabolic pathways.

Of course, the basic nutrient molecules—*carbohydrates*, *fats*, and *proteins* of the correct type—must be available to each cell to carry out these metabolic processes. Besides the basic nutrient molecules, cells also require small amounts of specific *vitamins* and *minerals* needed to produce the structural and functional components necessary for cellular metabolism.

METABOLISM

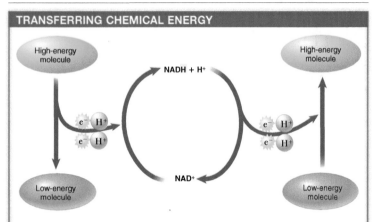

TRANSFERRING CHEMICAL ENERGY

The Role of Coenzymes in Transferring Chemical Energy.

The ability to transfer energy from molecule to molecule is, as you might imagine, essential to life. We have already discussed the critical role played by the nucleotide **adenosine triphosphate (ATP)** in transferring energy within living cells. ATP can accept energy from catabolic reactions and transfer that energy to energy-requiring anabolic reactions. Although we say that ATP is an "energy storage molecule," do not suppose that the energy is stored for very long periods. In fact, an ATP molecule exists for only a brief time before its last phosphate group is broken off and its energy is transferred to another molecule in some metabolic pathway. Long-term storage of energy can be accomplished only by nutrient molecules such as glucose, glycogen, and triglycerides.

In addition to ATP, various other energy transfer molecules are essential to human life. When atoms in a molecule absorb energy, some of their electrons may move outward to a higher energy level (shell). Electrons often become so energized that they leave the atom completely. As this occurs, pairs of "high-energy" electrons can be picked up and transferred to another molecule by an electron carrier such as **flavin adenine dinucleotide (FAD)** or **nicotinamide adenine dinucleotide (NAD).** The figure shows how NAD^+ (oxidized NAD) picks up a pair of energized electrons to become NADH. It should be noted here that electrons always travel with a proton (H^+) in the metabolic pathways described in this chapter. The electrons do not stay with the electron carrier for long, however. They are immediately transferred to molecules in another metabolic pathway, as the figure shows. In the cell, pairs of electrons (and their energy) can thus be transferred from pathway to pathway by NAD and FAD.

NAD and FAD, though very similar in function, do have their differences. One difference is that after NAD drops off its pair of high-energy electrons, three ATP molecules are generated and when FAD drops off its pair of electrons, only two ATP molecules are generated.

CARBOHYDRATES

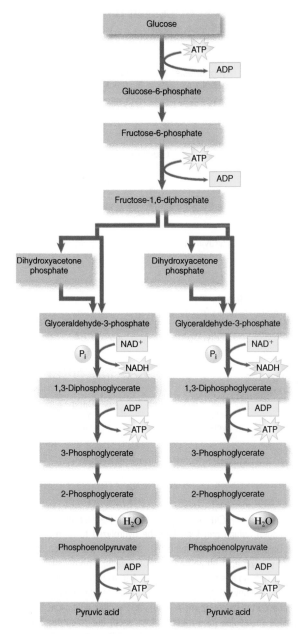

Glycolysis. The series of enzyme-catalyzed reactions that make up the portion of the catabolic pathway for carbohydrates is called *glycolysis*. *ADP,* Adenosine diphosphate; *ATP,* adenosine triphosphate; *NAD+,* oxidized nicotinamide adenine dinucleotide; *NADH,* reduced nicotinamide adenine dinucleotide; *Pi,* inorganic phosphate.

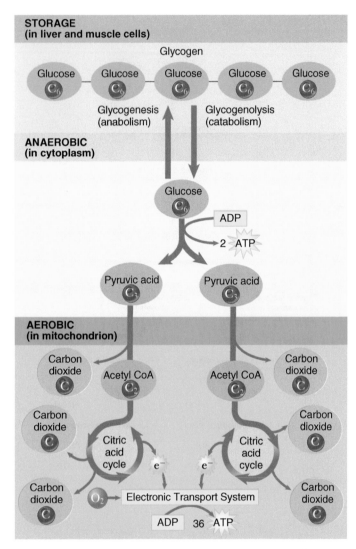

Catabolism of Glucose. Glucose may be stored in the liver and other tissues as the polymer glycogen, which can then later be hydrolyzed to form individual glucose molecules. Glycolysis splits one molecule of glucose (six carbon atoms) into two molecules of pyruvic acid (three carbon atoms each). The glycolytic pathway does not require oxygen, so it is termed *anaerobic.* A transition reaction removes a carbon dioxide molecule, converting each pyruvic acid molecule into a two-carbon acetyl group that is escorted by coenzyme A (CoA) into the citric acid cycle. There, two more carbon dioxide molecules (one carbon atom each) are released. The carbon and oxygen atoms in the original glucose molecule are thus released as waste products. However, the real metabolic prize is energy, which is released as the molecule is broken down. Because this part of the pathway requires oxygen, it is termed *aerobic.*

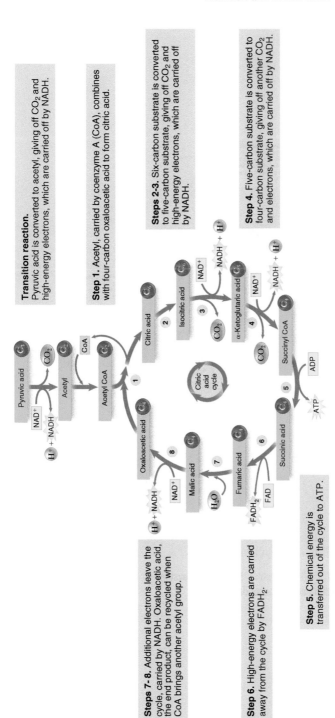

Transition reaction. Pyruvic acid is converted to acetyl, giving off CO_2 and high-energy electrons, which are carried off by NADH.

Step 1. Acetyl, carried by coenzyme A (CoA), combines with four-carbon oxaloacetic acid to form citric acid.

Steps 2-3. Six-carbon substrate is converted to five-carbon substrate, giving off CO_2 and high-energy electrons, which are carried off by NADH.

Step 4. Five-carbon substrate is converted to four-carbon substrate, giving off another CO_2 and electrons, which are carried off by NADH.

Steps 7-8. Additional electrons leave the cycle, carried by NADH. Oxaloacetic acid, the end product, can be recycled when CoA brings another acetyl group.

Step 6. High-energy electrons are carried away from the cycle by $FADH_2$.

Step 5. Chemical energy is transferred out of the cycle to ATP.

Citric Acid Cycle. Each pyruvic acid molecule is prepared to enter the citric cycle by the transition reaction, which yields a pair of high-energy electrons and a CO_2 molecule. The acetyl group that is thus formed is picked up by coenzyme A (CoA) and led into the citric acid cycle proper, which is described here as a recurring series of eight steps.

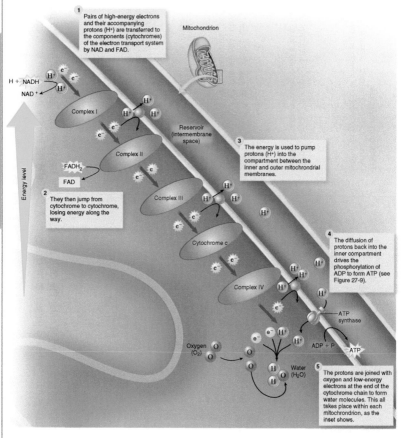

Electron Transport System (ETS). This system of energy transfer takes place entirely within each mitochondrion.

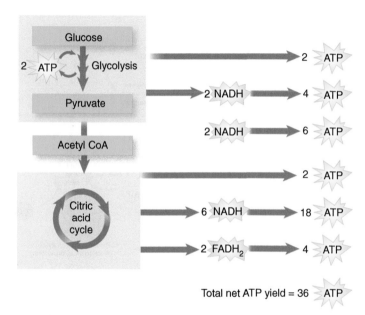

Total net ATP yield = 36 ATP

Energy Extracted From Glucose. Energy released from the breakdown of glucose is released mostly as heat, but some of it is transferred to a usable form—the high-energy bonds of adenosine triphosphate (ATP). In most human cells, one glucose molecule produces enough usable chemical energy to synthesize or "charge up" 36 ATP molecules. Some cells, such as heart and liver cells, shuttle electrons more efficiently and may be able to synthesize up to 38 ATP molecules. This represents an energy conversion efficiency of 38% to 44%, much better than the 20% to 25% typical of most machines.

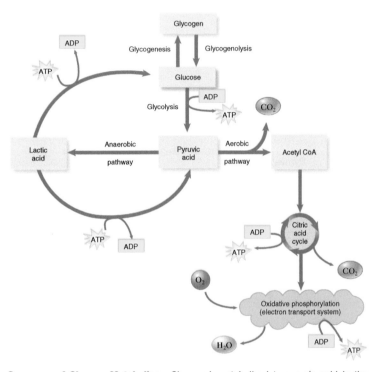

Summary of Glucose Metabolism. Glucose is catabolized to pyruvic acid in the process of **glycolysis**. If oxygen (O_2) is available, pyruvic acid is converted to **acetyl coenzyme A (acetyl-CoA)** and then enters the **citric acid cycle** and transfers energy to the maximum number of **adenosine triphosphate (ATP)** molecules via **oxidative phosphorylation** in the **electron transport system**. If O_2 is not available, pyruvic acid is converted to lactic acid, incurring an **O_2 debt.** The O_2 debt is later repaid when ATP produced via oxidative phosphorylation is used to convert lactic acid back into pyruvic acid or all the way back to glucose. If an excess of glucose exists, the cell may convert it to glycogen (**glycogenesis**). Later individual glucose molecules can be removed from the glycogen chain by the process of **glycogenolysis**. Although *nicotinamide-adenine dinucleotide (NAD)* and *flavin adenine dinucleotide (FAD)* play important roles in shuttling high-energy electrons between pathways, they have been left out of this diagram for the sake of simplicity.

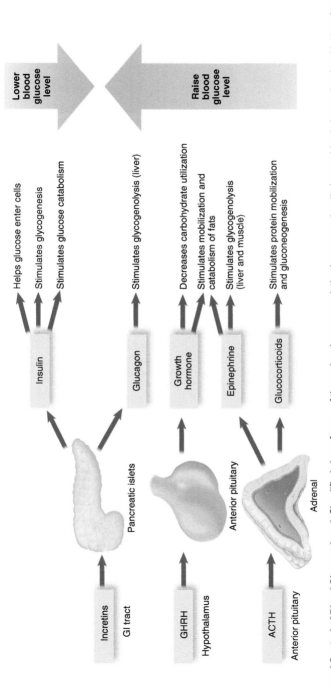

Hormonal Control of Blood Glucose Level. Simplified view of some of the major glucose-regulating hormones. Insulin lowers blood glucose level and is therefore hypoglycemic. Most hormones shown here raise blood glucose level and are called *hyperglycemic*, or *anti-insulin, hormones*.

PROTEINS

AMINO ACIDS

ESSENTIAL (INDISPENSABLE)	NONESSENTIAL (DISPENSABLE)
Histidine (His)*	Alanine (Ala)
Isoleucine (Ile)	Arginine (Arg)
Leucine (Leu)	Asparagine (Asn)
Lysine (Lys)	Aspartic acid (Asp)
Methionine (Met)	Cysteine (Cys)
Phenylalanine (Phe)	Glutamic acid (Glu)
Threonine (Thr)	Glutamine (Gln)
Tryptophan (Trp)	Glycine (Gly)
Valine (Val)	Proline (Pro)
	Selenocysteine (Sec)
	Serine (Ser)
	Tyrosine (Tyr)†

*Essential in infants and, perhaps, adult males.
†Can be synthesized from phenylalanine; therefore nonessential as long as phenylalanine is in the diet.

METABOLISM

NUTRIENT	ANABOLISM	CATABOLISM
Carbohydrates	Temporary excess changed into glycogen by liver cells in presence of insulin; stored in liver and skeletal muscles until needed and then changed back to glucose True excess beyond body's energy requirements converted into adipose tissue; stored in various fat depots of body	Oxidized, in presence of insulin, to yield energy (4.1 kcal per g) and wastes (carbon dioxide and water) $C_6H_{12}O_6 + 6\ O_2 \rightarrow$ Energy $+ 6\ CO_2 + 6\ H_2O$
Fats	Built into adipose tissue; stored in fat depots of body	Fatty acids Glycerol $\downarrow$ (beta-oxidation) $\downarrow$ (glycolysis) Acetyl CoA $\rightleftarrows$ Ketones Acetyl-CoA (tissues; citric acid cycle) $\downarrow$ Energy (9.3 kcal/g) $+ CO_2 + H_2O$
Proteins	Synthesized into tissue proteins, blood proteins, enzymes, hormones, etc.	Deaminated by liver, forming ammonia (which is converted to urea) and keto acids (which are either oxidized or changed to glucose or fat)

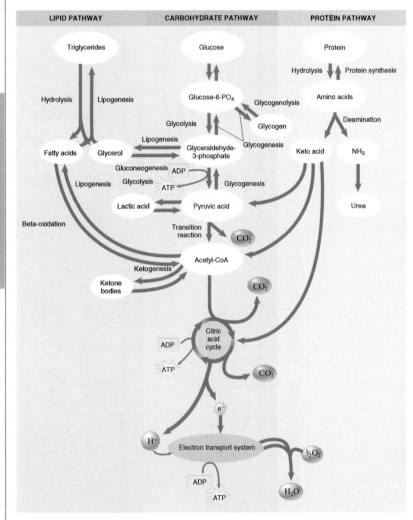

Summary of Metabolism. Notice the central role played by the citric acid cycle and electron transport system. Notice also how different molecules can be converted to forms that may enter other pathways. *ADP,* Adenosine diphosphate; *ATP,* adenosine triphosphate; *CoA,* coenzyme A.

REGULATING FOOD INTAKE

EXAMPLES OF APPETITE-REGULATING FACTORS*

OREXIGENIC FACTORS (STIMULATE APPETITE)	ANOREXIGENIC FACTORS (INHIBIT APPETITE)	SOURCE
	Leptin Interleukin 18 (IL-18)	Adipose tissue
Cortisol		Adrenal cortex
Ghrelin (GHRL)	Cholecystokinin (CCK) Glucagon-like peptide-1 (GLP-1) Oxyntomodulin (OXM) Peptide YY$_{3-36}$ (PYY$_{3-36}$)	GI tract
Endogenous opioid peptides (EOP) Galanin (GAL) Gamma-aminobutyric acid (GABA) Neuropeptide Y (NPY) Norepinephrine (NE) Orexins	Alpha-melanocyte–stimulating hormone (α-MSH) Cocaine- and amphetamine-regulated transcript (CART) Corticotropin-releasing hormone (CRH)	Hypothalamus
	Glucose	Liver
Emotions Environmental stimuli Food sensations Internal stimuli (e.g., blood temperature, glucose) Lifestyle choices and habits	Emotions Environmental stimuli Food sensations Internal stimuli (e.g., blood temperature, glucose) Lifestyle choices and habits	Nervous system[†]
	Insulin Pancreatic polypeptide (PP)	Pancreas

*Hormones, neurotransmitters, and other factors that affect feeding centers in the hypothalamus.
[†]Nervous factors not specifically hypothalamic in origin. *GI,* Gastrointestinal.

METABOLIC RATE

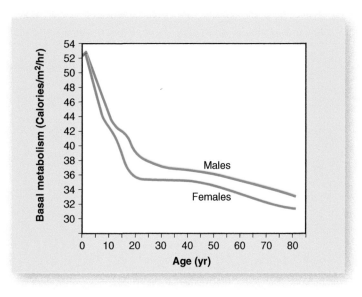

Basal Metabolic Rates Over the Life Span. The chart shows normal basal metabolic rates (BMRs) as function of age for each sex.

VITAMINS AND MINERALS

MAJOR VITAMINS

VITAMIN	DIETARY SOURCE	FUNCTIONS	SYMPTOMS OF DEFICIENCY
VITAMIN A	Green and yellow vegetables, dairy products, and liver	Maintains epithelial tissue and produces visual pigments	Night blindness and flaking skin
B-COMPLEX VITAMINS			
B$_1$ (thiamine)	Grains, meat, and legumes	Helps enzymes in the citric acid cycle	Nerve problems (beriberi), heart muscle weakness, and edema
B$_2$ (riboflavin)	Green vegetables, organ meats, eggs, and dairy products	Aids enzymes in the citric acid cycle	Inflammation of skin and eyes
B$_3$ (niacin)	Meat and grains	Helps enzymes in the citric acid cycle	Pellagra (scaly dermatitis and mental disturbances) and nervous disorders
B$_5$ (pantothenic acid)	Organ meat, eggs, and liver	Aids enzymes that connect fat and carbohydrate metabolism	Loss of coordination (rare), decreased gut motility
B$_6$ (pyridoxine)	Vegetables, meats, and grains	Helps enzymes that catabolize amino acids	Convulsions, irritability, and anemia
B$_9$ (folic acid)	Vegetables	Aids enzymes in amino acid catabolism and blood production	Digestive disorders and anemia
B$_{12}$ (cyanocobalamin)	Meat and dairy products	Involved in blood production and other processes	Pernicious anemia
Biotin (vitamin H)	Vegetables, meat, and eggs	Helps enzymes in amino acid catabolism and fat and glycogen synthesis	Mental and muscle problems (rare)
VITAMIN C (ascorbic acid)	Fruits and green vegetables	Helps in manufacture of collagen fibers; antioxidant	Scurvy and degeneration of skin, bone, and blood vessels
VITAMIN D (calciferol)	Dairy products and fish liver oil	Aids in calcium absorption	Rickets and skeletal deformity
VITAMIN E (tocopherol)	Green vegetables and seeds	Protects cell membranes from being destroyed; antioxidant	Muscle and reproductive disorders (rare)

MAJOR MINERALS

MINERAL	DIETARY SOURCE	FUNCTIONS	SYMPTOMS OF DEFICIENCY
Calcium (Ca)	Dairy products, legumes, and vegetables	Helps blood clotting, bone formation, and nerve and muscle function	Bone degeneration and nerve and muscle malfunction
Chlorine (Cl)	Salty foods	Aids in stomach acid production and acid-base balance	Acid-base imbalance
Cobalt (Co)	Meat	Helps vitamin B_{12} in blood cell production	Pernicious anemia
Copper (Cu)	Seafood, organ meats, and legumes	Involved in extracting energy from the citric acid cycle and in blood production	Fatigue and anemia
Iodine (I)	Seafood and iodized salt	Required for thyroid hormone synthesis	Goiter (thyroid enlargement) and decrease in metabolic rate
Iron (Fe)	Meat, eggs, vegetables, and legumes	Involved in extracting energy from the citric acid cycle and in blood production	Fatigue and anemia
Magnesium (Mg)	Vegetables and grains	Helps many enzymes	Nerve disorders, blood vessel dilation, and heart rhythm problems
Manganese (Mn)	Vegetables, legumes, and grains	Helps many enzymes	Muscle and nerve disorders
Phosphorus (P)	Dairy products and meat	Aids in bone formation and is used to make ATP, DNA, RNA, and phospholipids	Bone degeneration and metabolic problems
Potassium (K)	Seafood, milk, fruit, and meats	Helps muscle and nerve function	Muscle weakness, heart problems, and nerve problems
Selenium (Se)	Nuts, grains, meat, fish, mushrooms, eggs	Needed to make some amino acids; cofactor for enzymes	Heart muscle damage, cartilage degeneration, hypothyroidism
Sodium (Na)	Salty foods	Aids in muscle and nerve function and fluid balance	Weakness and digestive upset
Zinc (Zn)	Many foods	Helps many enzymes	Inadequate growth

Urinary System

The principal organs of the **urinary system** are the **kidneys,** which process blood and form urine as a waste to be excreted (removed from the body). The excreted urine travels from the kidney to the outside of the body via accessory organs: **ureters, urinary bladder,** and **urethra.**

Homeostasis of water and electrolytes, including pH, in body fluids depends largely on proper functioning of the kidneys. Each **nephron** within the kidney processes blood plasma in a way that adjusts its content to maintain a dynamic constancy of the internal environment of the body. Without renal processing, blood plasma characteristics would soon move out of their setpoint range.

EXCRETION

The urinary system's chief function is to regulate the volume and composition of body fluids and excrete unwanted material, but it is not the only system in the body that is able to excrete unneeded substances.

The table below compares the excretory functions of several systems. Although all of these systems contribute to the body's effort to remove wastes, only the urinary system can finely adjust the water and electrolyte balance to the degree required for normal homeostasis of body fluids.

SYSTEM	ORGAN	EXCRETION
Urinary	Kidney	Nitrogen compounds Toxins Water Electrolytes
Integumentary	Skin—sweat glands	Nitrogen compounds Electrolytes Water
Respiratory	Lung	Carbon dioxide Water
Digestive	Intestine	Digestive wastes Bile pigments Salts of heavy metals

Skin

Lungs
Liver
Kidneys
Large intestine
Bladder

ANATOMY OF THE URINARY SYSTEM

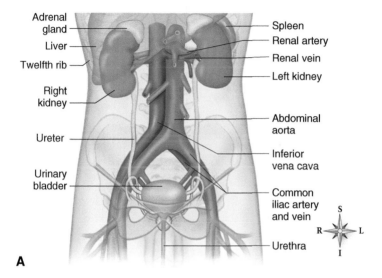

A

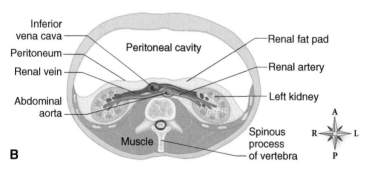

B

Location of Urinary System Organs. A, Anterior view of the urinary organs with the peritoneum and visceral organs removed. **B,** Horizontal (transverse) section of the abdomen showing the retroperitoneal position of the kidneys.

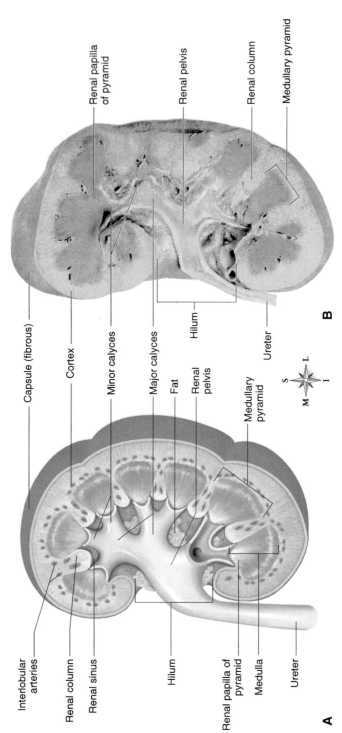

Internal Structure of the Kidney. A, Coronal section of the right kidney in an artist's rendering. **B,** Photo of a coronal section of a preserved human kidney.

Labels for A:
- Interlobular arteries
- Renal column
- Renal sinus
- Hilum
- Renal papilla of pyramid
- Medulla
- Ureter
- Capsule (fibrous)
- Cortex
- Minor calyces
- Major calyces
- Fat
- Renal pelvis
- Medullary pyramid

Labels for B:
- Renal papilla of pyramid
- Renal pelvis
- Renal column
- Medullary pyramid
- Minor calyces
- Major calyces
- Hilum
- Ureter

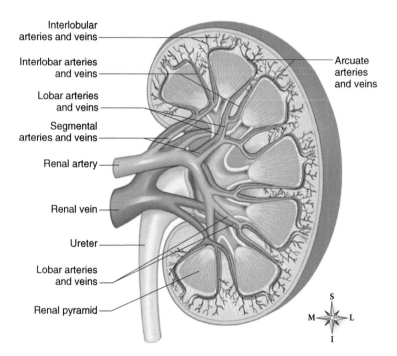

Interlobular arteries and veins

Interlobar arteries and veins

Lobar arteries and veins

Segmental arteries and veins

Renal artery

Renal vein

Ureter

Lobar arteries and veins

Renal pyramid

Arcuate arteries and veins

Circulation of Blood Through the Kidney. Diagram showing the major arteries and veins of the renal circulation.

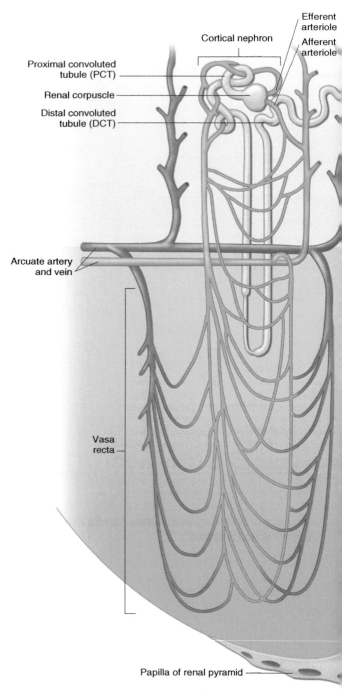

Efferent arteriole

Afferent arteriole

Cortical nephron

Proximal convoluted tubule (PCT)

Renal corpuscle

Distal convoluted tubule (DCT)

Arcuate artery and vein

Vasa recta

Papilla of renal pyramid

Blood Supply of Nephrons. Two types of nephrons (cortical and juxtaglomerular) are shown surrounded by the peritubular blood supply.

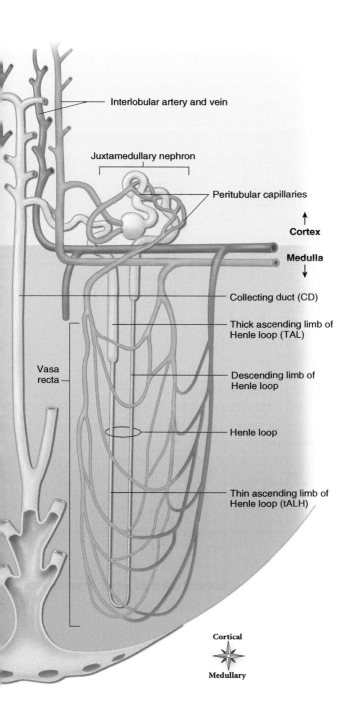

Interlobular artery and vein

Juxtamedullary nephron

Peritubular capillaries

Cortex

Medulla

Collecting duct (CD)

Thick ascending limb of Henle loop (TAL)

Vasa recta

Descending limb of Henle loop

Henle loop

Thin ascending limb of Henle loop (tALH)

Cortical

Medullary

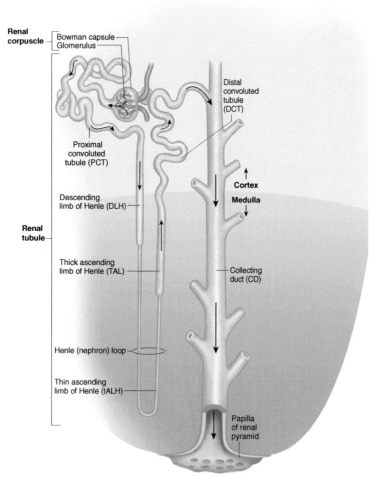

Renal corpuscle
- Bowman capsule
- Glomerulus

Distal convoluted tubule (DCT)

Proximal convoluted tubule (PCT)

Cortex

Medulla

Descending limb of Henle (DLH)

Renal tubule

Thick ascending limb of Henle (TAL)

Collecting duct (CD)

Henle (nephron) loop

Thin ascending limb of Henle (tALH)

Papilla of renal pyramid

Nephron. The nephron is the basic functional unit of the kidney. *Arrows* show the direction of flow within the nephron.

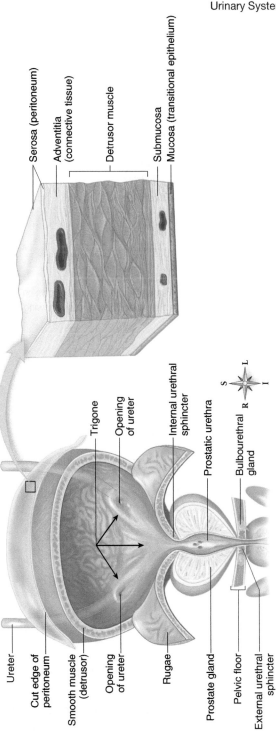

Serosa (peritoneum)

Adventitia (connective tissue)

Detrusor muscle

Submucosa

Mucosa (transitional epithelium)

Ureter

Cut edge of peritoneum

Smooth muscle (detrusor)

Opening of ureter

Rugae

Prostate gland

Pelvic floor

External urethral sphincter

Trigone

Opening of ureter

Internal urethral sphincter

Prostatic urethra

Bulbourethral gland

S
R — L
I

Structure of the Urinary Bladder. Frontal view of a dissected urinary bladder (male) in a fully distended state. *Inset* shows a cross section of the bladder wall, which has layers similar to those in other hollow abdominopelvic organs.

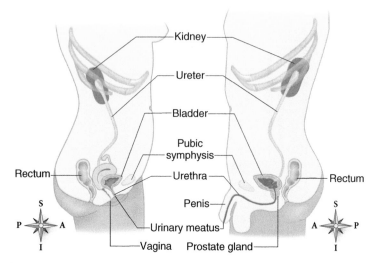

Sagittal View of the Urinary Tract. Female urinary system is shown on the reader's left and the male urinary system on the reader's right, each showing a distended (stretched) bladder.

PHYSIOLOGY OF THE URINARY SYSTEM

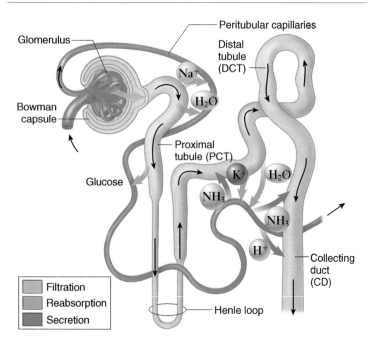

Overview of Urine Formation. The diagram shows the basic mechanisms of urine formation—filtration, reabsorption, and secretion—and where they occur in the nephron.

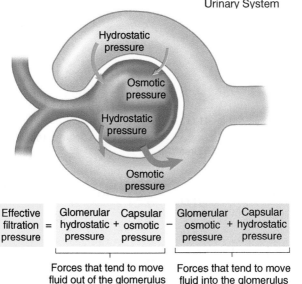

| Effective filtration pressure | = | Glomerular hydrostatic pressure | + | Capsular osmotic pressure | − | Glomerular osmotic pressure | + | Capsular hydrostatic pressure |

Forces that tend to move fluid out of the glomerulus | Forces that tend to move fluid into the glomerulus

Forces That Affect Glomerular Filtration. Effective filtration pressure (EFP) is determined by comparing the forces that push fluid into the capillary with those that push it out of the capillary.

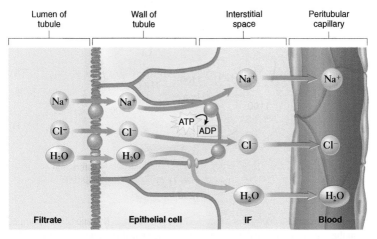

Mechanisms of Tubular Reabsorption. Sodium ions (Na^+) are pumped from the tubule cell to interstitial fluid (IF), thereby increasing the interstitial Na^+ concentration to a level that drives diffusion of Na^+ into blood. As Na^+ is pumped out of the cell, more Na^+ passively diffuses in from the filtrate to maintain an equilibrium of concentration. Enough Na^+ moves out of the tubule and into blood that an electrical gradient is established (blood is positive relative to the filtrate). Electrical attraction between oppositely charged particles drives diffusion of negative ions in the filtrate, such as chloride (Cl^-), into blood. As the ion concentration in blood increases, osmosis of water from the tubule occurs. Thus active transport of sodium creates a situation that promotes passive transport of negative ions and water.

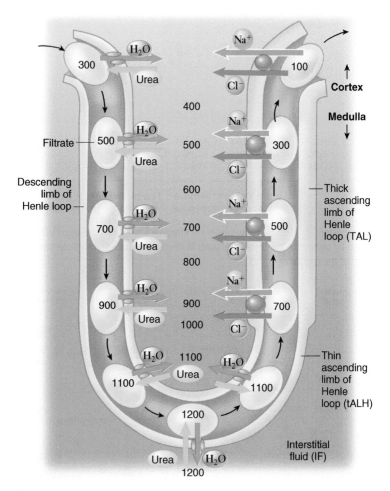

The Countercurrent Multiplier System in the Henle Loop. Na^+ and Cl^- are pumped from the ascending limb and moved into interstitial fluid (IF) to maintain high osmolality there. Because the salt content of the medullary IF increases, this is called a "multiplier" mechanism. Ion pumping also lowers the tubule fluid's osmolality by 200 mOsm, so fluid leaving the Henle loop is only 100 mOsm (hypotonic), as compared with 300 mOsm (isotonic) when it entered the loop. Numbers in the diagram are expressed in milliosmoles (mOsm).

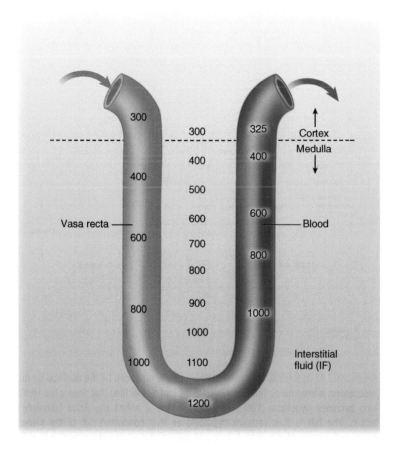

Countercurrent Exchange Mechanism in a Vas Rectum. Because a vas rectum forms a countercurrent loop, blood leaving the capillary bed has only a slightly higher solute content than when it entered. Thus the high osmolality of medullary tissue fluid is maintained. If peritubular blood instead traveled straight through the tissue, all excess solute in the medulla would be removed, and the osmolality of medullary interstitial fluid (IF) would be equivalent to that of the cortex. Numbers in the diagram are expressed in milliosmoles.

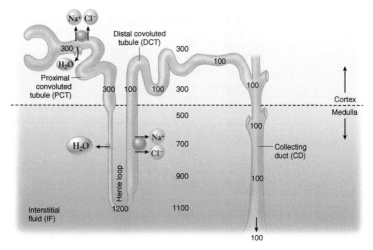

Production of Hypotonic Urine. Hypotonic urine is produced by the nephron by the mechanism shown here. The isotonic (300 mOsm) tubule fluid that enters the Henle loop becomes hypotonic (100 mOsm) by the time it enters the distal convoluted tubule. The tubule fluid remains hypotonic as it is conducted out of the kidney because the walls of the distal tubule and collecting duct are impermeable to H_2O, Na^+, and Cl^-. Values are expressed in milliosmoles.

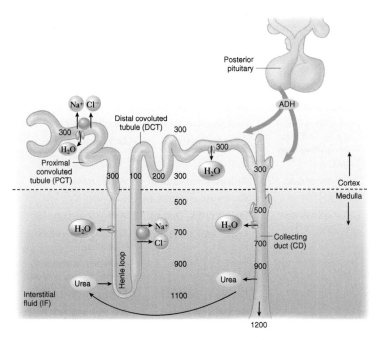

Production of Hypertonic Urine. Hypertonic urine can be formed when antidiuretic hormone (ADH) is present. ADH, a posterior pituitary hormone, increases the water permeability of the distal tubule and collecting duct. Thus hypotonic (100 mOsm) tubule fluid leaving the Henle loop can equilibrate first with the isotonic (300 mOsm) interstitial fluid (IF) of the cortex, then with the increasingly hypertonic (400 to 1200 mOsm) IF of the medulla. As H_2O leaves the collecting duct by osmosis, the filtrate becomes more concentrated with the solutes left behind. The concentration gradient causes urea to diffuse into the IF, where some of it is eventually picked up by tubule fluid in the descending limb of the Henle loop *(long arrow)*. This countercurrent movement of urea helps maintain a high solute concentration in the medulla. Values are expressed in milliosmoles.

SUMMARY OF NEPHRON FUNCTION

PART OF NEPHRON	FUNCTION	SUBSTANCE MOVED
Renal corpuscle	Filtration (passive)	Water
		Smaller solute particles (ions, glucose, etc.)
Proximal convoluted tubule (PCT)	Reabsorption (active)	Active transport: Na^+ Cotransport: glucose and amino acids
	Reabsorption (passive)	Diffusion: Cl^-, PO_4, urea, other solutes Osmosis: water
HENLE LOOP		
Descending limb (DLH) and thin ascending limb (tALH)	Reabsorption (passive)	Osmosis: water
	Secretion (passive)	Diffusion: urea
Thick ascending limb (TAL)	Reabsorption (active)	Active transport: Na^+
	Reabsorption (passive)	Diffusion: Cl^-
Distal convoluted tubule (DCT)	Reabsorption (active)	Active transport: Na^+
	Reabsorption (passive)	Diffusion: Cl^-, other anions
		Osmosis: water (only in the presence of ADH)
	Secretion (passive)	Diffusion: ammonia
	Secretion (active)	Active transport: K^+, H^+, some drugs
Collecting duct (CD)	Reabsorption (active)	Active transport: Na^+
	Reabsorption (passive)	Diffusion: urea
		Osmosis: water (only in the presence of ADH)
	Secretion (passive)	Diffusion: ammonia
	Secretion (active)	Active transport: K^+, H^+, some drugs

ADH, Antidiuretic hormone.

CHARACTERISTICS OF URINE

NORMAL CHARACTERISTICS

COLOR AND CLARITY

Normal urine: Should be clear; color varies with specific gravity

(Occasionally, normal urine may be cloudy because of high dietary levels of fat or phosphate.)

Dilute urine: Light yellow to yellow

Concentrated urine: Dark yellow to dark amber

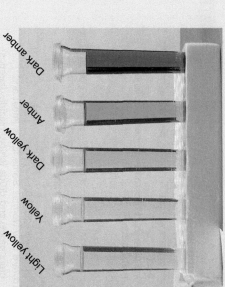

Light yellow

Yellow

Dark yellow

Amber

Dark amber

ABNORMAL CHARACTERISTICS

Abnormally colored urine may result from (1) pathologic conditions, (2) certain foods, and (3) numerous drugs:

1. Pathologic conditions (examples):
   Kidney cancer (hemorrhage)—red (RBCs)
   Bile duct obstruction (gallstones)—orange/yellow (bilirubin)
   Pseudomonas infection—green (bacterial toxins)

2. Foods (examples):
   Beets—red
   Rhubarb—brown
   Carrots—dark yellow

3. Drugs (examples):
   Pyridium (urinary tract analgesic)—orange
   Dilantin (anticonvulsant)—pink/red brown
   Dyrenium (diuretic)—pale blue

Cloudy urine may result from (examples):

1. Bacteria—active infection of urinary system organs

2. Blood cells
   RBCs—hemorrhage from kidney cancer
   WBCs—pus from urinary tract infection (UTI)

3. Casts—various types of tubelike clumps (blood cell, epithelial, hyaline, waxy, etc.) that form in diseased renal tubes

4. Proteinuria—(protein—usually albumin) in urine

5. Crystals—usually uric acid or phosphate/calcium oxalate in concentrated urine

Continued

CHARACTERISTICS OF URINE—cont'd

NORMAL CHARACTERISTICS	ABNORMAL CHARACTERISTICS
COMPOUNDS Mineral ions (for example, Na$^+$, Cl$^-$, K$^+$) Nitrogenous wastes: Ammonia, creatinine, urea, uric acid Urine pigment: Urochrome (product of bilirubin metabolism)	Ketones—generally acetone Protein—generally albumin Glucose Crystals—generally uric acid and phosphate or calcium oxalate Pigments—abnormal levels of bilirubin metabolites
ODOR Slight aromatic Some foods produce a characteristic odor (asparagus) Ammonia-like odor on standing may result from decomposition in stored urine	Strong, sweet, fruity (acetone) odor—uncontrolled diabetes mellitus Foul odor—urinary tract infections (UTI) Musty odor—phenylketonuria Maple syrup odor—congenital defect in protein metabolism
pH 4.6-8.0 (average, 6.0) Toward Low Normal: Some foods (meat and cranberries) and drugs (chlorothiazide diuretics) Toward High Normal: Some foods (citrus fruits, dairy products) and drugs (bicarbonate antacids)	High in alkalosis—kidneys compensate by excreting excess base Low in acidosis—kidneys compensate by excreting excess H$^+$
SPECIFIC GRAVITY Adult: 1.005-1.030 (usually 1.010-1.025) Elderly: Values decrease with age Newborn: 1.001-1.020	Above normal limits—glycosuria, proteinuria, dehydration, high solute load (may result in precipitation of solutes and kidney stone formation) Below normal limits—chronic renal diseases (inability to concentrate urine), overhydration

URINE COMPONENTS

TEST	NORMAL VALUES*	SIGNIFICANCE OF A CHANGE
ROUTINE URINALYSIS		
Acetone and acetoacetate	0	↑ during fasting ↑ in diabetic acidosis
Albumin	0-trace	↑ in hypertension ↑ in kidney disease ↑ after strenuous exercise (temporary)
Ammonia	20-70 mEq/L	↑ in liver disease ↑ in diabetes mellitus
Bile and bilirubin	—	↑ during obstruction of the bile ducts
Calcium	<150 mg/day	↑ in hyperparathyroidism ↓ in hypoparathyroidism
Color	Transparent yellow, straw-colored, or amber	Abnormal color or cloudiness may indicate blood in urine, bile, bacteria, drugs, food pigments, or high solute concentration
Odor	Characteristic slight odor	Acetone odor in diabetes mellitus (diabetic ketosis)
Osmolality	500-800 mOsm/L	↑ in dehydration ↑ in heart failure ↓ in diabetes insipidus ↓ in aldosteronism
pH	4.6-8.0	↑ in alkalosis ↑ during urinary infections ↓ in acidosis ↓ in dehydration ↓ in emphysema
Potassium	25-100 mEq/L	↑ in dehydration ↑ in chronic kidney failure ↓ in diarrhea or vomiting ↓ in adrenal insufficiency
Sodium	75-200 mg/day	↑ in starvation ↑ in dehydration ↓ in acute kidney failure ↓ in Cushing's syndrome
Creatinine clearance	100-140 ml/min	↑ in kidney disease
Creatine	1-2 g/day	↑ in infections ↓ in some kidney diseases ↓ in anemia (some forms)

Continued

URINE COMPONENTS—cont'd

TEST	NORMAL VALUES*	SIGNIFICANCE OF A CHANGE
Glucose	0	↑ in diabetes mellitus ↑ in hyperthyroidism ↑ in hypersecretion of adrenal cortex
Urea clearance	>40 ml blood cleared per min	↑ in some kidney diseases
Urea	25-35 g/day	↑ in some liver diseases ↑ in hemolytic anemia ↓ during obstruction of bile ducts ↓ in severe diarrhea
Uric acid	0.6-1.0 g/day	↑ in gout ↓ in some kidney diseases
MICROSCOPIC EXAMINATION		
Bacteria	<10,000/ml	↑ during urinary infections
Blood cells (RBC)	0-trace	↑ in pyelonephritis ↑ from damage by calculi ↑ in infection ↑ in cancer
Blood cells (WBC)	0-trace	↑ in infections
Blood cell casts (RBC)	0-trace	↑ in pyelonephritis
Blood cell casts (WBC)	0-trace	↑ in infection
Crystals	0-trace	↑ in urinary retention (Very large crystalline masses are called *calculi*.)
Epithelial casts	0-trace	↑ in some kidney disorders ↑ in heavy metal toxicity
Granular casts	0-trace	↑ in some kidney disorders
Hyaline casts	0-trace	↑ in some kidney disorders ↑ in fever

*Values vary with the analysis method used.

Fluid, Electrolyte, and Acid-Base Balance

16

The volume of fluid and the electrolyte levels inside the cells, in the interstitial spaces, and in the blood vessels all remain relatively constant when a condition of homeostasis exists. Fluid and electrolyte imbalance, then, means that both the total volume of water or level of electrolytes in the body or the amounts in one or more of its fluid compartments have increased or decreased beyond normal limits.

Acid-base balance refers to regulation of hydrogen ion concentration (pH) in the body fluids. Precise regulation of pH at the cellular level is necessary for survival. Even slight deviations from normal pH will result in pronounced, potentially fatal changes in metabolic activity.

FLUID AND ELECTROLYTE BALANCE

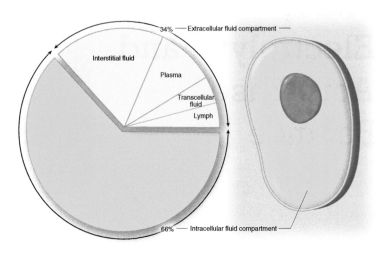

Distribution of Total Body Water.

COMMONLY USED ACRONYMS FOR BODY FLUIDS AND FLUID PRESSURES

ACRONYM	TERM	MEANING
BCOP	Blood colloid osmotic pressure	Force that draws water into the plasma (from the presence of colloid particles in plasma)
BHP	Blood hydrostatic pressure	Force of the blood pushing outward on blood vessel walls; blood pressure
ECF	Extracellular fluid	Any fluid outside cells, such as interstitial fluid (IF) or blood plasma
ICF	Intracellular fluid	Fluid inside the cell (cytosol)
IF	Interstitial fluid	Fluid between tissue cells
IFCOP	Interstitial fluid colloid osmotic pressure	Force that draws water out of the blood and into tissue spaces (from the presence of colloid particles in IF)
IFHP	Interstitial fluid hydrostatic pressure	Force (pressure) of the fluid between tissue cells

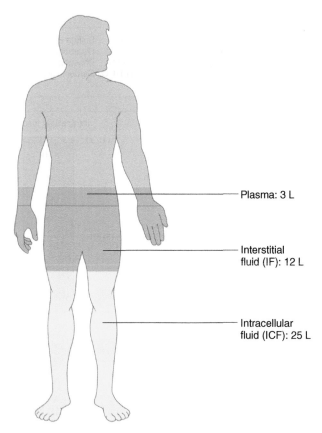

Plasma: 3 L

Interstitial
fluid (IF): 12 L

Intracellular
fluid (ICF): 25 L

Relative Volumes of Three Body Fluids. Values represent fluid distribution in a
young adult male.

VOLUMES OF BODY FLUID COMPARTMENTS*

BODY FLUID	INFANT	ADULT MALE	ADULT FEMALE
EXTRACELLULAR FLUID			
Plasma	4	4	4
Interstitial fluid	26	16	11
INTRACELLULAR FLUID	45	40	35
Total	75	60	50

*Percentage of body weight.

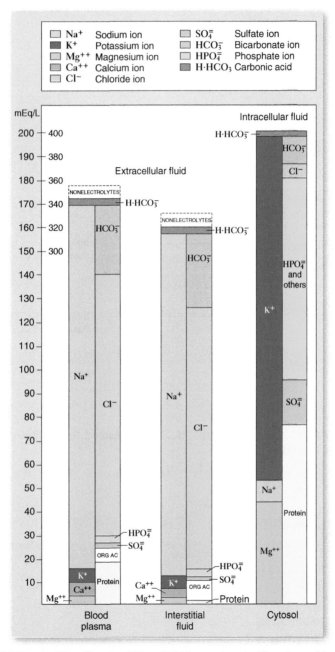

Chief Chemical Constituents of Three Fluid Compartments. The column of figures at the left (200, 190, 180, etc.) indicates the amount of cation or anion, whereas the figures on the right (400, 380, 360, etc.) indicate the sum of the cations and anions. *ORG AC,* Organic acid.

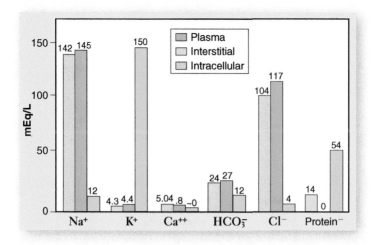

Electrolyte and Protein Concentrations in Body Fluid Compartments. This illustration compares individual electrolyte and protein concentrations in the three fluid compartments.

TYPICAL NORMAL VALUES (24 HOURS) FOR EACH PORTAL OF WATER ENTRY AND EXIT (WITH WIDE VARIATIONS)

INTAKE		OUTPUT	
Water in foods	700 ml	Lungs	350 ml
Ingested liquid	1500 ml	Skin	
Water formed by catabolism	200 ml	By diffusion	350 ml
		By sweat	100 ml
		Kidneys (urine)	1400 ml
		Intestines (in feces)	200 ml
Total	2400 ml		2400 ml

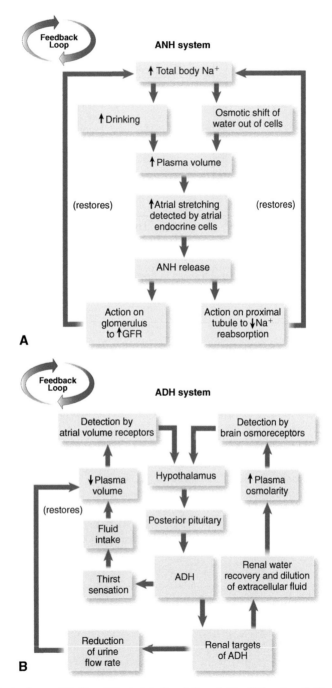

Mechanisms of Fluid and Electrolyte Regulation. A, The ANH system. **B,** The ADH system.

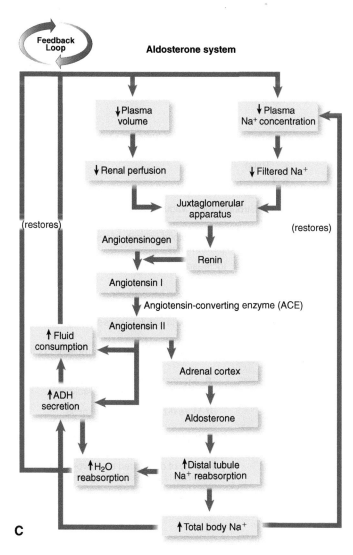

Mechanisms of Fluid and Electrolyte Regulation—cont'd. C, The aldosterone system. *ADH,* Antidiuretic hormone; *ANH,* atrial natriuretic hormone; *GFR,* glomerular filtration rate.

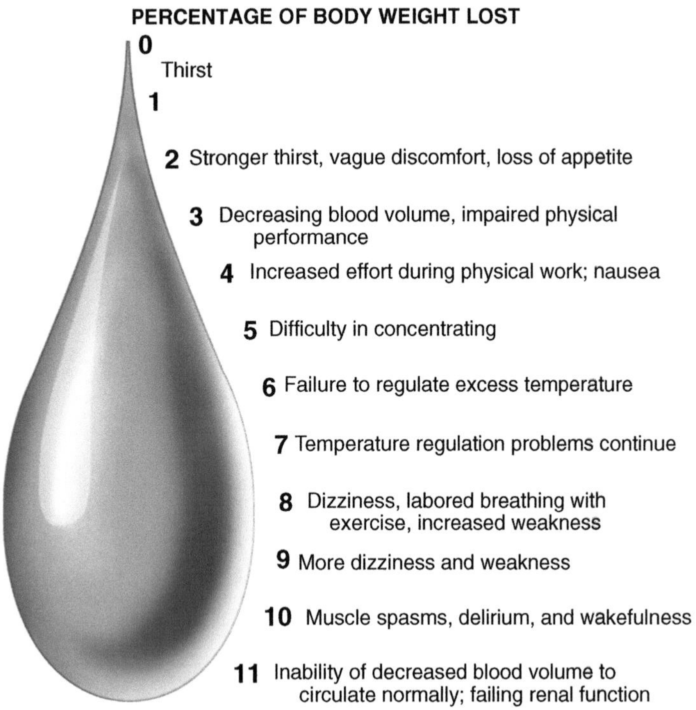

PERCENTAGE OF BODY WEIGHT LOST

0
Thirst

1

2 Stronger thirst, vague discomfort, loss of appetite

3 Decreasing blood volume, impaired physical performance

4 Increased effort during physical work; nausea

5 Difficulty in concentrating

6 Failure to regulate excess temperature

7 Temperature regulation problems continue

8 Dizziness, labored breathing with exercise, increased weakness

9 More dizziness and weakness

10 Muscle spasms, delirium, and wakefulness

11 Inability of decreased blood volume to circulate normally; failing renal function

The Effects of Dehydration.

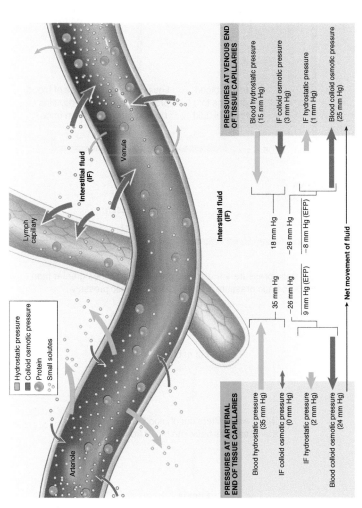

PRESSURES AT VENOUS END OF TISSUE CAPILLARIES

Blood hydrostatic pressure (15 mm Hg)

IF colloid osmotic pressure (3 mm Hg)

IF hydrostatic pressure (1 mm Hg)

Blood colloid osmotic pressure (25 mm Hg)

18 mm Hg

−26 mm Hg

−8 mm Hg (EFP)

← Net movement of fluid →

Interstitial fluid (IF)

Venule

Lymph capillary

Interstitial fluid (IF)

PRESSURES AT ARTERIAL END OF TISSUE CAPILLARIES

Blood hydrostatic pressure (35 mm Hg)

IF colloid osmotic pressure (0 mm Hg)

IF hydrostatic pressure (2 mm Hg)

Blood colloid osmotic pressure (24 mm Hg)

35 mm Hg

−26 mm Hg

9 mm Hg (EFP)

Arteriole

☐ Hydrostatic pressure
■ Colloid osmotic pressure
● Protein
∘ Small solutes

Forces that Affect Movement Between Fluid Compartments. *EFP*, Effective filtration pressure.

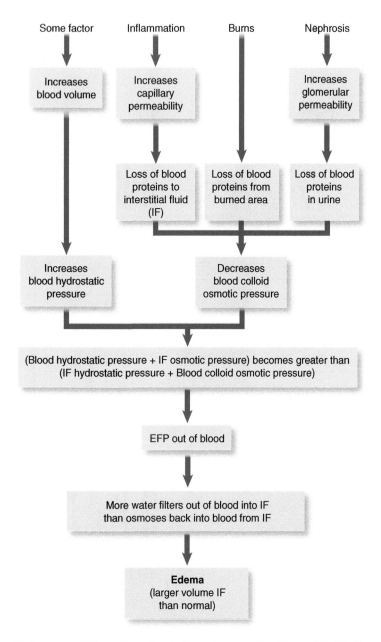

Mechanisms of Edema Formation in Some Common Conditions. *EFP,* Effective, or net, filtration pressure; *IF,* interstitial fluid.

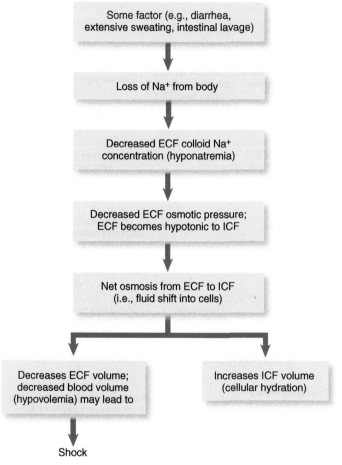

How Electrolyte Imbalance Leads to Fluid Imbalances. The schematic uses the example of sodium deficit (hyponatremia) and resulting hypovolemia (cellular hydration). *ECF,* Extracellular fluid; *ICF,* intracellular fluid.

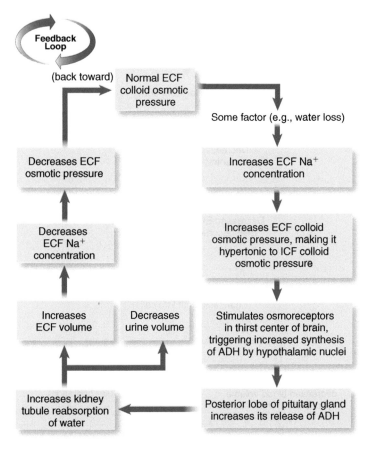

Antidiuretic Hormone (ADH) Mechanism for ECF Homeostasis. The ADH mechanism helps maintain homeostasis of extracellular fluid (ECF) colloid osmotic pressure by regulating its volume and thereby its electrolyte concentration, that is, mainly ECF Na^+ concentration. *ICF*, Intracellular fluid.

ACID-BASE BALANCE

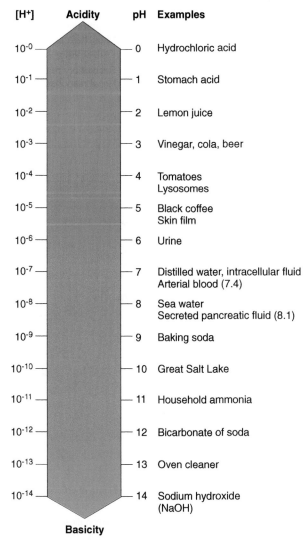

The pH Range. The pH value is shown on the right side of the scale, and the corresponding logarithmic value is on the left.

pH CONTROL SYSTEMS

TYPE	RESPONSE TIME	EXAMPLE
Chemical buffer systems	Immediate	Bicarbonate buffer system Phosphate buffer system Protein buffer system
Physiological buffer systems	Minutes Hours	Respiratory response system Renal response system

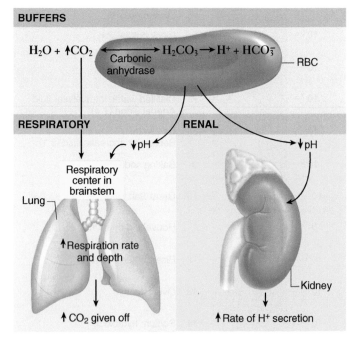

BUFFERS

$$H_2O + \uparrow CO_2 \xleftrightarrow[\text{Carbonic anhydrase}]{} H_2CO_3 \rightarrow H^+ + HCO_3^-$$ — RBC

RESPIRATORY   **RENAL**

$\downarrow$pH

Respiratory center in brainstem

Lung

$\uparrow$Respiration rate and depth

$\uparrow CO_2$ given off

$\downarrow$pH

Kidney

$\uparrow$Rate of H^+ secretion

Integration of pH Control Mechanisms. Elevated carbon dioxide (CO_2) levels result in increased formation of carbonic acid in red blood cells. The resulting increase in hydrogen ions, coupled with elevated CO_2 levels, results in an increase in respiratory rate and secretion of hydrogen ions (H^+) by the kidneys, thus helping regulate the pH of body fluids.

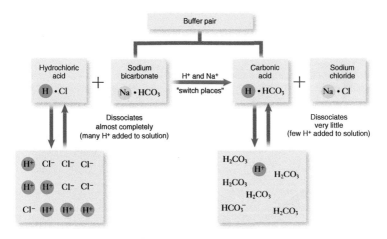

Buffering Action of Sodium Bicarbonate. Buffering of acid HCl by NaHCO₃. As a result of the buffer action, the strong acid (HCl) is replaced by a weaker acid (H • HCO₃). Note that HCl, as a strong acid, "dissociates" almost completely and releases more H⁺ than does H_2CO_3. Buffering decreases the number of H⁺ ions in the system.

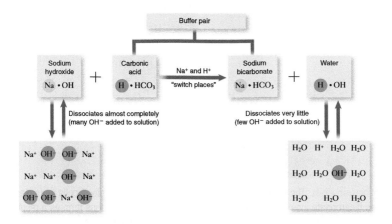

Buffering Action of Carbonic Acid. Buffering of the base NaOH by H_2CO_3. As a result of buffer action, the strong base (NaOH) is replaced by NaHCO₃ and H_2O. As a strong base, NaOH "dissociates" almost completely and releases large quantities of OH⁻. Dissociation of H_2O is minimal. Buffering decreases the number of OH⁻ ions in the system.

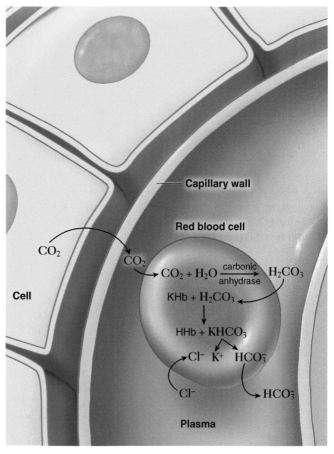

Chloride Shift. The concentration of chloride ions (Cl⁻) in red blood cells increases as bicarbonate ions (HCO₃⁻) diffuse out of the cell. Bicarbonate ions form as a result of the buffering of carbonic acid by the potassium salt of hemoglobin.

The hydrogen ions then diffuse into the tubular urine, where they displace basic ions (most often sodium) from a basic salt of a weak acid and thereby change the basic salt to an acid salt or to a weak acid that is eliminated in the urine. While this is happening, the displaced sodium or other basic ion diffuses into a tubule cell. Here, it combines with the bicarbonate ion left over from the carbonic acid dissociation to form sodium bicarbonate. The sodium bicarbonate then diffuses—is reabsorbed—into the blood. Consider the various results of this mechanism. Sodium bicarbonate (or other basic bicarbonate) is conserved for the body. Instead of all the basic salts that filter out of glomerular blood, leaving the body in the urine, considerable amounts are recovered into peritubular capillary blood. In addition, extra hydrogen ions are added to the urine and thereby eliminated from the body. Both the reabsorption of base bicarbonate into blood and the excretion of hydrogen ions into urine tend to increase the ratio of the bicarbonate buffer pair B • $HCO_3/H • HCO_3$ (BB/CA) present in blood. This automatically increases blood pH. In short, kidney tubule base bicarbonate reabsorption and hydrogen ion excretion both tend to alkalinize blood by acidifying urine.

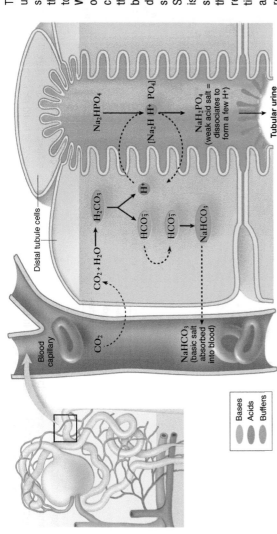

Acidification of Urine and Conservation of Base by Distal Renal Tubule Excretion of Hydrogen Ions (H^+). A decrease in blood pH accelerates the renal tubule ion-exchange mechanisms that acidify urine and conserve blood's base, thereby tending to increase blood pH back to normal. Distal and collecting tubules secrete hydrogen ions into the urine in exchange for basic ions, which they reabsorb. Note in the figure that carbon dioxide diffuses from tubule capillaries into distal tubule cells, where the enzyme carbonic anhydrase accelerates the combining of carbon dioxide with water to form carbonic acid. The carbonic acid dissociates into hydrogen ions and bicarbonate ions.

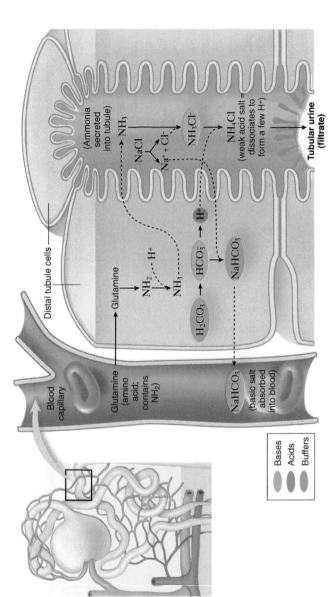

Acidification of Urine by Tubule Excretion of Ammonia (NH_3). An amino acid (glutamine) moves into the tubule cell and loses an amino group (NH_2) to form ammonia, which is secreted into urine. In exchange, the tubule cell reabsorbs a basic salt (mainly $NaHCO_3$) into blood from urine. Renal tubule excretion of hydrogen and ammonia is controlled at least in part by the blood pH level. A decrease in blood pH accelerates tubule excretion of both hydrogen and ammonia. An increase in blood pH produces the opposite effects.

ACID-BASE IMBALANCES

All of the **buffer pairs** in body fluids play an important role in acid-base balance. However, only in the **bicarbonate system** can the body regulate quickly and precisely the levels of both chemical components in the buffer pair. Carbonic acid levels can be regulated by the respiratory system and bicarbonate ion by the kidneys. A 20:1 ratio of base bicarbonate to carbonic acid (BB:CA) will, according to the *Henderson-Hasselbalch equation,* maintain acid-base balance and normal blood pH. Therefore, from a clinical standpoint, disturbances in acid-base balance depend on the relative quantities of carbonic acid and base bicarbonate in the extracellular fluid. Two types of disturbances, metabolic and respiratory, can alter the proper ratio of these components. Metabolic disturbances affect the bicarbonate element, and respiratory disturbances affect the carbonic acid element of the buffer pair.

Metabolic and respiratory acidosis, for example, are separate and very different types of acid-base imbalances. Both are treated by the intravenous infusion of solutions containing sodium lactate. The infused lactate ions are metabolized by liver cells and converted to bicarbonate ions. This therapy helps replace the depleted bicarbonate reserves required to restore acid-base balance in metabolic acidosis. In respiratory acidosis the additional bicarbonate ions function to offset elevated carbonic acid levels.

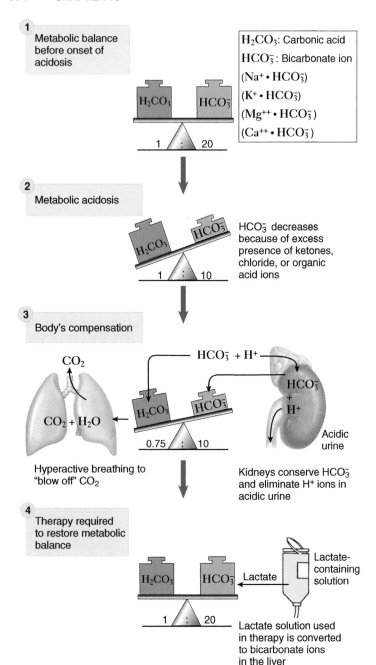

1

Metabolic balance before onset of acidosis

H_2CO_3: Carbonic acid
HCO_3^-: Bicarbonate ion
$(Na^+ \cdot HCO_3^-)$
$(K^+ \cdot HCO_3^-)$
$(Mg^{++} \cdot HCO_3^-)$
$(Ca^{++} \cdot HCO_3^-)$

H_2CO_3 HCO_3^-

1 : 20

2

Metabolic acidosis

H_2CO_3 HCO_3^-

1 : 10

HCO_3^- decreases because of excess presence of ketones, chloride, or organic acid ions

3

Body's compensation

$HCO_3^- + H^+$

CO_2

$CO_2 + H_2O$

H_2CO_3 HCO_3^-

0.75 : 10

HCO_3^- + H^+

Acidic urine

Hyperactive breathing to "blow off" CO_2

Kidneys conserve HCO_3^- and eliminate H^+ ions in acidic urine

4

Therapy required to restore metabolic balance

H_2CO_3 HCO_3^- Lactate

Lactate-containing solution

1 : 20

Lactate solution used in therapy is converted to bicarbonate ions in the liver

Metabolic Acidosis.

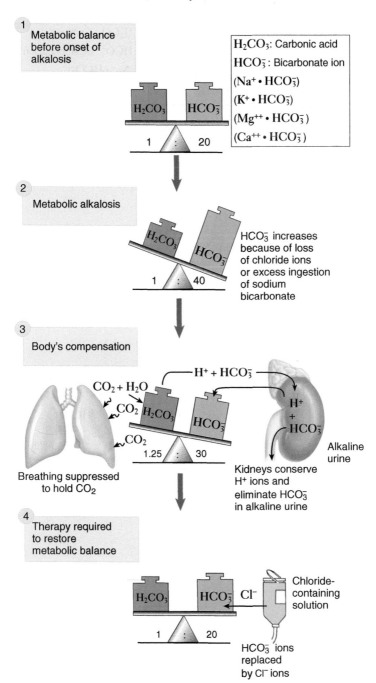

Metabolic Alkalosis.

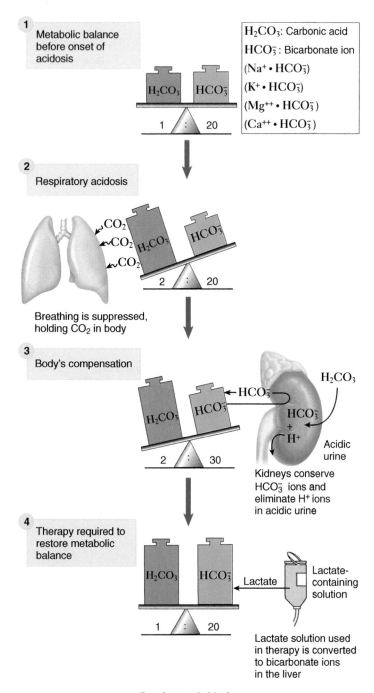

1 Metabolic balance before onset of acidosis

H_2CO_3: Carbonic acid
HCO_3^-: Bicarbonate ion
$(Na^+ \cdot HCO_3^-)$
$(K^+ \cdot HCO_3^-)$
$(Mg^{++} \cdot HCO_3^-)$
$(Ca^{++} \cdot HCO_3^-)$

H_2CO_3 HCO_3^-

1 : 20

2 Respiratory acidosis

CO_2
CO_2
CO_2
H_2CO_3 HCO_3^-

2 : 20

Breathing is suppressed, holding CO_2 in body

3 Body's compensation

H_2CO_3 HCO_3^- ← HCO_3^-

2 : 30

H_2CO_3

HCO_3^- + H^+

Acidic urine

Kidneys conserve HCO_3^- ions and eliminate H^+ ions in acidic urine

4 Therapy required to restore metabolic balance

H_2CO_3 HCO_3^- ← Lactate

1 : 20

Lactate-containing solution

Lactate solution used in therapy is converted to bicarbonate ions in the liver

Respiratory Acidosis.

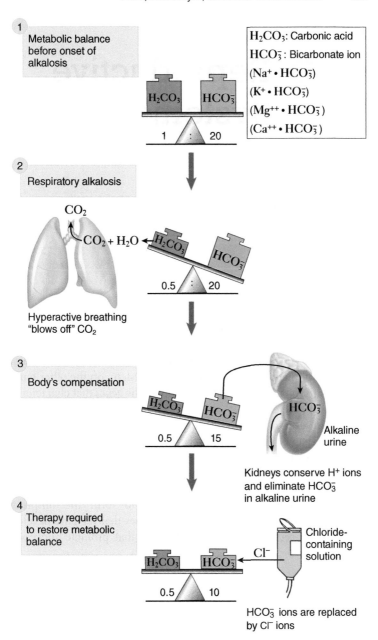

1 Metabolic balance before onset of alkalosis

H_2CO_3: Carbonic acid
HCO_3^-: Bicarbonate ion
$(Na^+ \cdot HCO_3^-)$
$(K^+ \cdot HCO_3^-)$
$(Mg^{++} \cdot HCO_3^-)$
$(Ca^{++} \cdot HCO_3^-)$

H_2CO_3 HCO_3^-

1 : 20

2 Respiratory alkalosis

CO_2

$CO_2 + H_2O$ H_2CO_3 HCO_3^-

0.5 : 20

Hyperactive breathing "blows off" CO_2

3 Body's compensation

H_2CO_3 HCO_3^- HCO_3^-

0.5   15

Alkaline urine

Kidneys conserve H^+ ions and eliminate HCO_3^- in alkaline urine

4 Therapy required to restore metabolic balance

H_2CO_3 HCO_3^- Cl^- Chloride-containing solution

0.5   10

HCO_3^- ions are replaced by Cl^- ions

Respiratory Alkalosis.

17

Reproductive Systems

The importance of **reproductive system** function is notably different from that of any other organ system of the body. Ordinarily, systems function to maintain the relative stability and survival of the individual organism (homeostasis). The reproductive system, on the other hand, ensures survival not of the individual but of the *genes* that characterize the human species.

In both sexes, organs of the reproductive system are adapted for the specific sequence of functions that are concerned primarily with transferring genes to a new generation of offspring. A male reproductive system in one parent and a female reproductive system in another parent are needed to reproduce.

Besides producing the cells needed to form the offspring, each reproductive system produces hormones that regulate development of the secondary sex characteristics that promote successful reproduction.

MALE REPRODUCTIVE SYSTEM

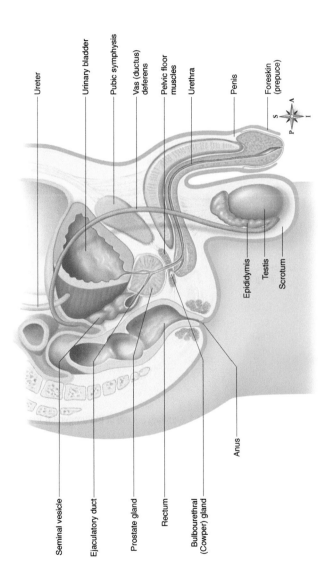

Ureter

Urinary bladder

Pubic symphysis

Vas (ductus) deferens

Pelvic floor muscles

Urethra

Penis

Foreskin (prepuce)

Seminal vesicle

Ejaculatory duct

Prostate gland

Rectum

Bulbourethral (Cowper) gland

Anus

Epididymis

Testis

Scrotum

Male Reproductive Organs. Sagittal section of inferior abdominopelvic cavity showing placement of male reproductive organs.

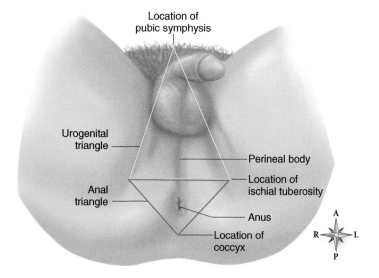

Male Perineum. Inferior view. Sketch showing outline of the urogenital triangle *(red)* and anal triangle *(blue)*.

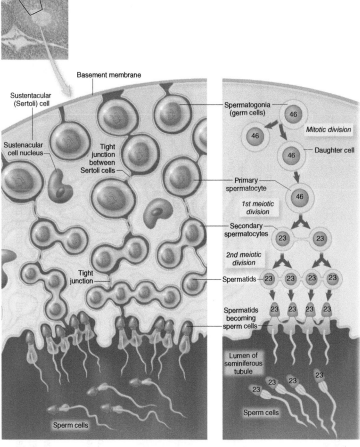

Spermatogenesis. First, spermatogonia in the outer rim of the seminiferous tubule produce daughter cells by mitotic division. These daughter cells, each with 46 chromosomes, become primary spermatocytes. A primary spermatocyte then undergoes meiotic division I to form two secondary spermatocytes, each with a haploid number of chromosomes (23). Each of the two secondary spermatocytes undergoes meiotic division II to form a total of four spermatids. Spermatids then differentiate to form heads and tails, eventually becoming mature spermatozoa—all with 23 chromosomes. Recall the role of the sustentacular, or Sertoli, cells, which support the developing male gametes structurally (by physically supporting them) and functionally (by releasing nutrients to them and by secretion of the hormone inhibin).

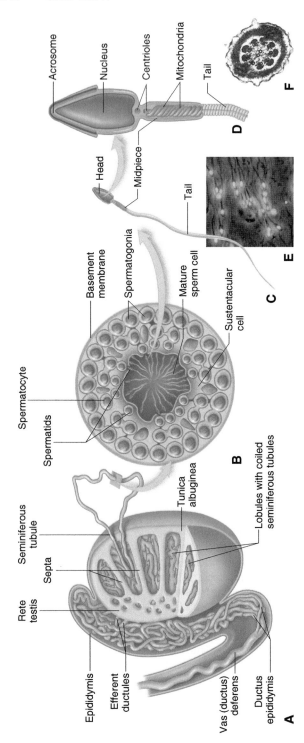

Development and Structure of Sperm. A, View of testis and seminiferous tubules. **B,** Spermatid cells in a seminiferous tubule. **C,** Mature sperm. **D,** Enlarged view of head and midpiece. **E,** Micrograph of sperm that shows taken-up nuclear material that glows with a fluorescent dye. **F,** Electron micrograph (EM) of a cross section of sperm tail showing nine double microtubules arranged around two single central microtubules.

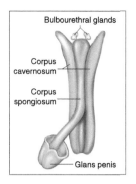

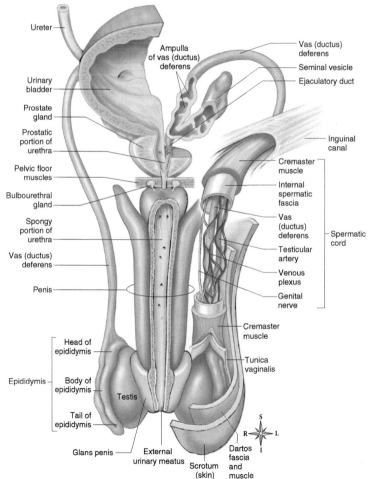

The Male Reproductive System. Illustration showing the testes, epididymis, vas (ductus) deferens, and glands of the male reproductive system in an isolation/ dissection format.

MALE REPRODUCTIVE HORMONES

HORMONE	SOURCE	TARGET	ACTION
Dehydroepiandrosterone (DHEA)	Adrenal gland, testis, other tissues	Converted to other hormones	Eventually converted to estrogens, testosterone, or both
Estrogen	Testis (interstitial cells), liver, other tissues	Testis (spermatogenic tissue), other tissues	Role of estrogen in men is still uncertain; may play role in spermatogenesis, inhibition of gonadotropins, male sexual behavior and partner preference
Follicle-stimulating hormone (FSH)	Anterior pituitary (gonadotroph cells)	Testis (spermatogenic tissue)	Gonadotropin; promotes development of testes and stimulates spermatogenesis
Gonadotropin-releasing hormone (GnRH)	Hypothalamus (neuroendocrine cells)	Anterior pituitary (gonadotroph cells)	Stimulates production and release of gonadotropins (FSH and LH) from anterior pituitary
Inhibin	Testis (sustentacular cells)	Hypothalamus Anterior pituitary (gonadotroph cells)	Inhibits GnRH secretion by the hypothalamus and FSH production in the anterior pituitary
Luteinizing hormone (LH)	Anterior pituitary (gonadotroph cells)	Testis (interstitial cells)	Gonadotropin; stimulates production of testosterone by interstitial cells of testis
Testosterone	Testis (interstitial cells)	Spermatogenic cells, skeletal muscle, bone, other tissues	Stimulates spermatogenesis, stimulates development of primary and secondary sexual characteristics, promotes growth of muscle and bone (anabolic effect)

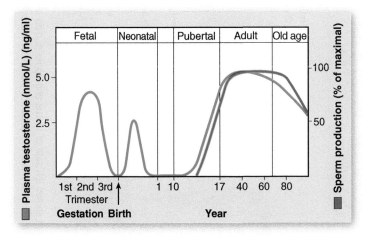

Testosterone Levels and Sperm Production. Plasma testosterone levels *(red line)* rise during fetal development, when it stimulates early development of male sexual organs. Testosterone rises again briefly around the time of birth, which facilitates descent of the testes into the scrotum. Then at puberty, testosterone rises enough to support sperm production *(blue line)* and later tapers off in advanced old age.

FEMALE REPRODUCTIVE SYSTEM

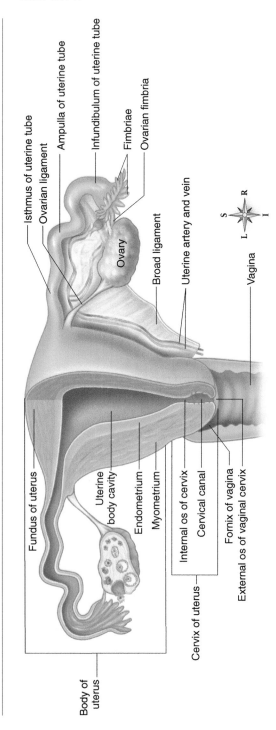

Internal Female Reproductive Organs. Posterior view. Diagram shows left side of uterus and upper portion of the vagina, and the left uterine tube and ovary in a frontal section. The broad ligament has been removed from the posterior surface of the uterus and adjacent structures.

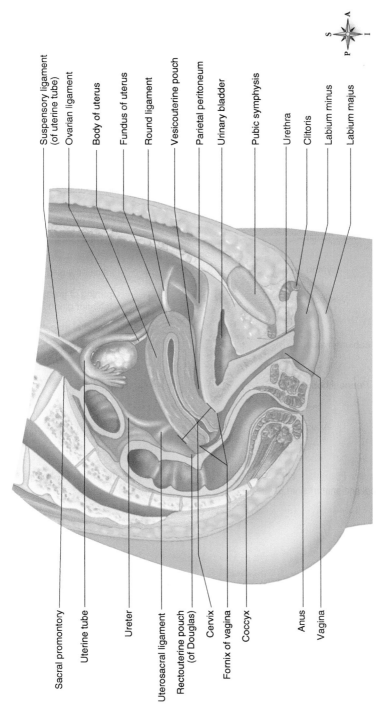

Suspensory ligament (of uterine tube)
Ovarian ligament
Body of uterus
Fundus of uterus
Round ligament
Vesicouterine pouch
Parietal peritoneum
Urinary bladder
Pubic symphysis
Urethra
Clitoris
Labium minus
Labium majus

Sacral promontory
Uterine tube
Ureter
Uterosacral ligament
Rectouterine pouch (of Douglas)
Cervix
Fornix of vagina
Coccyx
Anus
Vagina

Female Reproductive Organs. A, Diagram (sagittal section) of pelvis showing location of female reproductive organs.

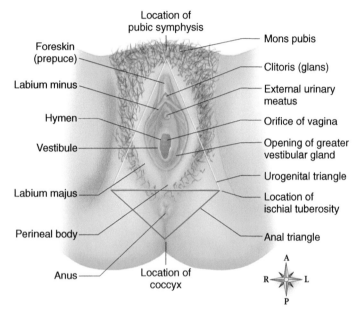

Female Perineum. Inferior view. Sketch showing outline of the urogenital triangle *(red)* and anal triangle *(blue)*.

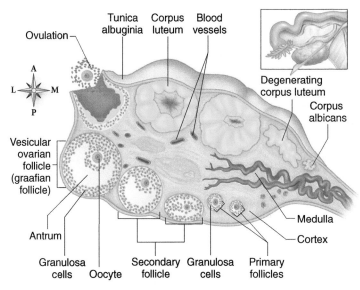

Stages of Ovarian Follicle Development. Artist's rendition shows the successive stages of ovarian follicle and oocyte development. Begin with the first stage (*primary follicle*) and follow around clockwise to the final stage that is labeled *degenerating corpus luteum*. Remember, however, that all the stages shown occur over time to a *single* follicle, and the presence of all these stages at a single point in time is an artificial construct for learning purposes only.

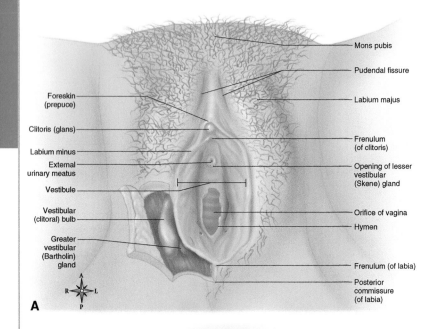

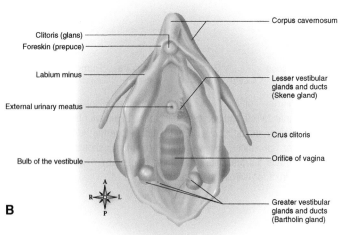

Vulva (Pudendum). A, Sketch showing major features of the external female genitals (genitalia). **B,** Sketch showing the full structure of the clitoris, which in life is mostly hidden by overlying external tissue.

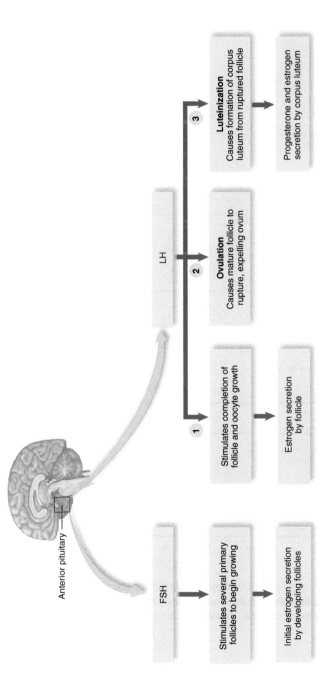

The Primary Effects of Gonadotropins on the Ovaries. Follicle-stimulating hormone (FSH) gets its name from the fact that it triggers development of primary ovarian follicles and stimulates follicular cells to secrete estrogens. Luteinizing hormone (LH) has several effects on ovaries: (1) LH acts as a synergist to FSH to enhance its effects on follicular development and secretion; (2) LH presumably triggers ovulation—hence it is called "the ovulating hormone"; and (3) LH has a luteinizing effect (for which the hormone was named); FSH is also necessary for luteinization.

Anterior pituitary

FSH

Stimulates several primary follicles to begin growing

Initial estrogen secretion by developing follicles

LH

1 Stimulates completion of follicle and oocyte growth

Estrogen secretion by follicle

2 **Ovulation** Causes mature follicle to rupture, expelling ovum

3 **Luteinization** Causes formation of corpus luteum from ruptured follicle

Progesterone and estrogen secretion by corpus luteum

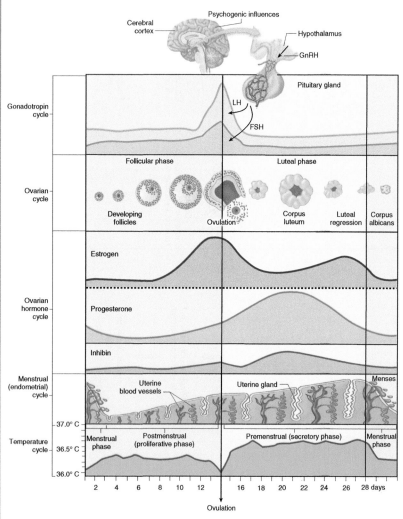

Female Reproductive Cycles. This diagram illustrates the interrelationships among the cerebral, hypothalamic, pituitary, ovarian, and uterine functions throughout a standard 28-day menstrual cycle. The variations in basal body temperature are also illustrated.

SOME FEMALE REPRODUCTIVE HORMONES

HORMONE	SOURCE	TARGET	ACTION
Dehydroepiandrosterone (DHEA)	Adrenal gland, ovary, other tissues	Converted to other hormones	Eventually converted to estrogens, testosterone, or both
Estrogens (including estradiol [E₂] and estrone)	Ovary and placenta (small amounts in other tissues)	Uterus, breast, other tissues	Stimulates development of female sexual characteristics, breast development, bone and nervous system maintenance
Follicle-stimulating hormone (FSH)	Anterior pituitary (gonadotroph cells)	Ovary	Gonadotropin; promotes development of ovarian follicle; stimulates estrogen secretion
Gonadotropin-releasing hormone (GnRH)	Hypothalamus (neuroendocrine cells)	Anterior pituitary (gonadotroph cells)	Stimulates production and release of gonadotropins (FSH and LH) from anterior pituitary
Human chorionic gonadotropin (hCG)	Placenta	Ovary	Stimulates secretion of estrogen and progesterone during pregnancy
Inhibin	Ovary	Hypothalamus Anterior pituitary (gonadotroph cells)	Inhibits GnRH production in the hypothalamus and FSH production in the anterior pituitary
Luteinizing hormone (LH)	Anterior pituitary (gonadotroph cells)	Ovary	Gonadotropin; triggers ovulation; promotes development of corpus luteum
Oxytocin (OT)	Posterior pituitary	Uterus and mammary glands	Stimulates uterine contractions; stimulates ejection of milk into ducts of mammary glands; involved in social bonding
Progesterone	Ovary and placenta	Uterus, mammary glands, other tissues	Helps maintain proper conditions for pregnancy
Prolactin (PRL) (lactogenic hormone)	Anterior pituitary (lactotroph cells)	Mammary glands (alveolar secretory cells)	Promotes milk secretion
Relaxin	Placenta	Uterus and joints	Inhibits uterine contractions during pregnancy and softens pelvic joints to facilitate childbirth
Testosterone	Adrenal glands, ovaries	Nervous tissue, bone tissue, other tissues	May affect mood, sex drive, learning, sleep, protein anabolism, other functions

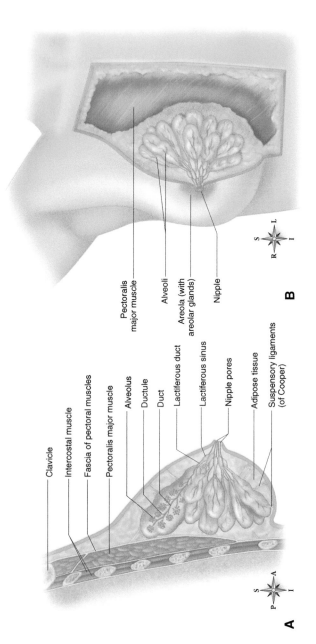

Clavicle
Intercostal muscle
Fascia of pectoral muscles
Pectoralis major muscle

Alveolus
Ductule
Duct
Lactiferous duct
Lactiferous sinus
Nipple pores
Adipose tissue
Suspensory ligaments (of Cooper)

Pectoralis major muscle
Alveoli
Areola (with areolar glands)
Nipple

A

B

The Female Breast. A, Sagittal section of a lactating breast. Notice how the glandular structures are anchored to the overlying skin and to the pectoral muscles by the suspensory ligaments of Cooper. Each lobule of glandular tissue is drained by a lactiferous duct that eventually opens through the nipple. **B,** Anterior view of a lactating breast. Overlying skin and connective tissue have been removed from the medial side to show the internal structure of the breast and underlying skeletal muscle. In nonlactating breasts, the glandular tissue is much less prominent, with adipose tissue making up most of each breast.

HORMONES THAT SUPPORT MILK PRODUCTION

CATEGORY	ROLE IN LACTATION	HORMONES
Mammogenic hormones	Promote tissue growth and development	↑ estrogens ↑ growth hormone (GH) ↑ insulin-like growth factor (IGF-I) ↑ insulin ↑ cortisol ↑ prolactin (PRL) ↑ relaxin ↑ epidermal growth factor (EGF)
Lactogenic hormones	Initiate milk production by secretory cells of alveolus	↑ prolactin (PRL) ↑ placental lactogen (hPL) ↑ cortisol ↑ insulin ↑ insulin-like growth factor (IGF-I) ↑ thyroid hormones (T_3, T_4) ↑ growth hormone (GH) ↓ estrogens ↓ progesterone
Galactokinetic hormones	Promote milk ejection by stimulating myoepithelial cells surrounding alveoli	↑ oxytocin (OT) ↑ antidiuretic hormone (ADH) (vasopressin [AVP])
Galactopoietic hormones	Maintain milk production (after it has already started)	↑ prolactin (PRL) ↑ cortisol ↑ insulin ↑ insulin-like growth factor (IGF-I) ↑ thyroid hormones (T_3, T_4)

18

Growth, Development, and Genetics

Before a new human life can begin, some preliminary processes must occur. Of utmost importance is the production of mature gametes, or sex cells, by each parent. **Spermatozoa,** gametes of the male parent, are produced by a process called *spermatogenesis*. **Ova,** gametes of the female parent, are produced by a process called *oogenesis*.

The sexual union of a male and female may result in fusion of the gametes of the two adults to form the first cell of the offspring. Thus genetic information from two different individuals is now united in a new and unique way.

The first cell of the offspring—the **zygote**—quickly divides again and again to eventually produce a mass of cells that will hopefully implant in the wall of the mother's uterus. The offspring and mother biologically connect to each other so that the mother's physiological mechanisms can sustain the offspring until its own systems are developed sufficiently.

After many weeks of growth and development—including *histogenesis* and *organogenesis* of a full complement of diverse tissues and organs—delivery of the offspring occurs. This event is one of a continuing series of changes: *infancy, childhood, puberty, adolescence, adulthood, senescence,* and *death*.

At some point in adolescence or adulthood, many of us have the opportunity to complete the "circle of life" by passing some of the **genetic code** we received from our parents on to yet another human generation.

GROWTH AND DEVELOPMENT

A New Human Life

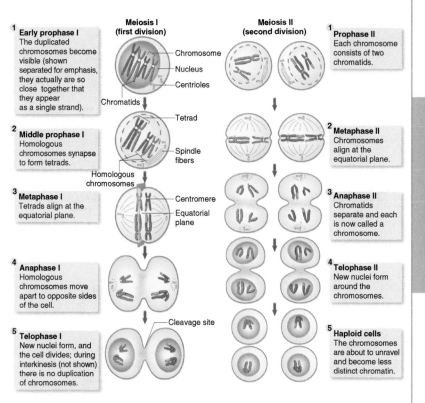

1 Early prophase I
The duplicated chromosomes become visible (shown separated for emphasis, they actually are so close together that they appear as a single strand).

2 Middle prophase I
Homologous chromosomes synapse to form tetrads.

3 Metaphase I
Tetrads align at the equatorial plane.

4 Anaphase I
Homologous chromosomes move apart to opposite sides of the cell.

5 Telophase I
New nuclei form, and the cell divides; during interkinesis (not shown) there is no duplication of chromosomes.

**Meiosis I
(first division)**

Chromosome
Nucleus
Centrioles
Chromatids
Tetrad
Spindle fibers
Homologous chromosomes
Centromere
Equatorial plane
Cleavage site

**Meiosis II
(second division)**

1 Prophase II
Each chromosome consists of two chromatids.

2 Metaphase II
Chromosomes align at the equatorial plane.

3 Anaphase II
Chromatids separate and each is now called a chromosome.

4 Telophase II
New nuclei form around the chromosomes.

5 Haploid cells
The chromosomes are about to unravel and become less distinct chromatin.

Meiotic Cell Division. Meiosis is a series of events that involves two separate division processes called *meiosis I* and *meiosis II*. Notice that four daughter cells, each with the haploid number of chromosomes, are produced from each parent cell that enters meiotic cell division. For simplicity's sake, only four chromosomes are shown in the parent cell instead of the usual 46.

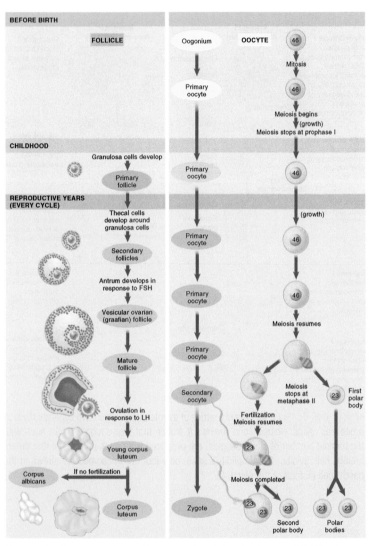

Oogenesis. Production of a mature ovum (oocyte) and subsequent fertilization are shown on the right as a series of cell divisions and on the left as a series of changes in the ovarian follicle. *FSH,* Follicle-stimulating hormone; *LH,* luteinizing hormone.

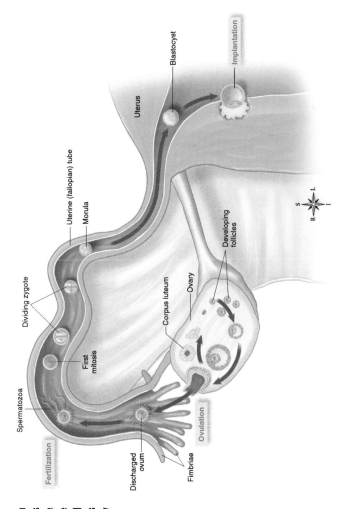

Fertilization and Implantation. At ovulation, an ovum is released from the ovary and begins its journey through the uterine tube. While in the tube, the ovum unites with a sperm to form the single-celled zygote. After a few days of rapid mitotic division, a ball of cells called a *morula* is formed. After the morula develops into a hollow ball called a *blastocyst*, implantation occurs.

Prenatal Period

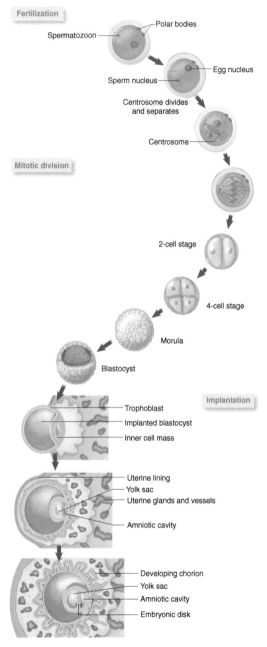

From Fertilization to Implantation and Development of the Yolk Sac. Rapid growth of uterine glands and vessels covers the developing blastocyst at the time of implantation.

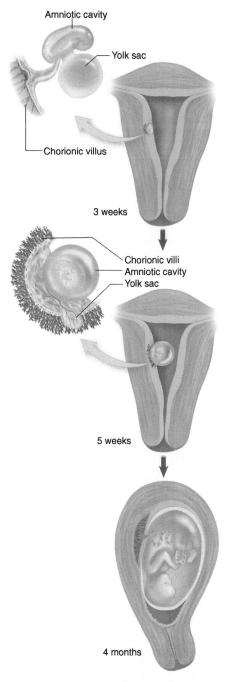

Development of the Chorion and Amniotic Cavity to 4 Months of Gestation.

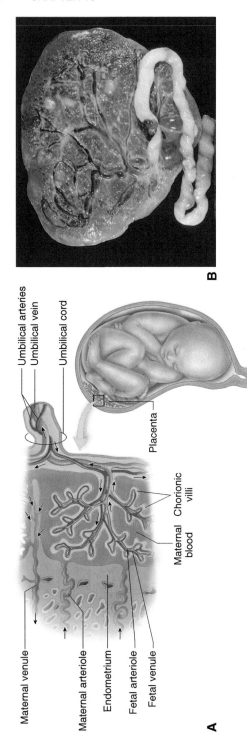

Structural Features of the Placenta. The close proximity of the fetal blood supply and the maternal blood supply permits diffusion of nutrients and other substances. The placenta also forms a thin barrier that prevents diffusion of most harmful substances. No mixing of fetal and maternal blood occurs. **A,** Diagram showing a cross section of the placental structure. **B,** Photograph of a normal, full-term placenta (fetal side) showing the branching of the placental blood vessels and umbilical cord.

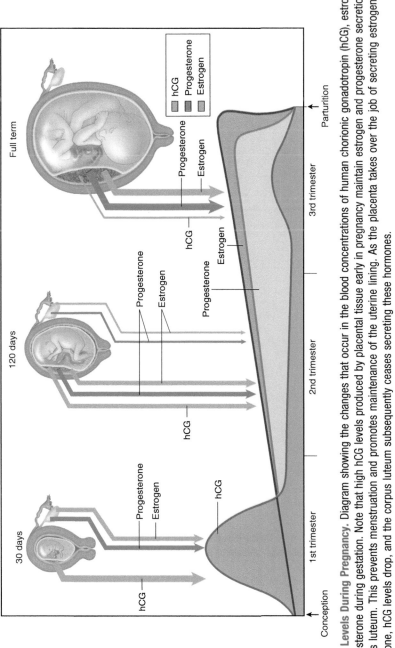

Hormone Levels During Pregnancy. Diagram showing the changes that occur in the blood concentrations of human chorionic gonadotropin (hCG), estrogen, and progesterone during gestation. Note that high hCG levels produced by placental tissue early in pregnancy maintain estrogen and progesterone secretion by the corpus luteum. This prevents menstruation and promotes maintenance of the uterine lining. As the placenta takes over the job of secreting estrogen and progesterone, hCG levels drop, and the corpus luteum subsequently ceases secreting these hormones.

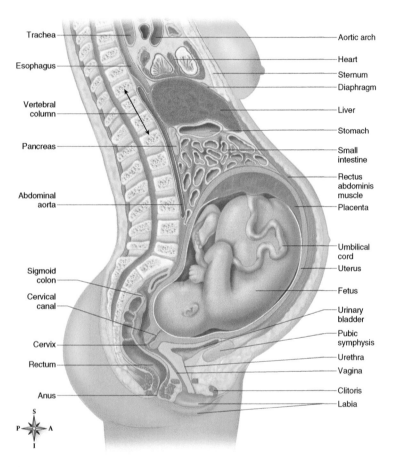

Trachea

Esophagus

Vertebral column

Pancreas

Abdominal aorta

Sigmoid colon

Cervical canal

Cervix

Rectum

Anus

Aortic arch

Heart

Sternum

Diaphragm

Liver

Stomach

Small intestine

Rectus abdominis muscle

Placenta

Umbilical cord

Uterus

Fetus

Urinary bladder

Pubic symphysis

Urethra

Vagina

Clitoris

Labia

Full-Term Pregnancy. Notice that the mother's organs are being pushed by the developing fetus, placenta, and uterus and that the woman's center of gravity is now shifted forward.

Postnatal Period

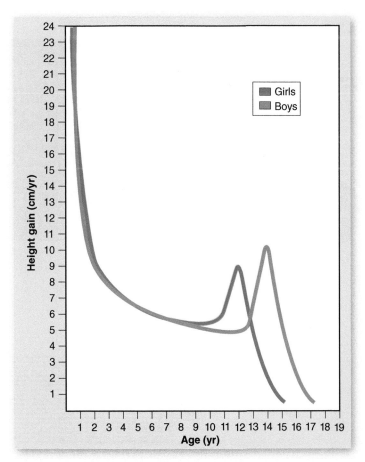

Growth in Height. The graph shows typical patterns of gain in height from birth to adulthood for girls and boys. Notice the rapid gain in height during the first few years, a period of slower growth, then another burst of growth during adolescence—finally ending at the beginning of adulthood.

GENETICS

Chromosomes and Genes

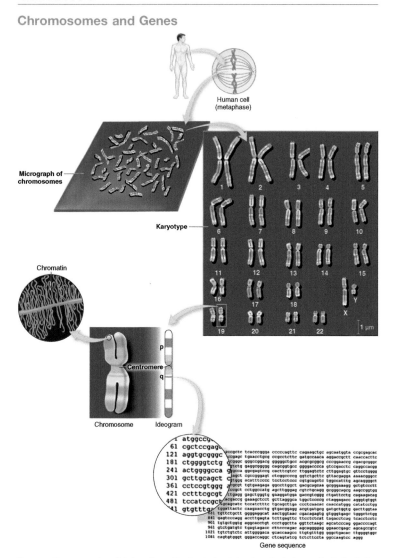

Human Genome. A cell taken from the body is stained and photographed. A photograph of nuclear chromosomes is then cut and pasted, arranging each of the 46 chromosomes into numbered pairs of decreasing size to form a chart called the *karyotype*. Each chromosome is a coiled mass of chromatin (DNA). In this figure, differentially stained bands in each chromosome appear as different, bright colors. Such bands are useful as reference points when identifying the locations of specific genes within a chromosome. The staining bands are also represented on an ideogram, or simple graph, of the chromosome as reference points to locate specific genes. The genes themselves are usually represented as the actual sequence of nucleotide bases, abbreviated as *a, c, g,* and *t*. In this figure, the sequence of one exon (segment) of a gene called *GPI* from chromosome 19 is shown. Each of the different images in this figure can be thought of as a different type of "genetic map."

Meiosis

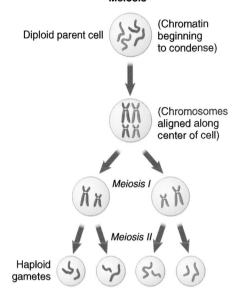

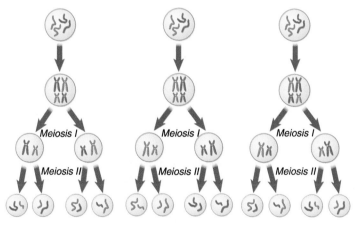

Meiosis and the Principle of Independent Assortment. In meiosis, a series of two divisions results in the production of gametes with one half the number of chromosomes of the original parent cell. In both meiotic divisions shown here, the original cell has four chromosomes and the gametes each have two chromosomes. During the first division of meiosis, pairs of similar chromosomes line up along the cell's equator for even distribution to daughter cells. Because different pairs assort independently of each other, four (2^2) different alignments of chromosomes can occur. Because human cells have 23 pairs of chromosomes, more than 8 million (2^{23}) different combinations are possible.

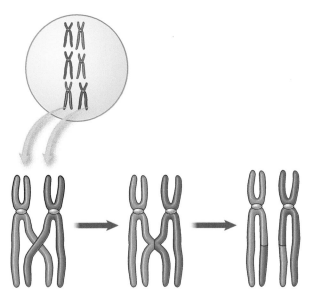

Crossing Over. Genes (or linked groups of genes) from one chromosome are exchanged with matching genes in the other chromosome of a pair during meiosis.

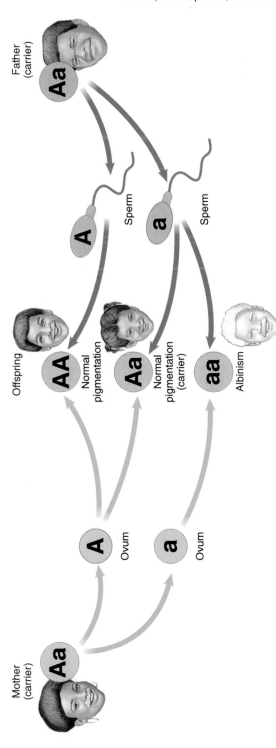

Inheritance of Albinism. Albinism is a recessive trait, producing abnormalities only in those with two recessive genes (a). Presence of the dominant gene (A) prevents albinism.

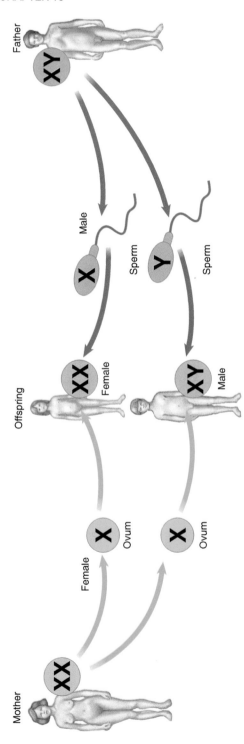

Sex Determination. The presence of the Y chromosome specifies maleness. In the absence of a Y chromosome, an individual develops into a female.

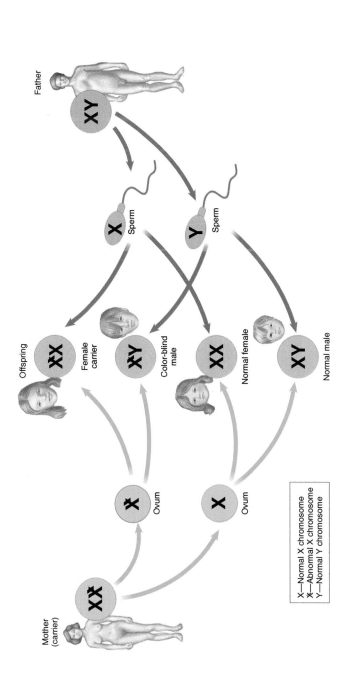

Sex-Linked Inheritance. Some forms of color blindness involve recessive X-linked genes. In this case, a female carrier of the abnormal gene can produce male children who are color blind.

Medical Genetics

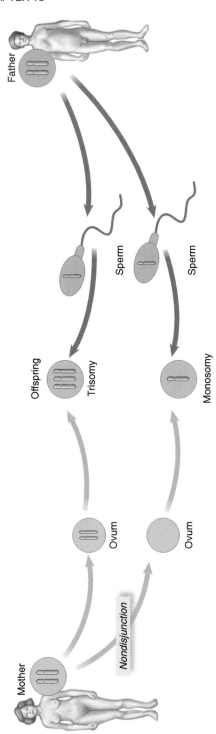

Effects of Nondisjunction. Nondisjunction, failure of a chromosome pair to separate during gamete production, may result in trisomy or monosomy in the offspring.

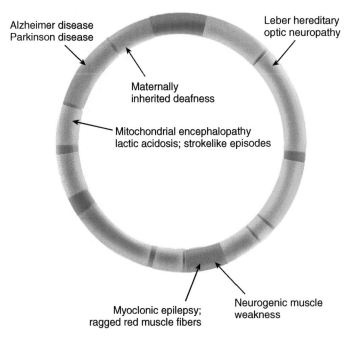

Map of Mitochondrial DNA (mtDNA). Ideogram showing locations of some mtDNA genes associated with various diseases.

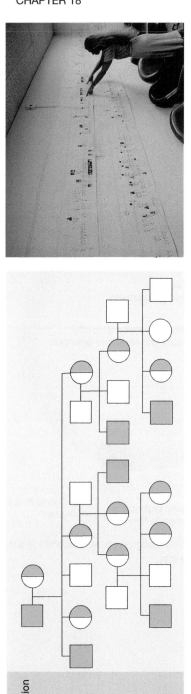

Pedigree. A, Pedigrees chart the genetic history of family lines. Squares represent males, and circles represent females. Fully shaded symbols indicate affected individuals, partly shaded symbols indicate carriers, and unshaded symbols indicate unaffected noncarriers. Roman numerals indicate the order of generations. This pedigree reveals the presence of an X-linked recessive trait. **B,** This huge pedigree compiled by Dr. Nancy Wexler of Columbia University and the Hereditary Disease Foundation traces Huntington disease (HD) over several generations of a large family in Venezuela. Dr. Wexler and other researchers collaborated in using information from this pedigree, along with techniques of molecular biology, to find the gene responsible for this disease and develop a test to detect the presence of the gene before the disease becomes apparent. Dr. Wexler became interested in this disease after her mother's death from HD.

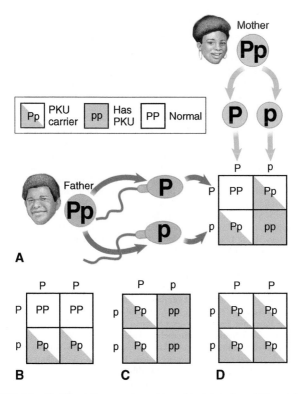

Punnett Square. The Punnett square is a grid used to determine relative probabilities of producing offspring with specific gene combinations. Phenylketonuria (PKU) is a recessive disorder caused by the gene *p. P* is the normal gene. **A,** Possible results of cross between two PKU carriers. Because one in four of the offspring represented in the grid have PKU, a genetic counselor would predict a 25% chance that this couple will produce a PKU baby at each birth. **B,** Cross between a PKU carrier and a normal noncarrier. **C,** Cross between an individual with PKU and a PKU carrier. **D,** Cross between an individual with PKU and a normal noncarrier.

Credits

Anatomical Position and Bilateral Symmetry. Copyright Kevin Patton, Lion Den Inc, Weldon Spring, MO. Nine Regions of the Abdominopelvic Cavity. Barbara Cousins. Division of the Abdomen into Four Quadrants. Barbara Cousins. RNA Interference. Modified from Pollard T, Earnshaw W: Cell biology, revised reprint, international edition, 1e, Philadelphia, 2004, Saunders. Hair Follicle Micrograph. © copyright by David Scharf 1986. Structure of Nails. Courtesy Christine Olekyk. Vertebral Column. Inset from Williams P: Gray's anatomy, 38e, Philadelphia, Churchill Livingstone, 1996. Right Scapula. B courtesy of Vidic B, Suarez FR: Photographic atlas of the human anatomy, St Louis, 1984, Mosby. Left Coxal (Hip) Bone. From Abrahams P, Marks S, Hutchings R: McMinn's color atlas of human anatomy, 5e, Philadelphia, 2003, Mosby. Cerebellum. Inset from Abrahams P, Marks S, Hutchings R: McMinn's color atlas of human anatomy, 5e, Philadelphia, 2003, Mosby. EEG. From Chipps EM, Clanin NJ, Campbell VG: Neurologic disorders, St Louis, 1992, Mosby. Adaptation of Sensory Receptors. Modified from Guyton A, Hall J: Textbook of medical physiology, 11e, Philadelphia, 2006, Saunders. Ophthalmoscopic View of the Retina. From Newell FW: Ophthalmology: principles and concepts, 7e, St Louis, 1992, Mosby. Formation of Prostaglandin and Related Molecules. Modified from Hinson J, Raven P: The endocrine system, Edinburgh, 2007, Churchill Livingstone. Results of Cross-matching Different Combinations (Types) of Donor and Recipient Blood. Inset from Belcher AE: Blood disorders, St Louis, 1993, Mosby. Vasomotor Effects on Blood Pressure. Modified from Boron W, Boulpaep E: Medical physiology, updated version, 1e, Philadelphia, Saunders, 2005. Stroke Volume. Modified from Rhoades R, Pflanzer R: Human physiology, 3e, Philadelphia, 1995, Perennial. Venous Valves. Modified from McCance K, Huether S: Pathophysiology, 4e, St Louis, 2002, Mosby. Lymphatic Drainage of the Head and Neck. From Seidel HM, Ball JW, Dains JE, Benedict GW: Mosby's guide to physical examination, 6e, St Louis, 2006, Mosby. Lymphatic Drainage of the Breast. From Seidel HM, Ball JW, Dains JE, Benedict GW: Mosby's guide to physical examination, 6e, St Louis, 2006, Mosby. Clonal Selection Theory. From Abbas A, Lichtman A: Cellular and molecular immunology, 5e, Philadelphia, 2003, Saunders. Lymphocyte Functions. From Abbas A, Lichtman A: Cellular and molecular immunology, 5e, Philadelphia, 2003, Saunders. Stages of the Adaptive Immune Response. From Abbas A, Lichtman A: Cellular and molecular immunology, 5e, Philadelphia, 2003, Saunders. Spirometer. Modified from Boron W, Boulpaep E: Medical physiology, updated version, 1e, Philadelphia, 2005, Saunders. Flow-Volume Loops. Adapted from Davies A, Moores C: The respiratory system, Edinburgh, 2004 Churchill-Livingstone. Ducts That Carry Bile from the Liver and Gallbladder. Inset from Abrahams P, Marks S, Hutchings R: McMinn's coloring atlas of human anatomy, 5e, Philadelphia, 2003, Saunders. Location of Urinary System Organs. A from Barbara Cousins. Internal Structure of the Kidney. B from Abrahams P, Marks S, Hutchings R: McMinn's coloring atlas of human anatomy, 5e, Philadelphia, 2003, Saunders. Nephron. Adapted from Brundage DJ: Renal disorders, Mosby's clinical nursing series, St Louis, 1992, Mosby. Characteristics of Urine. Bonewit-West K: Clinical procedures for medical assistants, 8e, St Louis, Saunders, 2011. Effects of Dehydration. Modified from Mahan LK, Escott-Stump S; Krause's food, nutrition and diet therapy, 12e, St Louis, 2007, Saunders. Development and Structure of Sperm. E from Lennart Nilsson/TT. F from Stevens A, Lowe J: Human histology, 3e, Philadelphia, 2005, Mosby. Male Reproductive System. Barbara Cousins. Testosterone Levels and Sperm Production. Adapted from Guyton A, Hall J: Textbook of medical physiology, 11e, Philadelphia, 2006, Saunders. MRI Scan, Female Pelvic Viscera. B from Moses K, Nava P, Banks J, Peterson D: Moses atlas of clinical gross anatomy, Philadelphia, 2005, Mosby. Structural Features of the Placenta. B from Cotran R, Kumar V, Collins T: Robbins pathologic basis of disease, 6e, Philadelphia, 1999, Saunders. Hormone Levels during Pregnancy. B modified from Hinson J, Raven P, The endocrine system, Edinburgh, 2007, Churchill Livingstone. Growth in Height. B modified from Mahan LK, Escott-Stump S; Krause's food, nutrition and diet therapy, 12e, St Louis, 2007, Saunders. Pedigree. B courtesy Nancy S. Wexler, PhD, Columbia University.

Index

Page numbers followed by "f"
indicate figures, "t" indicate
tables, and "b" indicate boxes.

TABLE 1   WORD PARTS COMMONLY USED AS PREFIXES

Word Part	Meaning
a-	without, not
a[d]-	toward
all[o]-	[an]other, different
an-	without, not
ante-	before
anti-	against, resisting
auto-	self
bi-	two, double
circum-	around
co-, con-	with, together
contra-	against
de-	down from, undoing
dia-	across, through
dipl-	twofold, double
dys-	bad, disordered, difficult
ectop-	displaced
ef-	away from
em-, en-	in, into
endo-	within
epi-	upon
eu-	good
ex-, exo-	out of, out from
extra-	outside of
hapl-	single
hem-, hemat-	blood
hemi-	half
hom(e)o-	same, equal
hyper-	over, above
hypo-	under, below
infra-	below, beneath
inter-	between
intra-	within
iso-	same, equal
macro-	large
mega-	large, million(th)
mes-	middle
meta-	beyond, after
micro-	small, millionth
milli-	thousandth
mono-	one (single)
neo-	new
non-	not
oligo-	few, scanty
ortho-	straight, correct, normal
para-	by the side of, near
per-	through
peri-	around, surrounding
poly-	many
post-	after
pre-	before
pro-	first, promoting
quadr-	four
re-	back again
retro-	behind
semi-	half
sub-	under
super-, supra-	over, above, excessive
trans-	across, through
tri-	three, triple

TABLE 2   WORD PARTS COMMONLY USED AS SUFFIXES

Word Part	Meaning
-al, -ac	pertaining to
-algia	pain
-aps, -apt	fit, fasten
-arche	beginning, origin
-ase	signifies an enzyme
-blast	sprout, make
-centesis	a piercing
-cide	to kill
-clast	break, destroy
-crine	release, secrete
-ectomy	a cutting out
-emesis	vomiting
-emia	refers to blood condition
-flux	flow
-gen	creates, forms
-genesis	creation, production
-gram*	something written
-graph(y)*	to write, draw
-hydrate	containing H_2O (water)
-ia, -sia	condition, process
-iasis	abnormal condition
-ic, -ac	pertaining to
-in	signifies a protein
-ism	signifies "condition of"
-itis	signifies "inflammation of"
-lemma	rind, peel
-lepsy	seizure
-lith	stone, rock
-logy	study of
-lunar	moon, moonlike
-malacia	softening
-megaly	enlargement
-metric, -metry	measurement, length
-oid	like, in the shape of
-oma	tumor
-opia	vision, vision condition
-oscopy	viewing
-ose	signifies a carbohydrate (especially sugar)
-osis	condition, process
-ostomy	formation of an opening
-otomy	cut
-penia	lack
-philic	loving
-phobic	fearing
-phragm	partition
-plasia	growth, formation
-plasm	substance, matter
-plasty	shape, make
-plegia	paralysis
-pnea	breath, breathing
-(r)rhage, -(r)rhagia	breaking out, discharge
-(r)rhaphy	sew, suture
-(r)rhea	flow
-some	body
-tensin, -tension	pressure
-tonic	relating to pressure, tension
-tripsy	crushing
-ule	small, little
-uria	refers to urine condition

*A term ending in -graph refers to an apparatus that results in a visual or recorded representation of biological phenomena, whereas a term ending in -graphy is the technique or process of using the apparatus. A term ending in -gram is the record itself. For example, in electrocardiography, an electrocardiograph is used to produce an electrocardiogram.